JOYCE ADAMS, CMT

SAUNDERS OPHTHALMOLOGY WORD BOOK

W.B. SAUNDERS COMPANY
Harcourt Brace Jovanovich, Inc.
Philadelphia London Toronto Montreal Sydney Tokyo

W. B. SAUNDERS COMPANY
Harcourt Brace Jovanovich, Inc.

The Curtis Center
Independence Square West
Philadelphia, PA 19106

Library of Congress Cataloging-in-Publication Data

Adams, Joyce.
Saunders ophthalmology word book / Joyce Adams.
p. cm.
ISBN 0-7216-3672-1
1. Ophthalmology—Dictionaries. I. Title.
[DNLM: 1. Eye Diseases—abbreviations. 2. Eye Diseases—terminology. 3. Ophthalmology—abbreviations. 4. Ophthalmology—terminology. WW 15 A214s]
RE21.A33 1991
617.7'03—dc20
DNLM/DLC
91-17561

Editor: Margaret M. Biblis
Designer: Ellen Bodner-Zanolle
Production Manager: Bill Preston
Manuscript Editor: W. B. Saunders Staff

SAUNDERS OPHTHALMOLOGY WORD BOOK ISBN 0-7216-3672-1

Printed in the United States of America

Last digit is the print number: 9 8 7 6 5 4 3 2 1

*I would like to thank Robert and Leslie Adams
for their invaluable contribution to my eight-year endeavor.
Special thanks go to Helen McDonell, who sparked the interest.*

CONTENTS

SECTION ONE

SECTION TWO

SECTION THREE

SECTION FOUR

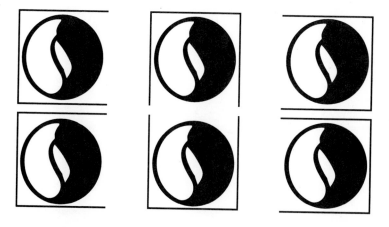

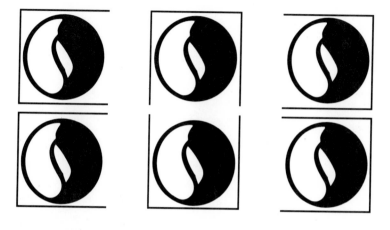

SECTION ONE

ABBREVIATIONS

a

A — accommodation
AA — amplitude of accommodation
AACG — acute angle closure glaucoma
AAMD — atrophic age-related macular degeneration
AC — anterior chamber
AC ratio — accommodation ratio
ACAT — age-related cataract
Acc — accommodation
ACG — angle-closure glaucoma
ACS — Alcon Closure System
ADV — adenovirus
AHM — anterior hyaloid membrane
AIDS — acquired immunodeficiency syndrome
AMO — Allergan Medical Optics
AMPPE — acute multifocal placoid pigment epitheliopathy
APD — afferent pupillary defect
ARC — AIDS-related complex
ARC — abnormal retinal correspondence
ARC — anomalous retinal correspondence
As.M. — myopic astigmatism
Ast. — astigmatism
ATD — aqueous tear deficiency
AV ratio — arteriovenous ratio
Ax — axis of cylindric lens

b

BAT — Brightness Acuity Test
BI — base-in prism
BO — base-out prism
BSS — balanced salt solution
BSV — binocular single vision
BU — base-up prism
BUT — breakup time
BVA — best-corrected visual acuity

c

CAT scan — computerized axial tomography
cc — with correction
CF — counting fingers
CME — cystoid macular edema
CMI — cell-mediated immunity
CMI — cytomegalic inclusion disease
CNS — central nervous system
CO_2 — carbon dioxide
COAG — chronic open-angle glaucoma
CPC — central posterior curve
CPEO — chronic progressive external ophthalmoplegia
CRA — central retinal artery
CRAO — central retinal artery occlusion
CRV — central retinal vein
CRVO — central retinal vein occlusion
CT — cover test

CT scan — computerized tomography scan
Cx — axis of cylindric lens
Cyl — cylindric lens or cylinder

d

D — diopter
D&N — distance and near
DDH — dissociated double hypertropia
DNCB — dinitrochlorobenzene
DUSN — diffuse unilateral subacute neuroretinitis
DVA — distance visual acuity
DVD — dissociated vertical deviation

e

E — esophoria
ECCE — extracapsular cataract extraction
EKC — epidemic keratoconjunctivitis
ELISA — enzyme-linked immunosorbent assay
ENG — electronystagmography
EOG — electro-oculogram
EOG — electro-oculography
EOM — extraocular muscles
EOM — extraocular movement
EOMI — extraocular movements intact
ERG — electroretinogram
ERG — electroretinography
ERPM — early receptor potential mottling
ET — esotropia
EW — Edinger-Westphal

f

FB — foreign body
fc — foot-candles
fpa — far point of accommodation

g

GPC — giant papillary conjunctivitis
gt — gutta (drop)
gtt — guttae (drops)
Guttat. — guttatim (drop by drop)

h

H — hyperphoria
HCL — hard contact lens
Hg — mercury
HM/3ft — hand motion at 3 feet
HM — hand movements
HSV — herpes simplex virus
HT — hypertropia

i

I/A — irrigation and aspiration
ICCE — intracapsular cataract extraction
ICD — intercanthal distance
ICE — iridocorneal epithelial syndrome
IK — interstitial keratitis
INO — internuclear ophthalmoplegia
IO — inferior oblique
IOL — intraocular lens
IOM — intraocular muscles
ION — ischemic optic neuropathy
IOP — intraocular pressure
IPD — interpupillary distance
IR — inferior rectus
IRMA — intraretinal microvascular abnormalities

j

J — joule(s)
JXG — juvenile xanthogranuloma

k

KCS — keratoconjunctivitis sicca
KP — keratitic precipitates
KW — Keith-Wagener changes

l

LE — left eye
LGB — lateral geniculate body
LGN — lateral geniculate nucleus
LHT — left hypertropia
LKP — lamellar keratoplasty
LP — light perception
LR — lateral rectus

m

MG — Marcus Gunn pupil
mJ — millijoules
MLF — medial longitudinal fasciculus
mmHg — millimeters of mercury
MR — medial rectus
MRI scan — magnetic resonance imaging scan
MVK — Massachusetts Vision Kit
MVS — Massachusetts XII Vitrectomy System

n

N — nasal
N. — cranial nerve

N.II — optic nerve
N.III — oculomotor nerve
N.IV — trochlear nerve
N.V — trigeminal nerve
N.VI — abducent nerve
Nd — neodymium
NLP — no light perception
nm — nanometer
NPA — near point accommodation
NPC — near point of convergence
NRC — normal retinal correspondence
NSAID — nonsteroidal anti-inflammatory drugs
nsec — nanosecond
Nv. — naked vision
NVA — near visual acuity

O

OD — oculus dexter (right eye)
ODN — ophthalmodynamometry
OHT — ocular hypertension
OKN — optokinetic nystagmus
OPG — oculopneumoplethysmography
OS — oculus sinister (left eye)
OU — oculi unitas (both eyes)
OU — oculi uterque (each eye)
OWS — overwear syndrome

P

p.o. — by mouth
p.r.n. — as needed
P&C — prism and cover test
PAM — Potential Acuity Meter
PAN — periarteritis nodosa
PAN — periodic alternating nystagmus
PAS — periodic-acid Schiff
PAS — peripheral anterior synechia
PAT — prism adaptation test
PC — posterior chamber
PCIOL — posterior chamber intraocular lens
PCLI — posterior chamber lens implant
PD — pupillary distance
PD — prism diopter
PDR — proliferative diabetic retinopathy
PE — pigment epithelium
PEK — punctate epithelial keratopathy
PEO — progressive external ophthalmoplegia
PERG — pattern-evoked electroretinogram
PERLA — pupils equal, reactive to light and accommodation
PERRLA — pupils equal, round, reactive to light and accommodation
PGC — pontine gaze center
PHM — posterior hyaloid membrane

PHPV — persistent hyperplasia of primary vitreous
PI — peripheral iridectomy
PKP — penetrating keratoplasty
PKU — phenylketonuria
PMMA — polymethyl methacrylate
PN — periarteritis nodosa
POHS — presumed ocular histoplasmosis syndrome
PP — punctum proximum of convergence
PPMD — posterior polymorphic dystrophy
PPRF — paramedian pontine reticular formation
PR — presbyopia
PRP — panretinal photocoagulation
PRRE — pupils round, regular, and equal
PSC — posterior subcapsular cataract
PSP — progressive supranuclear palsy
PVR — proliferative vitreoretinopathy
PXE — pseudoxanthoma elasticum

q

q. — every, each
q.a.m. — every morning
q.d. — every day
q.h. — every hour
q2h — every two hours
qhs — hour of sleep (at bedtime)
q.i.d. — four times a day
ql — as much as desired
qm — every morning
qn — every night
qod — every other day

r

R&R — recession-resection, recess-resect
RAPD — relative afferent pupillary defect
RD — retinal detachment
REM — rapid eye movements
RK — radial keratotomy
RLF — retrolental fibroplasia
RP — retinitis pigmentosa
RPE — retinal pigment epithelium

s

S — spherical lens
SBV — single binocular vision
sc — without correction
SCL — soft contact lens
SFP — simultaneous foveal perception
SMD — senile macular degeneration
SMP — simultaneous macular perception

SO — superior oblique
SOF — superior orbital fissure
SPC — simultaneous prism and cover test
sph. — sphere
SPK — superficial punctate keratitis
SR — superior rectus
SRNV — subretinal neovascularization
SSPE — subacute sclerosing panencephalitis

t

t.i.d. — three times a day
TAP — tension by applanation
TN — tension
TOD — tension of right eye (tension oculus dextra)
TOS — tension of left eye (tension oculus sinister)
TPI — treponema pallidum immobilization
TVA — true visual acuity

u

UGH — uveitis glaucoma hyphema

V

VA — visual acuity
VECP — visual evoked cortical potential
VEP — visual evoked potential
VER — visual evoked response
VF — visual field
VOD — vision of right eye (visio oculus dextra)
VOR — vestibulo-ocular response
VOS — vision of left eye (visio oculus sinister)
VOU — vision of both eyes (visio oculus uterque)
VSR — venous stasis retinopathy

X

X — exophoria
x — axis of Fick
X(T) — intermittent exotropia
XT — exotropia

SECTION TWO

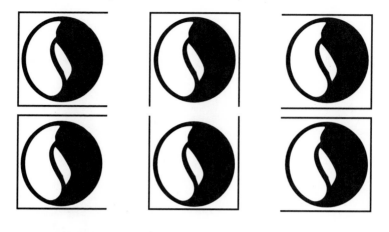

PHARMACOLOGICAL

a

AC eye drops
acetazolamide
Acetonide
acetylcholine chloride
Achromycin
ACTH
Acyclovir
Adapettes
Adapt
adenine arabinoside
Adrenalin
Adsorbocarpine
Adsorbonac
Adsorbotear
Aerosporin
Akarpine
Akorn
AKWA Tears
AK-Chlor
AK-Cide
AK-Con
AK-Con-A
AK-Dex
AK-Dilate
AK-Fluor
AK-Homatropine
AK-Lor
AK-Mycin
AK-NaCl
AK-Nefrin
AK-Neo-Cort
AK-Pentolate
AK-Poly-Bac
AK-Pred
AK-Rinse
AK-Spore
AK-Sporin
AK-Sulf
AK-Sulf Forte
AK-Taine
AK-Tate
AK-Tracin
AK-Trol
AK-Vernacon
AK-Zol
Albalon A
Albalon Liquifilm
Alcaine
Alclear
Alconefrin
Alidase
Almocarpine
Almocetamide
Alpha Chymar
alpha-chymotrypsin
Alphadrol
amikacin
Amikin
amphotericin B
ampicillin
Amvisc
Anacel
Ancef
Aosept
Apraclonidine
Aqua-Flow
Aqua-Tears
Aquasonic 100 gel
ARA-A
Argyrol
Aristocort
Aristospan
Artificial Tears
Atropair
atropine
Atropisol
Aureomycin

b

B.N.P.
Baciguent

bacitracin
bacitracin zinc
Bacticort
balanced salt solution (BSS)
Baldex
Basol-S
Beer's collyrium
Benazol
Betadine
Betagan
Betaxolol
Betoptic
Biomydrin
Biotic-O
Blairex System
Blefcon
Bleph
Bleph-10 Liquifilm
Bleph-10 S.O.P.
Blephamide
Blink-N-Clean
Blinx
BoilnSoak
Brevital
BSS — balanced salt solution
BSS Plus
bupivacaine

C

Carbacel
carbachol
Carbacholine
carbenicillin
Carbocaine
Carcholin
Catarase
cefazolin
Celestone
Cellu-Visc
cephalothin
Cetamide
Cetapred
Cetazol
Chloracol
chloramphenicol
Chlorofair
Chloromyxin
Chloroptic
Chymar
chymotrypsin
Ciba Vision Cleaner
Clean-N-Soak
Clean-N-Soakit
Clean-N-Stow
Clear Eyes
Clerz 2
clindamycin
cocaine hydrochloride
Colforsin
colistin
collyrium
Coly-Mycin S
Comfort Drops
Comfort Tears
CooperVision balanced salt solution
Coracin
Cort-Dome
Cortef
cortisol
cortisone
Cortisporin
Cyclogyl
Cyclomydril
cyclopentolate

d

Dacriose
Dalcaine

Daranide
De-Stat
Decadron
deferoxamine
Degest-2
Delta-Cortef
Deltasone
demecarium
Dendrid
Depo-Medrol
Dexacidin
Dexair
dexamethasone
Dexasporin
Dexsone
dextran
Diamox Sequels
diazepam
dichlorphenamide
Dilatair
dipivefrin
Dorsacaine
Doryl
Dual-Wet
Duo-Flow
Duolube
Duracare
Duralone
Duranest
Duratears
Durazyme
Dynosol

e

E Carpine
E Pilo
E Pilo-1
E Pilo-2
E Pilo-3
E Pilo-4
E Pilo-6
Echodide
Econochlor
Econopred
edrophonium
Efricel
Enuclene
ephedrine
Epicar
Epifrin
Epinal
epinephrine
Epitrate
Eppy/N
erythrocin
erythromycin
eserine
Estivin
Eye-Cool
Eye-Drops
Eye-Mo
Eye-Sed
Eye-Stream
Eye Wash
Eye-Zine

f

F Cortef
Feldman buffer solution
Flex-Care
Flexsol
Florinef
Floropryl
flucytosine
Fluor-I-Strip
Fluor-Op
Fluoracaine
Fluorescein
Fluorescite
Fluoresoft

Fluorets
Fluorexon
fluorometholone
Fluress
FML Forte
Freeman's solution
Ful-Glo-Strips
Funduscein
Funduscein -10
Funduscein -25
Fungizone

g

Gantrisin
Garamycin
Gel Clean
Genoptic
Gentacidin
Gentafair
Gentak
gentamicin
Gentrasul
Glaucon
glycerin
glycerol
Glyrol
Gonak
Gonio Gel
Goniosol

h

Healon
HEPES buffer
Herplex Liquifilm
Hexadrol
hexylcaine
HMS
Homatrocel
homatropine hydrobromide
Humorsol
Hy-Flow
hyaluronidase
Hydeltrasol
hydrocortisone
Hydronol
Hypersal
Hypoclear
Hypotears

i

I-Chlor
I-Drops
I-Gent
I-Homatrine
I-Liqui Tears
I-Lube
I-Naphline
I-Neocort
I Neospor
I-Paracaine
I-Parescein
I-Pentolate
I-Phrine
I-Picamide
I-Pilopine
I-Pred
I-Prednicet
I-Rescein
I-Rinse
I-Sol
I-Sulfacet
I-Sulfalone
I-Trol
I-Tropine

I-Wash
I-White
idoxuridine
Ilotycin
Indocin
indomethacin
Inflamase Forte
Innovar
insulin
Intersol
Iocare
Iri-Sol
Irigate
Ismotic
Isocaine
Isoflurophate
Isopto Alkaline
Isopto Atropine
Isopto Carbachol
Isopto Carpine
Isopto Cetamide
Isopto Cetapred
Isopto Eserine
Isopto Frin
Isopto Homatropine
Isopto Hyoscine
Isopto P-ES
Isopto Plain
Isopto Prednisolone
Isopto Sterofrin
Isopto Tears
isosorbide
Isuprel

k

K Sol preservation solution
Kainair
Keflin
Kefzol
Kenacort
Kenalog
ketoconazole

l

Lacri-Lube
Lacril
Lacrisert
Lacrivial
Lauro
Lavoptik Eye Wash
LC-65
Lens Clear
Lens Fresh
Lens Mate
Lens Plus
Lens Wet
levo-epinephrine
lidocaine
Lidoject
Lincocin
lincomycin
Liquifilm
Lite-Pred
Lubrifair
Lyteers

m

M-Rinse
Mallazine
mannitol
Marcaine
Marlin Salt System II
Maxidex
Maxitrol

McCarey-Kaufman medium
Medrol
medrysone
methacholine
methicillin
Methopto
Methulose
Metimyd
Metreton
Metycaine
miconazole
Microsponge
Milroy Artificial Tears
Miocel
Miochol
Miostat
Mira
MiraFlow
MiraSept
MiraSol
MK medium — McCarey-Kaufman medium/solution
Moisture Drops
Murine Plus
Muro's 128
Muro's Opcon
Muro's Opcon A
Muro's Tears
Murocel
Murocoll-2
Mycitracin
Mycostatin
Mydfrin
Mydramide
Mydrapred
Mydriacyl
Mydriafair
Mytrate

n

Nafazair
naphazoline
Naphcon-A
Naphcon Forte
Naptazane
Natacyn
natamycin
Natural Tears
Neo-Cobefrin
Neo-Cortef
Neo-Delta Cortef
Neo Dexair
Neo-Flow
Neo-Hydeltrasol
Neo-Medrol
Neo-Polycin
Neo-Synephrine
Neo-Synephrine Cocaine mixture 50:50
Neo-Tears
NeoDecadron
neomycin
Neosporin
neostigmine
Neotal
Neotricin
Neptazane
Nervocaine
Nesacaine
Nizoral
Normol
Novocain
Nulicaine

O

Ocu-Bath
Ocu-Caine
Ocu-Carpine
Ocu-Chlor
Ocu-Cort
Ocu-Dex

Ocu-Drop
Ocu-Lone
Ocu-Lube
Ocu-Meter
Ocu-Mycin
Ocu-Pentolate
Ocu-Phrin
Ocu-Pred A
Ocu-Pred Forte
Ocu-Sol
Ocu-Spor B
Ocu-Spor G
Ocu-Sul 10
Ocu-Sul 15
Ocu-Sul 30
Ocu-Tears
Ocu-Trol
Ocu-Tropic
Ocu-Tropine
Ocu-Zoline
Ocuclear
Ocudose
Ocufen
Ocugestrin
Oculaid
Oculinum
Ocumeter
Ocumycin
Ocusert Pilo-20
Ocusert Pilo-40
Ocusoft
Ocutricin
One Solution
Op-Thal-Zin
Opcon
Opcon A
Ophacet
Ophtha PS
Ophthacet
Ophthaine
Ophthalgan
Ophthel
Ophthetic
Ophthochlor
Ophthocort
Opt-Ease
Optacon
Optacryl
Optef
Opti-Bon
Opti-Clean II
Opti-Pure
Opti-Soft
Opti-Tears
Opti-Zyme
Opticrom
Optigene
Optimyd
Optised
Optisoap
Optrex
Or Topic-M
Oratrol
Osmitrol
Osmoglyn
oxacillin
oxytetracycline

p

P.V. Carpine Liquifilm
Panmycin
Paredrine
penicillin
penicillin G
Pentolair
phenacaine
Phenoptic
Phenylzin
pHisoHex
Pilocar
pilocarpine
Pilocel
Pilofrin
Pilokair

Pilomiotin
Pilopine gel 4%
Piloptic
Pliagel
Poly Pred
Polycycline
polymyxin
Polysporin
Pontocaine
povidone
Pred Forte
Pred G
Pred Mild
Predair A
Predair Forte
Predamide
Predate
Prednefrin
prednisolone
Predsulfair
Predulose
Preflex
Prefrin A
Prefrin Liquifilm
Prefrin Z Liquifilm
Presert
prilocaine
probenicid
procaine
ProFree GP
Propine
PV Carpine

r

Refresh
Renu
RO Optho
Rose bengal

S

saline solution
Schirmer strips
scopolamine
Sensitive Eyes
Sensorcaine
Septicon
Septra
Sereine
Silaclean
silver nitrate
Soaclens
Soakare
Sof/Pro Clean
Soflens
Soft Mate
Solu-Cortef
Solu-Medrol
Soothe Eye
Soquette
Spectrocin
Staphcillin
Statrol
Stay-Brite
Stay-Wet
Steclin
Sterane
Sterapred
Stoxil
streptomycin
Sulf 10
Sulfacel 15
Sulfair 10
Sulfair Forte
Sulphrin
Sulpred
Sulten-10
Suprofen
Surgisol

Sus-Phrine
Swim Eye

t

Tear-Efrin
Tearfair
Teargard
Teargen
Tearisol
Tears Naturale
Tears Plus
Tears Renewed
Tegretol
Tensilon
Terg-A-Zyme
Terra-Cortril
Terramycin
tetracaine
Tetracon
tetracycline
Tetracyn
Tetrasine
THC
thimerosal
timolol
Timoptic Ocudose
Tobradex
tobramycin
Tobrex
Total
Tramacort
Tri-Ophtho
triamcinolone
trifluridine
Triple-Gen
Trisol
tromethamine
Tropicacyl
tropicamide
Trump solution
Twenty/Twenty drops
Tyzine

u

Ultra Tears
Ultracaine
Ultrapred
Ultrazyme
Unisol
Uviban

v

vancomycin
Vasocidin
VasoClear
VasoClear A
Vasocon A
Vasocon Regular
Vasosulf
Velva Kleen
Vernacel
vidarabine
Vira-A
Viroptic
Visalens
Viscoat
Visculose
Visine A.C.
Vit-a-Drops

W

Wet-N-Soak
Wydase

X

Xylocaine

Z

Zephiran
zinc bacitracin
zinc sulfate
Zincfrin
Zolyse
Zovirax

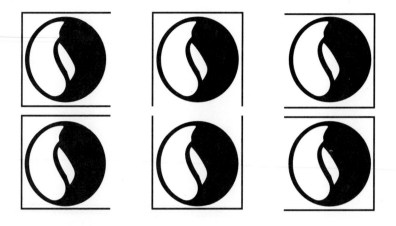

SECTION THREE

MEDICAL TERMINOLOGY

a

A — accommodation
A scan ultrasonography
AA — amplitude of accommodation
AACG — acute angle-closure glaucoma
AAMD — atrophic age-related macular degeneration
ab externo filtering operation
Abadie's sign
abaissement
abducens
  a. facial paralysis
  a. nerve
  a. palsy
  a. paralysis
abduct
abducted
abduction
abductor muscles
aberrant regeneration
aberration
  chromatic a.
  distantial a.
  regeneration a.
  spherical a.
aberrometer
abiotrophy
ablatio retinae
ablation
ablepharia
ablepharon
ablepharous
ablephary
ablepsia
ablepsy
abnormal
  a. harmonious retinal correspondence
abnormal *(continued)*
  a. retinal correspondence
  a. unharmonious retinal correspondence
abrader
  Howard a.
abrasio corneae
abrasion
  conjunctival a.
  corneal a.
abrin
abscess
  corneal a.
  lacrimal a.
  orbital a.
  ring a.
  vitreous a.
abscessed
abscesses
abscessus siccus corneae
abscission
  corneal a.
absence
absent guttata
absolute
  a. accommodation
  a. glaucoma
  a. hemianopia
  a. hyperopia
  a. scotoma
  a. strabismus
absorbable suture
absorption
abtorsion
abutted
abutting
AC/A ratio — accommodation convergence ratio
AC — anterior chamber
AC ratio — accommodation ratio
acanthocytosis
acanthosis

ACAT — age-related cataract
accessory
 a. fibers
 a. nucleus
 a. organs of eye
accidental image
accommodation
 absolute a.
 binocular a.
 esodeviation a.
 estropia a.
 excessive a.
 iridoplegia a.
 negative a.
 positive a.
 range a.
 reflex a.
 relative a.
 subnormal a.
Accommodation Rule
accommodative
 a. asthenopia
 a. convergence
 a. cyclophoria
 a. effort syndrome
 a. esotropia
 a. palsy
 a. spasm
 a. strabismus
 a. target
accommodometer
Accugel lens
acetylcholine receptor antibody level
ACG — angle-closure glaucoma
achloropsia
achroacytosis
achromat
achromatic
 a. lens
 a. perimetry
 a. threshold
 a. vision
achromatism
achromatopia
achromatopic
achromatopsia
acid burns
acid-fast bacilli
acidophilic adenoma
acne
 a. ciliaris
 a. conjunctivitis
 a. rosacea keratitis
acorea
acorn-shaped eye implant
acoustic
acoustical
 a. conductive gel
 a. hollowing
 a. shadowing
 a. sonolucent
acquired
 a. astigmatism
 a. esotropia
 a. immunodeficiency syndrome
 a. retinoschisis
acritochromacy
acrocephalosyndactylia of Apert
acromegalic habitus
acrylic
ACS needle
actinic
 a. conjunctivitis
 a. keratitis
 a. retinitis
actinomycosis
active pterygium
Acuiometer
acuity
 Vernier a.
 visual a.
 a. visual projector
Acuscan Transducer 400
acute

acute *(continued)*
  a. angle-closure glaucoma
  a. congestive conjunctivitis
  a. congestive glaucoma
Adams'
  ectropion
  operation
adaptation
  color a.
  dark a.
  light a.
  photopic a.
  retinal a.
  scotopic a.
adaptometer
  color a.
adduct
adducted
adduction
adductor muscles
adenocarcinoma
adenologaditis
adenophthalmia
adenoviral
adenovirus
adherence syndrome
adherent cataract
adhesion
adhesive syndrome
Adie's
  pupil
  syndrome
  tonic pupil
adipose body
aditus orbitae
adjustable sutures
Adler's operation
adnerval
adneural
adnexa
  a. oculi
adnexal
adolescent cataract
adrenergic blocking drug
adrenoleukodystrophy
Adson's forceps
adtorsion
ADV — adenovirus
advancement
  capsular a.
  a. flap
  a. procedure
Aebli's corneal scissors
aerial haze
aerosol keratitis
afferent
  a. defect
  a. limb
  a. nerve
  a. pupil defect
  a. pupillary defect
aftercataract
  a. bur
afterimage test
aftervision
against motion
against-the-rule astigmatism
agglutinins
aggregates
aggregation
aglaucopsia
Agnew's
  canaliculus knife
  canthoplasty
  keratome
  operation
  tattooing needle
agnosia
agonist muscle
agraphia
Agrikola's
  lacrimal sac retractor
  operation
  refractor

Agrikola's
  tattooing needle
Aicardi's syndrome
AIDS-related retinitis
air
  a. block glaucoma
  a. bubble
  a. cannula
  a. injection cannula
air-fluid exchange
air-puff tonometer
Aker's lens pusher
akinesia
  O'Brien's a.
  retrobulbar a.
  supraorbital a.
  Van-Lint's a.
akinesis
akinetic
aknephascopia
ala minor ossis sphenoidalis
Alabama-Green needle holder
alacrima
alar
albedo retinae
albinism
  localized a.
  ocular a.
  oculocutaneous a.
  partial a.
  tyrosinase-negative a.
  tyrosinase-positive a.
albinoidism
  oculocutaneous a.
  punctate oculocutaneous a.
albinotic fundus
albipunctate fundus
Albright's disease
albuginea oculi
albugo
Alcon's
  aspiration

Alcon's *(continued)*
  cautery
  cryophake
  Cryosurgical System
  hand cautery
  I-knife
  irrigation/aspiration unit
  Microsponge
  phacoemulsification
  surgical knife
  suture
  vitrectomy probe
Alexander's law
Alexander-Ballen retractor
alexia
  optical a.
  subcortical a.
alexic
Alfonso's
  guarded bur
  speculum
algorithm
aliquot
alkali burns
alkaline phosphatase
alkaptonuria
allele
Allen's
  cyclodialysis
  implant
  operation
  orbital implant
Allen-Barker forceps
Allen-Braley
  forceps
  implant
Allen-Burian trabeculotome
Allen-Schiotz tonometer
Allen-Thorpe
  gonioscopic prism
  lens
Allergan Humphrey
  laser

Allergan Humphrey *(continued)*
perimeter
refractor
Allergan
lensometer
Medical Optics photokeratoscope
allergic
a. conjunctivitis
a. pannus
allesthesia
visual a.
alligator
a. scissors
a. tears
allograft
allokeratoplasty
allophthalmia
Allport's
cutting bur
operation
all-transretinal
Aloe reading unit
alopecia
a. areata
a. orbicularis
Alpar implant
alpha hemolytic
alpha-chymotrypsin
a. cannula
a. glaucoma
Alport's syndrome
Alström's syndrome
Alström-Olsen syndrome
Alsus' operation
alternate cover-uncover test
alternate day esotropia
alternating
a. cross-eyes
a. esotropia
a. exotropia
a. mydriasis

alternating *(continued)*
a. strabismus
a. sursumduction
a. tropia
altitudinal
a. defect
a. field
a. hemianopsia
Alvis'
curet
operation
spud
Alvis-Lancaster sclerotome
amacrinal
amacrine cells
amaurosis
albuminuric a.
Burn's a.
cat's eye a.
a. centralis
cerebral a.
a. congenita of Leber
congenital a.
diabetic a.
a. fugax
hysteric a.
intoxification a.
Leber's a.
a. partialis fugax
reflex a.
saburral a.
toxic a.
uremic a.
a. nystagmus
amaurotic pupil
ambient
ambiopia
amblyope
amblyopia
alcoholic a.
ametropic a.
anisometric a.
arsenic a.

amblyopia *(continued)*
astigmatic a.
color a.
a. crapulosa
crossed a.
a. cruciata
deprivation a.
a. ex anopsia
exertional a.
functional a.
hysterical a.
irreversible a.
nocturnal a.
organic a.
postmarital a.
quinine a.
reflex a.
refractive a.
reversible a.
strabismic a.
suppression a.
tobacco a.
toxic a.
traumatic a.
uremic a.
amblyopiatrics
amblyopic
amblyoscope
major a.
amelanotic
ameliorate
ameliorated
Amenabar's
capsule forceps
counterpressor
discission hook
iris retractor
lens loop
American Hydron
American Medical Optics
American Optical photocoagulator
ametrometer
ametropia
axial a.
curvature a.
index a.
position a.
refractive a.
ametropic amblyopia
amino aciduria
Ammon's
canthoplasty
operation
amnesic color blindness
Amoils'
cryoextractor
cryopencil
cryophake
cryoprobe
cryosurgical unit
refractor
amorphous corneal dystrophy
amotio retinae
amphamphoterodiplopia
amphodiplopia
amphoterodiplopia
amplitude
a. of accommodation
a. of convergence
a. of fusion
AMPPE — acute multifocal placoid pigment epitheliopathy
ampulla
a. canaliculi lacrimalis
a. ductus lacrimalis
a. of lacrimal canal
a. of lacrimal duct
ampullae
Amsler's
aqueous transplant needle
chart
corneal graft
grid test

Amsler's *(continued)*
marker
needle
operation
scleral marker
amyloid corneal degeneration
amyloidosis
anaclasis
anaglyph test
anagnosasthenia
Anagnostakis' operation
analgesia
a. permeation
surface a.
anangioid disk
anaphoria
anaphylactic conjunctivitis
anastigmatic
anastomoses
anastomosis
anatomic
a. equator
a. substrate
anatropia
anatropic
anchor
anchored
anchoring suture
Andersen's syndrome
Andogsky's syndrome
Anel's operation
anencephaly
anergy
anesthesia
intraorbital a.
modified Van Lint's a.
O'Brien's a.
orbital a.
retrobulbar a.
topical a.
Van Lint's a.
aneuploides
aneurysm
aneurysm *(continued)*
miliary a.
orbital a.
Angelucci's
operation
syndrome
angiodiathermy
angiogram
angiography
fluorescein a.
angioid
a. choroidal streaks
a. retinal streaks
angiokeratoma
a. corporis diffusum universale
diffuse a.
angioma
angiomatosis
cerebroretinal a.
a. of retina
angiopathia retinae juvenilis
angiopathy
angiophakomatosis
angioscotoma
angioscotometry
angiospasm
angle
a. of aberration
alpha a.
anomaly a.
anterior chamber a.
a. of aperture
biorbital a.
a.-closure glaucoma
convergence a.
critical a.
a. of deviation
a. of direction
elevation a.
filtration a.
gamma a.
a. of incidence

angle *(continued)*
iridial a.
iridocorneal a.
a. of iris
Jacquart's a.
kappa a.
lambda a.
lateral a.
limiting a.
medial a.
meter a.
minimum separable a.
minimum visible a.
minimum visual a.
ocular a.
open-a. glaucoma
optic a.
recession-a. glaucoma
refraction a.
squint a.
visual a.

angled
a. capsule forceps
a. counterpressor
a. discission hook
a. iris hook and IOL dialer
a. iris retractor
a. left/right cannula
a. lens loop
a. nucleus removal loop
a. probe
a. suction tube
a. Vico manipulator

angor ocularis

angstrom

angular
a. blepharitis
a. distance
a. gyrus
a. iridocornealis
a. oculi lateralis
a. oculi medialis

angulated iris spatula

angulus
a. iridis
a. iridocornealis
a. oculi lateralis
a. oculi medialis

anhidrosis

anicteric

aniridia

Anis' irrigating vectis

aniseikonia

aniseikonic

anisoaccommodation

anisochromatic

anisocoria contraction

anisometric amblyopia

anisometrope

anisometropia

anisometropic

anisometropsia

anisophoria

anisopia

anisotropal

anisotrophy

ankyloblepharon
a. filiforme adnatum
a. totale

ankylosing spondylitis

annular
a. corneal graft
a. plexus
a. scleritis
a. scotoma
a. staphyloma
a. synechia
a. ulcer

annulus
a. ciliaris
a. of conjunctiva
a. iridis major
a. iridis minor
a. tendineus communis
a. of Zinn

annulus
a. zinnii
anomalies
coloboma a.
facial a.
anomalopia
anomaloscope
anomalous
a. disks
a. retinal correspondence
a. trichromatism
a. trichromatopsia
anomaly
Axenfeld's a.
developmental a.
Peter's a.
Rieger's a.
anoopsia
anophoria
anophthalmia
anophthalmos
anophthalmus
anopia
anopsia
anorthopia
anorthoscope
anotropia
antagonist
contralateral a.
ipsilateral a.
antecubital vein
anterior
a. axial developmental cataract
a. capsule shagreen
a. chamber cannula
a. chamber irrigating vectis
a. chamber irrigator
a. chamber paracentesis
a. chamber reaction
a. chamber synechiae scissors

anterior *(continued)*
a. chamber tap
a. choroiditis
a. ciliary arteries
a. corneal staphyloma
a. embryotoxon
a. epithelium corneae
a. focal point
a. knee of von Willebrand
a. lens
a. limiting lamina
a. lip
a. megalophthalmos
a. pole
a. pyramidal cataract
a. scleritis
a. sclerotomy
a. segment sleeve
a. staphyloma
a. symblepharon
a. synechia
a. uveitis
anteroposterior axis of Fick
Anthony's orbital compressor
anticholinesterase
antifungal
antigen
antigenicity
antihyaluronidase
anti-inflammatories
anti-inflammatory
antilens protein antibodies
antimelanoma
antimetabolites
antimetropia
antimongoloid slant
antinuclear factor
antisuppression exercise
antitonic
antiviral
antixerophthalmic
Anton-Babinski syndrome

Anton's
symptom
syndrome
antophthalmic
antrophose
anulus. *See annulus*
A-O applanation tonometer
A-O binocular indirect ophthalmoscope
A-O Ful-Vue diagnostic unit
A-O lensometer
A-O Project-O-Chart
A-O Reichert Instruments
aortic arch syndrome
A-pattern esotropia
A-pattern exotropia
A-pattern strabismus
APD — afferent pupillary defect
Apert's
disease
syndrome
aperture
orbital a.
apex
aphacia
aphacic
aphacos
aphake
aphakia
aphakic
a. correction
a. spectacles
aphasia
visual a.
aphose
aphotesthesia
aphotic
aphthous-like
aphthous ulcers
apical
a. clearance
a. cone
a. radius
apical
a. zone
apices
aplanatic focus
aplanatism
aplasia
lacrimal nucleus a.
macular a.
punctum a.
retinal a.
aponeurosis
apoplectic
a. glaucoma
a. retinitis
apoplexy
retinal a.
apparatus
ciliary a.
lacrimal a.
a. lacrimalis
a. suspensorius lentis
appearance
beaten-metal a.
ground-glass a.
mottled a.
spongy a.
appendage of the eye
applanation
a. pressure
a. tonometer
a. tonometry
applanometer
applicator
Gifford's a.
apposition
apraxia
aqua oculi
Aquaflex
aqueocapsulitis
aqueous
a. chamber
a. flare
a. humor

aqueous *(continued)*
    a. outflow
    a. paracentesis
    plasmoid a.
    a. tear deficiency
    a. transplant needle
    a. veins
AR 1000 refractor
arachnodactyly
arachnoid
    a. hemorrhage
    a. sheath
arachnoiditis
    optochiasmatic a.
arborescent cataract
arborization pattern
arc and bowl perimeters
arc flash conjunctivitis
arc
    a. of contact
    nuclear a.
    a. perimeter
    a. perimetry
    a. scotoma
    xenon a.
ARC — abnormal retinal correspondence
ARC — AIDS-related complex
ARC — anomalous retinal correspondence
arcade
arch
    orbital a.
    Salus a.
    superciliary a.
    supraorbital a.
arcuate
    a. course
    a. field defects
    inferior a. bundle
    a. nerve fiber bundle
    a. retinal folds
    a. scotoma
arcuate *(continued)*
    superior a. bundle
    superior a. scotoma
arcus
    a. adiposus
    a. corneae
    a. cornealis
    a. juvenilis
    a. lipoides corneae
    a. palpebralis inferior
    a. palpebralis superior
    a. parieto-occipitalis
    a. senilis
    a. superciliaris
area
    Brodmann's a.
    a. centralis
    a. of critical definition
    a. martegiani
    mirror a.
    Panum's a.
areflexia
areolar central choroiditis
argamblyopia
argema
argon
    a. blue
    Britt pulsed a. laser
    Coherent 920 a. laser
    a. green
    a. laser photocoagulation
    LPK-80 II a. laser
    Ophthalas a. laser
    Sharplan a. laser
Argyll-Robertson Instruments
Argyll-Robertson
    operation
    pupil
argyria
argyriasis
argyrism
argyrosis
ariboflavinosis

aridosiliculose cataract
aridosiliquate
Arion's
  operation
  sling
Arlt's
  disease
  epicanthus repair
  eyelid repair
  line
  loop
  operation
  pterygium
  scoop
  sinus
  trachoma
  triangle
Arlt-Jaesche
  excision
  operation
  recessus
  sinus
  trachoma
arrachement
Arrowhead's operation
Arroyo's
  cataract extraction
  dacryostomy
  encircling suture
  expressor
  forceps
  implant
  keratoplasty
  operation
  protector
  sign
  tenotomy
  trephine
Arruga's
  cataract extraction
  dacryostomy
  encircling suture
  expressor

Arruga's *(continued)*
  implant
  keratoplasty
  lacrimal trephine
  lens
  needle holder
  retractor
  tenotomy
  trephine
Arruga-Berens operation
Arruga-Moura-Brazil implant
arterial circle
arteriola
  a. macularis inferior
  a. macularis superior
  a. medialis retinae
  a. nasalis retinae inferior
  a. nasalis retinae superior
  a. temporalis retinae inferior
  a. temporalis retinae superior
arteriolar
  a. attenuation
  a. narrowing
  a. nicking
arteriole
  inferior macular a.
  medial a. of retina
  nasal a. of retina
  superior macular a.
  temporal a. of retina
arteriosclerosis
arteriovenous
  a. aneurysm
  a. crossings
  a. ratio
arteritis
  cranial a.
  giant cell a.
  idiopathic a. of Takayasu
  temporal a.
artery

artery *(continued)*
- anterior ciliary a.
- anterior conjunctival a.
- central retinal a.
- copper-wire a.
- corkscrew a.
- episcleral a.
- infraorbital a.
- lacrimal a.
- long ciliary a.
- ophthalmic a.
- posterior ciliary a.
- posterior conjunctival a.
- short ciliary a.
- short posterior ciliary a.
- supraorbital a.
- tarsal a.
- zygomatico-orbital a.

arthro-ophthalmopathy

artifact

artifactiously

artifactual

artificial
- a. eye
- a. pupil
- a. silk keratitis
- a. tears

As.M. — myopic astigmatism

Ascher's
- glass
- rod
- syndrome

Ascon Instruments

Aseptron II

ash leaf spots

aspheric
- a. cornea
- a. lens
- a. lenticular area
- a. viewing lens

aspirator
- Cavitron a.
- Cooper a.

aspirator *(continued)*
- Kelman a.
- Nugent a.
- SITE a.

Assi's cannula

Ast. — astigmatism

asteroid
- a. hyalitis
- a. hyalosis

asthenocoria

asthenometer

asthenope

asthenopia
- accommodative a.
- muscular a.
- nervous a.
- retinal a.
- tarsal a.

asthenopic

astigmagraph

astigmagraphic error

astigmatic
- a. axis
- a. clock
- a. dial

astigmatism
- acquired a.
- against the rule a.
- compound a.
- compound myopic a.
- congenital a.
- corneal a.
- direct a.
- hypermetropic a.
- hyperopic a.
- inverse a.
- irregular a.
- lenticular a.
- mixed a.
- myopic a.
- oblique a.
- physiological a.
- regular a.

astigmatism *(continued)*
- simple a.
- simple myopic a.
- total a.
- with the rule a.

astigmatometer
astigmatometry
astigmatoscope
astigmia
astigmic
astigmometer
astigmometry
astigmoscope
astigmoscopy
astrocyte
astrocytic
asymmetric
- a. refractive errors
- a. surgery

asymmetry
- chromatic a.

at distance and near
at near
ataxia
- ocular a.

ataxia-telangiectasia syndrome
ATD — aqueous tear deficiency
Athens suture spreader
atheroembolism
atheroma
athetosis
- pupillary a.

Atkin's lid block
Atkinson's
- corneal scissors
- needle
- retrobulbar needle
- sclerotome
- single-bevel, blunt-tip needle
- 25-G short curved cystotome
- tip peribulbar needle

atonia
atonic
atopic
- a. conjunctivitis
- a. dermatitis
- a. eczema

Atraloc suture
atresia
- a. iridis
- tilting lens a.

atretoblepharia
atretopsia
atrophia
- a. bulbi
- a. bulborum hereditaria
- a. choroideae et retinae
- a. dolorosa
- a. gyrata

atrophic
- a. excavation
- a. macular degeneration

atrophy
- Behr's a.
- bow-tie a.
- bulbus a.
- choroidal a.
- consecutive a.
- essential a. of iris
- Fuchs' a.
- gray a.
- gyrate a.
- hemifacial a.
- Kjer's dominant a.
- Leber's a.
- linear subcutaneous a.
- optic a.
- primary optic a.
- Schnabel's a.
- secondary optic a.
- senile a.
- subcutaneous fat a.
- tabelic a.

atropine conjunctivitis

atropinism
atropinization
attention reflex
attenuation
attollens aurem
autoantibodies
autofluorescence
autofunduscope
autofunduscopy
autogenous
  a. dermis fat graft
  a. fibronectin
autograft
autoimmune demyelination
autokeratometer
autokeratoplasty
autokinesis visible light
automated
  a. hemisphere perimeter
  a. refractor
  a. trephine
autonomic nervous system
auto-ophthalmoscope
auto-ophthalmoscopy
Auto-Plot
auto-refractor
autosomal
  a. dominant trait
  a. dominant vitellirupture
  a. recessive inheritance
Autoswitch System
auxiometer
AV crossing defect
AV ratio — arteriovenous ratio
avascular
Avit handpiece
avulsion
A-wave
awl
  lacrimal a.
  Mustarde a.
axanthopsia
Axenfeld's

Axenfeld's *(continued)*
  anomaly
  loop
  syndrome
axial
  a. ametropia
  a. cataract
  a. chamber
  a. fusiform developmental cataract
  a. hyperopia
  a. length
  a. myopia
  a. view
axillary cataract
axis
  anteroposterior a.
  a. bulbi externus
  a. bulbi internus
  external a. of eye
  frontal a.
  geometric a.
  internal a. of eye
  lens a.
  a. lentis
  longitudinal a.
  ocular a.
  a. oculi externa
  a. oculi interna
  a. of Fick
  optic a.
  optical a.
  a. opticus
  principal a.
  pupillary a.
  sagittal a.
  secondary a.
  vertical a.
  visual a.
  Y a. of Fick
  Z a. of Fick
Axisonic II ultrasound
axometer

axon
axonal loss
axonometer
axoplasm
axoplasmic
  a. flow
  a. stasis
  a. transport
Ayer's chalazion forceps
Ayerst Instruments
azotemia

b

B-Scan
background retinopathy
Backhaus' syndrome
bacterial conjunctivitis
Badal's operation
Baer's nystagmus
bag
  capsular b.
Bagley-Wilmer expressor
Bagolini's lens
Bahn's spud
Bailey's lacrimal cannula
Bailliart's
  goniometer
  ophthalmodynamometer
  ophthalmoscope
balanced salt solution
balding the limbus
Balint's syndrome
ball
  ice b.
  Pinky b.
  snow b.
  Super Pinky b.
Ballen-Alexander orbital retractor
Ballet's sign
Bamatter's syndrome
band
  encircling b.
  keratitis b.
  silicone b.
  zonular b.
band-shaped keratitis
bandage
  binocle b.
  binocular b.
  Borsch b.
  b. contact lens
  b. lens
  monocular b.
  b. scissors
Bangerter's
  iris spatula
  pterygium operation
bank keratitis
Banner's enucleation snare
bar reader
Bárány's sign
Bard's sign
Bard-Parker
  keratome
  knife
  razor
  trephine
Bardelli's lid ptosis operation
Bardet-Biedl syndrome
bare scleral technique
baring of the blind spot
Barkan's
  double cyclodialysis operation
  goniolens
  gonioscopic lens
  goniotomy knife
  goniotomy operation
  infant implant
  knife
  light
  operation

Barkan-Cordes linear cataract operation
Baron-Bietti syndrome
Barraquer's
- cannula
- corneal dissector
- enzymatic zonulolysis operation
- erysiphake
- eye shield
- implant
- iris scissors
- irrigator spatula
- keratomileusis operation
- knife
- lens
- needle
- needle carrier
- needle holder
- operation
- razor blade breaker
- scissors
- shield
- spatula
- speculum
- trephine
- vitreous strand scissors
- zonulolysis

Barraquer-Colibri speculum
Barraquer-DeWecker scissors
Barraquer-Krumeich test
Barraquer-Vogt needle
Barré's signs
barred distortion
barrel distortion
Barrie-Jones canaliculodacryorhinostomy operation
barrier
- blood aqueous b.

Barrier
- drapes
- Phaco Extracapsular Pack

Barrier
- sheet

Barrio operation
Barron's epikeratophakia trephine
basal
- b. choroid
- b. ciliary body
- b. encephalocele
- b. lamina
- b. ophthalmoplegia

base
- b. curve
- vitreous b.

base-down prism
base-in prism
base-out prism
base-up prism
baseball lens
Basedow's disease
basement membrane
basic exotropia
basket-style scleral supporter speculum
basophil
basophilic adenoma
Bassen-Kornzweig syndrome
Basterra's operation
BAT — Brightness Acuity Test
bathomorphic
Batten-Mayou disease
Bausch-Lomb-Thorp slit lamp
bay
- lacrimal b.

BD — base-down prism
beading
Béal's
- conjunctivitis
- syndrome

beam scatter
bear tracks
Beard's knife
Beard-Cutler operation

beaten-copper appearance
Beaupre's forceps
Beaver's
- blade
- cryoextractor
- discission blade
- keratome
- knife
- ocu-curved cystotome

Beaver-Lundsgaard blade
Beaver-Okamura blade
Beaver-Zeigler blade
Becker's
- corneal section spatulated scissors
- goniogram

Becker-Park speculum
Beckerscope Binocular Microscope
bed
bedewing
- b. of cornea
- b. to wet

Beebe's loupe
Beer's
- cataract knife
- collyrium
- knife
- operation

Behçet's
- disease
- syndrome

Behr's
- atrophy
- disease
- pupil
- syndrome

Bekhterev's nystagmus
Bell's
- erysiphake
- palsy
- phenomenon
- reflex

Bellows' cryoextractor
belly
- b. of muscle
- b. of pterygium

belonoskiascopy
Benedict's
- orbit operation
- syndrome

Bennett's forceps
Benson's disease
bent blunt needle
Béraud's valve
Bercovici's wire lid speculum
Berens'
- cataract knife
- corneal dissector
- corneal transplant scissors
- corneoscleral punch
- dilator
- electrode
- expressor
- forceps
- glaucoma knife
- implant
- iridocapsulotomy scissors
- keratome
- keratoplasty knife
- lens loop
- lid everter
- marking caliper
- muscle clamp
- muscle forceps
- operation
- orbital compressor
- Pinhole and Dominance Test
- prism bar
- pterygium transplant operation
- ptosis knife
- punch
- retractor

Berens' *(continued)*
scissors
scleral hook
sclerectomy operation
spatula
speculum
suturing forceps
test object
Three Character Test
tonometer
Berens-Rosa implant
Berens-Smith cul-de-sac restoration
Berens-Tolman ocular hypertension indicator
Bergmeister's papilla
Berke's
clamp
forceps
lid everter
operation
ptosis
Berkeley Bioengineering
bipolar cautery
brass scleral plug
infusion terminal port
mechanized scissors
Ocutome
Berke-Motais operation
Berlin's
disease
edema
Berman's
foreign body locator
localizer
Bernheimer's fibers
Berry's circle
Bertel's position
besiclometer
Best's
disease
vitelliform macular dystrophy
best-corrected
vision
visual acuity
beta
b. hemolytic
b. radiation
Bethke's iridectomy
Bianchi's valve
Biber-Haab-Dimmer degeneration
Bicap Biometric
biconcave lens
biconvex lens
bicoronal
b.i.d. — twice a day
Bielschowsky's
disease
head-tilt test
operation
phenomenon
strabismus
three-step, head-tilt test
Bielschowsky-Jansky disease
Bielschowsky-Lutz-Cogan syndrome
Bietti's
dystrophy
syndrome
bifixation
bifocal
b. fixation
b. glasses
bifoveal fixation
bifurcation
bilaminar membrane
bilateral
b. hemianopia
b. strabismus
binasal
b. hemianopia
b. quadrant fields
Binkhorst's
collar stud lens implant

Binkhorst's *(continued)*
four-loop iris fixated implant
two-loop lens
Binkhorst-Fyodorov lens
binocle bandage
binocular
b. accommodation
b. bandage
b. depth perception
b. diplopia
b. dressing
b. eye patch
b. field
b. fixation
b. fusion
b. hemianopia
b. indirect ophthalmoscope
b. loupe
b. parallax
b. polyopia
b. rivalry
b. strabismus
b. vision
b. visual acuity
binocularity
binoculus
binophthalmoscope
binoscope
biometric ruler
biomicroscope slit lamp
biomicroscopy
Bio-Pen
biophotometer
Biophysic Laser
biopsy
Bioptic
camera
microscope
Telescope System
Bio-Rad Lab
biorbital angle
bipolar
b. cells
b. cone
b. giant
b. rod
biprism applanation tonometer
biprong muscle marker
Birch-Harmon irrigator
Birch-Hirschfeld
entropion operation
lamp
birdshot
b. retinochoroidopathy
b. retinopathy
b. spot
birefractive
birefringent
Birkhauser test chart
Birks Mark II Instruments
micro cross-action holder
micro push/pull
micro spatula
micro trabeculectomy scissors
push/pull spatula
birth trauma
Bishop's tendon tucker
Bishop-Harmon
anterior chamber irrigator
bladebreaker
cannula
forceps
irrigator
knife
Superblade
Bishop-Peter tendon tucker
bite
bitemporal hemianopsia
bithermal caloric stimulation
bitoric contact lens
Bitot's spots

Bjerrum's
- scotoma
- scotometer
- screen
- sign

black
- b. braided nylon suture
- b. cataract
- b. cornea
- b. reflex
- b. silk sling suture
- b. sunburst

blade
- Bard-Parker b.
- Beaver's b.
- Beaver-Lundsgaard b.
- Beaver-Okamura b.
- Beaver-Zeigler b.
- bent blunt b.
- Berens' b.
- broken razor b.
- Castroviejo's razor
- CooperVision Surgeon-Plus Ultra Thin b.
- Curdy's b.
- Curdy-Hebra b.
- diamond-dusted knife b.
- GS-9 b.
- Hebra's b.
- Hoskin's razor fragment b.
- Keeler's retractable b.
- Lange's b.
- Martinez corneal trephine b.
- McPherson-Wheeler b.
- miniature b.
- MVR b.
- myringotomy b.
- razor b.
- replaceable b.
- Scheie's b.
- Superblade No.75 b.

blade *(continued)*
- trephine b.
- V-lance b.

bladebreaker
- Barraquer's razor b.
- knife b.
- Swiss b.
- Troutman's b.

Blair's
- epicanthus repair
- head drape
- operation
- retractor
- stiletto

blanching

blank spot

Blasius's lid flap operation

Blaskovics'
- canthoplasty operation
- flap
- inversion of tarsus operation
- lid operation
- tarsectomy

Blaskovics-Berke ptosis

Blaskovics-Doyen

blastomycosis

Blatt's operation

Blaydes' forceps

blear eye

bleb
- b. cup
- filtering b.
- iron leaking b.
- leaking b.

Blenderm tape

blenorrhea
- b. adultorum
- inclusion b.
- b. neonatorum

blenorrheal conjunctivitis

blepharadenitis

blepharal

blepharectomy
blepharelosis
blepharism
blepharitis
- b. angularis
- b. ciliaris
- eczematoid b.
- b. marginalis
- nonulcerative b.
- seborrheic b.
- b. squamosa
- squamous seborrheic b.
- b. ulcerosa

blepharoadenitis
blepharoadenoma
blepharoatheroma
blepharochalasis
blepharochromidrosis
blepharoclonus
blepharoconjunctivitis
- acne rosacea b.
- angular b.
- bacterial b.
- chronic b.
- b. Moraxella lacunata
- b. vaccinia

blepharodiastasis
blepharoncus
blepharopachynsis
blepharophimosis
- epicanthus b.
- b. inversus
- b. ptosis syndrome

blepharoplast
blepharoplasty
blepharoplegia
blepharoptosis
blepharopyorrhea
blepharorrhaphy
blepharospasm
- essential b.
- symptomatic b.

blepharosphincterectomy
blepharostat
- McNeill-Goldman b.

blepharostenosis
blepharosynechia
blepharotomy
blepharoxysis
Blessig-Iwanoff cyst
Blessig's
- cyst
- groove

blind
- color b.
- b. reflex

blind spot
- b.s. enlargement
- b.s. of Mariotte
- b.s. reflex
- b.s. syndrome

blindness
- amnesic color b.
- blue b.
- Bright's b.
- color b.
- concussion b.
- cortical psychic b.
- day b.
- eclipse b.
- electric light b.
- epidemic b.
- flash b.
- flight b.
- functional b.
- green b.
- legal b.
- letter b.
- mind b.
- moon b.
- night b.
- note b.
- object b.
- psychic b.
- red b.
- river b.

blindness *(continued)*
- snow b.
- soul b.
- syllabic b.
- b. test
- total b.
- twilight b.
- yellow b.

blink
- b. adequacy
- b. inadequacy
- b. reflex

Bloch-Stauffer syndrome
Bloch-Sulzberger syndrome
block
- Atkin's lid b.
- ciliovitrectomy b.
- modified Van Lint's b.
- O'Brien's b.
- pupillary b.
- retrobulbar b.
- Van Lint's b.

blond fundi
blood
- b. agar
- b. barrier
- b. lipids
- b. reflux
- retinal b.

blot and dot hemorrhages
blotchy positive staining
blown pupil
blow-out fracture
blue
- b. blindness
- b. cataract
- b. cone monochromatism
- b. dot cataract
- b. line
- b. nevus
- b. sclera
- b. spot

blunt needle
blur
- b. and clear exercise
- b. point
- b. zone

blurring of vision
B-mode handpiece
BO — base-out prism
boat hook
- Katena b.h.

bobbing
Boberg-Ans lens implant
Bodkin's thread holder
bodies. *See body*
body
- adipose b.
- ciliary b.
- colloid b.
- cystoid b.
- Elschnig's b.
- Hassall's b.
- Henle's b.
- Hensen's b.
- hyaloid b.
- intracytoplasmic inclusion b.
- Landolt's b.
- lenticular b.
- Lewy's b.
- Lipschultz b.
- nigroid b.
- Prowazek-Greeff b.
- Prowazek-Halberstaedter b.
- trachoma b.
- vitreous b.

Boeck's sarcoid
boggy edema
Böhm's operation
bolster
bolus
bombé
- b. configuration

bombé
- iris b.

Bonaccolto's
- forceps
- monoplex orbital implant
- orbital implant
- scleral ring
- trephine
- vitreous

Bonaccolto-Flieringa
- operation
- scleral ring

bone
- b. punch
- b. spicules
- b. trephine

bone-biting
- forceps
- punch
- trephine

Bonn's forceps
Bonnet's enucleation operation
Bonnet-Dechaume-Blanc syndrome
Bonnier's syndrome
Bonzel's
- blood staining of cornea
- operation

boomerang-shaped lesion
border
- orbital b. of sphenoid bone

Bores twist fixation ring
Borsch's bandage
Borthen's iridostasis operation
Bossalino's blepharoplasty operation
Boston's trephine
bottlemaker's cataract
botulism
Botvin-Bradford enucleator
bouche de tapir
bougie
boule
bound-down muscle
bounding
- b. mydriasis
- b. pupil

bouquet of Rochon-Duvigneaud
Bourneville's disease
Bovie's
- cautery
- electrocautery unit
- electrosurgical unit
- retinal detachment unit
- wet field cautery

bovied
Bowen's disease
Bowman's
- cataract needle
- lamina
- layer
- membrane
- muscle
- needle
- operation
- probe
- stop needle
- tube
- zone

bowstring
bow tie
- b.t. atrophy
- b.t. knot

boxcarring
Boyce's needle holder
Boyd's
- implant
- operation
- orbital implant
- zone

Boyden's chamber technique
Boynton's needle holder
Bozzi's foramen
brachium conjunctiva
brachymetropia

brachymetropic
Bracken's
  cannula
  effect
  forceps
braid
  b. effect
  b. strabismus
braided
  b. silk suture
  b. vicryl suture
Brailey's operation
brain cortex
brain stem
branch vein occlusion
brass scleral plug
Brawley's retractor
Brawner's orbital implant
brawny scleritis
breadth of accommodation
break
  b. in retinal integrity
  b. point
break-up time
Brickner's sign
bridge
  b. coloboma
  b. pedicle flap
  b. operation
Bridge's operation
bridle suture
Briggs' strabismus operation
Bright's
  blindness
  disease
  eye
Brightness Acuity Test
bright-sense
Britt's
  argon/krypton laser
  BL-12 laser
  pulsed argon laser
Brodmann's area
Brombach's perimeter
Bromley's foreign body operation
Bronson's foreign body removal operation
Bronson-Magnion
  eye magnet
  forceps
Bronson-Park speculum
Bronson-Turner foreign body locator
Bronson-Turz
  refractor
  retractor
brown cataract
Brown's
  sterile adhesive
  syndrome
Brown-Dohlman Silastic corneal implant
Brown-Pusey corneal trephine
brucellosis
Bruch's membrane
Bruchner's test
Brücke's
  fibers
  lens
  muscle
  tunica nervea
bruit
brunescent cataract
brush
  Barraquer's sable b.
  Haidinger's b.
  Thomas' b.
Brushfield's spots
B-scan ultrasonogram
B-scan ultrasonography
BSS — balanced salt solution
BU — base-up prism
bubble
  Chamber's sterile adhesive b.

bubble
- Expo B.

buckle
- choroid b.
- encircling b.

buckling
- b. choroid
- b. sclera

budding yeast cells
Budinger's blepharoplasty operation
Buettner-Parel vitreous cutter
buffered formaldehyde
buffy coat
bufilcon A
build-up implant
bulb of the eye
bulbar
bulbocapnine
bulbus
- b. oculi

bull's eye
- macular lesion
- maculopathy
- retinopathy

bulla
- ethmoid b.
- b. ethmoidalis cavinasi
- b. ethmoidalis ossis
- b. ossea

bullae
bulldog clamp
Buller's shield
bullosa
bullosus
bullous
- b. detachment
- b. keratopathy

bullular canal
Bumke's pupil
bundle
- Drualt's b.
- maculopapular b.

bundle
- nerve b.

Bunge's evisceration spoon
Bunker's implant
buphthalmia
buphthalmos
buphthalmus
bur
- after-cataract b.
- Alfonso's guarded b.
- Allport's cutting b.
- Burwell's b.
- corneal b.
- corneal foreign body b.
- cutting b.
- lacrimal sac b.
- Storz's corneal b.
- Yazujian's b.

Burch's
- caliper
- evisceration operation
- pick
- tendon tucker

Burch-Greenwood tucker
Burch-Lester speculum
buried drusen
Burns' amaurosis
burns were made
Burow's flap operation
Burr's
- butterfly needle
- corneal ring
- silicone button

Burwell's bur
Busacca's nodules
BUT — breakup time
butterfly macular dystrophy
button
- corneal b.

buttonholed
button tip manipulator
butyl cyanoacrylate
Buzzi's operation

BVA - best corrected visual acuity
B-VAT acuity tester
b-wave
Byron Smith ectropion operation

C

cabufocon A
Cairn's
  operation
  trabeculectomy
calcarine fissure
calcific band keratopathy
calcium
  c.-containing opacities
  c. deposition
  c. emboli
  c. salts
calculi
calculus
Caldwell's view
Caldwell-Waters view
Calhoun's needle
Calhoun-Hagler
  lens extraction operation
  lens needle
Calhoun-Merz needle
caliculus ophthalmicus
caligo
  c. corneae
  c. lentis
  c. pupillae
calipers
  Berens's marking c.
  Burch's c.
  Castroviejo's c.
  Green's c.
  Jameson's c.

calipers *(continued)*
  John Green c.
  Stahl's c.
  Thorpe's c.
  Thorpe-Castroviejo c.
Callahan's
  fixation forceps
  lens loop
  operation
Callender's cell type classification
Calmette's ophthalmoreaction
caloric testing
caloric-induced nystagmus
calotte
calvaria
camera
  c. bulbi anterior
  c. bulbi posterior
  c. lucida
  c. obscura
  c. oculi
  c. oculi anterior
  c. oculi posterior
  c. vitrea bulbi
Campbell's
  refractor
  retractor
  slit lamp
campimeter
campimetry
Campodonico's operation
canal
  bullular c.
  Campodonico's c.
  central c.
  ciliary c.
  Cloquet's c.
  ethmoid c.
  Ferrein's c.
  Fontana's c.
  Hannover's c.
  hyaloid c.

canal *(continued)*
- infraorbital c.
- lacrimal c.
- Lauth's c.
- nasal c.
- nasolacrimal c.
- c. of Nuck
- optic c.
- orbital c.
- Petit's c.
- Schlemm's c.
- scleral c.
- scleroticochoroidal c.
- Sondermann's c.
- c. of Stilling
- supraciliary c.
- supraoptic c.
- supraorbital c.
- tarsal c.
- zygomaticofacial c.
- zygomaticotemporal c.

canalicular scissors
canaliculi
canaliculitis
canaliculodacryocystostomy
canaliculodacryorhinostomy
canaliculorhinostomy
canaliculum
canaliculus
- c. infraorbitalis opticus
- c. lacrimalis
- c. rod and suture

canalis
- c. hyaloideus
- c. opticus

cancrum nasi
candela
Candida albicans
candidal
- c. conjunctivitis
- c. endophthalmitis
- c. keratitis
- c. uveitis

candle wax drippings
cannula
- air injection c.
- alpha-chymotrypsin c.
- angled left/right c.
- anterior chamber c.
- Assi's c.
- Bailey's lacrimal c.
- Barraquer's c.
- Bishop-Harmon c.
- Bracken's c.
- Castroviejo's cyclodialysis c.
- cyclodialysis c.
- DeLavega's vitreous aspirating c.
- double irrigating/aspirating c.
- Drews' c.
- Fasenella's lacrimal c.
- Galt's aspirating c.
- Gans' c.
- Gass' cataract aspirating c.
- Gills' double Luer-Lok c.
- Goldstein's c.
- goniotomy knife c.
- Gormley's double c.
- Heyner's double c.
- Hilton's self-retaining infusion c.
- iris hook c.
- irrigating/aspirating c.
- Johnson's double c.
- J-shaped irrigating/aspirating c.
- Karickhoff's double c.
- Keeler-Keislar lacrimal c.
- Kelman's cyclodialysis c.
- Klein's curved c.
- knife c.
- Kraff's cortex c.
- lacrimal c.

cannula *(continued)*
- liquid vitreous aspirating c.
- Maumenee's goniotomy knife c.
- Moncrieff's c.
- O'Gawa's cataract aspirating c.
- Oaks' double straight c.
- Packo pars plana c.
- Pearce's coaxial irrigating/aspirating c.
- Peczon's irrigating/aspirating c.
- Randolph's cyclodialysis c.
- reel aspiration c.
- Roper's alpha-chymotrypsin c.
- Scheie's anterior chamber c.
- self-retaining irrigating c.
- side port c.
- Simcoe's double c.
- Steriseal disposable c.
- Swet's goniotomy knife c.
- Tenner's lacrimal c.
- Thomas' c.
- two-way cataract aspirating c.
- Ulanday's double c.
- Veirs' c.
- VISCOFLOW c.
- Welsh's cortex stripper c.
- Welsh's flat olive tip double c.
- Wergland's double c.

Canon fundus camera

Cantelli's sign

canthal
- c. raphe
- c. tendon

canthectomy

canthi

canthitis

cantholysis

canthomeatal

canthopexy

canthoplasty

canthorrhaphy

canthotomy

canthus
- inner c.
- lateral c.
- medial c.
- outer c.

capillary
- c. bed
- c. hemangioma
- c. lumen
- c. lumina
- c. plexus

capsid

capsitis

capsula
- c. bulbi
- c. lentis

capsular
- c. bag
- c. debris
- c. exfoliation syndrome

capsular-zonular

capsule
- anterior lens c.
- Bonnet's c.
- crystalline c.
- c. fragment spatula
- ocular c.
- c. of lens
- c. polisher
- Tenon's c.

capsule polisher
- Kraff's c.p. curet
- Terry Silicone c.p.

capsulectomy
capsulitis
capsulolenticular cataract
capsulorrhexis
capsulotome
    Darling's c.
capsulotomy
    c. scissors
    Darling's c.
capture
    iris c.
    pupillary c.
carbonic anhydrase inhibitors
carcinoma
    epidermoid c.
    metastatic c.
cardinal
    c. direction of gaze
    c. point
    c. position
cardiopharyngioma
Cardona's
    corneal prosthesis forceps
    corneal prosthesis trephine
    fiberoptic diagnostic lens
    focalizing fundus lens implant
    gonio-focalizing lens implant
    threading forceps
Carl Zeiss Instruments
carotid
    c. artery
    c. cavernous fistula
Cartella's eye shield
Carter's
    operation
    sphere
    sphere introducer
cartilage
    central c.
    ciliary c.
    palpebral c.
    tarsal c.
caruncle
    epicanthus c.
    lacrimal c.
caruncula lacrimalis
caruncular papilloma
Casanellas' lacrimal operation
case
    trial c.
caseating tubercles
Casey's operation
Caspar's ring opacity
Castallo's
    retractor
    speculum
Castroviejo's
    acrylic implant
    anterior synechia
    aspirator
    blade
    bladebreaker
    caliper
    capsule forceps
    capsulotomy
    clip, scleral shortening
    compressor
    corneal dissector
    corneal holding forceps
    corneal scissors with inside stop
    corneal section scissors
    corneal transplant marker
    corneal transplant scissors
    corneal transplant trephine
    corneoscleral punch
    cyclodialysis cannula

Castroviejo's *(continued)*
cyclodialysis spatula
discission knife
double end spatula
electro-keratotome
enucleation snare
erysiphake
fixation forceps
forceps
implant
iridectomy
iridocapsulotomy scissors
iridotomy
keratectomy
keratome
keratoplasty scissors
knife
lacrimal dilator
lacrimal sac probe
lens loupe
lens spoon
lid clamp
lid retractor
mini-keratoplasty
needle holder
orbital aspirator
punch
radial iridotomy
razor blade
refractor
retractor
scissors
scleral shortening clip
sclerotome
snare
spatula
speculum
spoon
suturing forceps
synechiae scissors
trephine
twin knife

Castroviejo's
vitreous aspirating needle
Castroviejo-Arruga forceps
Castroviejo-Galezowski dilator
Castroviejo-Kalt needle holder
Castroviejo-Scheie cyclodiathermy operation
CAT scan — computerized axial tomography scan
cat
c. scratch fever
"cat cry" syndrome — cri-du-chat syndrome
cat. ext. — cataract extraction
cat's eye
amaurosis
pupil
reflex
syndrome
catadioptric
cataphoria
mature c.
cataplexy
cataract
adherent c.
adolescent c.
aminoaciduria c.
annular c.
anterior c.
anterior axial c.
anterior axial embryonal c.
anterior polar c.
anterior pole c.
anterior pyramidal c.
arborescent c.
aridosiliculose c.
aridosiliquate c.
c. aspirating needle
c. aspiration
atopic c.
axial c.

cataract *(continued)*
- axial embryonal c.
- axial fusiform c.
- axillary c.
- black c.
- blue c.
- blue dot c.
- bony c.
- bottlemaker's c.
- brown c.
- brunescent c.
- calcareous c.
- capsular c.
- capsulolenticular c.
- central c.
- cerulean c.
- cheesy c.
- choroidal c.
- complete congenital c.
- complicated c.
- concussion c.
- congenital c.
- contusion c.
- copper c.
- coralliform c.
- coronary c.
- cortical c.
- cortical spokes c.
- crystalline c.
- cuneiform c.
- cupuliform c.
- cystic c.
- dendritic c.
- dermatogenic c.
- developmental c.
- diabetic-osmotic c.
- diffuse c.
- dilacerated c.
- disk-shaped c.
- dry-shelled c.
- electric c.
- embryonal nuclear c.
- embryonic c.

cataract *(continued)*
- embryopathic c.
- evolutional c.
- extraction c.
- fibrinous c.
- fibroid c.
- flap operation c.
- floriformis c.
- fluid c.
- furnacemen c.
- fusiform c.
- galactose c.
- general c.
- glassblower c.
- c. glasses
- glaucomatous c.
- gray c.
- green c.
- hard c.
- heat-ray c.
- hedger c.
- heterochromic c.
- hook-shaped c.
- hypermature c.
- hypocalcemic c.
- hypoglycemic c.
- immature c.
- incipient c.
- infantile c.
- infrared c.
- intumescent c.
- irradiation c.
- juvenile c.
- knife c.
- lacteal c.
- lamellar c.
- lamellar zonular perinuclear c.
- lenticular c.
- life-belt c.
- lightning c.
- c. mask ring
- mature c.

cataract *(continued)*
- membranous c.
- metabolic c.
- milky c.
- mixed c.
- morgagnian c.
- myotonic dystrophy c.
- naphthalinic c.
- needle c.
- nuclear c.
- nutritional deficiency c.
- O'Brien's c.
- osmotic c.
- overripe c.
- partial c.
- pear c.
- c. pencil
- perinuclear c.
- peripheral c.
- pisciform c.
- polar c.
- posterior polar c.
- postinflammatory c.
- prematurity c.
- presenile c.
- primary c.
- probe c.
- progressive c.
- puddler c.
- punctate c.
- pyramidal c.
- radiation c.
- reduplication c.
- ring form congenital c.
- ripe c.
- rubella c.
- sanguineous c.
- secondary c.
- sedimentary c.
- senescent c.
- senile nuclear sclerotic c.
- senile sclerotic c.
- shaped c.

cataract *(continued)*
- sideratic c.
- siliculose c.
- siliquose c.
- snowflake c.
- snowstorm c.
- Soemmering's ring c.
- soft c.
- spindle c.
- spurious c.
- stationary c.
- stellate c.
- subcapsular c.
- sugar c.
- sunflower c.
- supranuclear c.
- sutural c.
- syndermatotic c.
- syphilitic c.
- tetany c.
- thermal c.
- total c.
- toxic c.
- traumatic c.
- tremulous c.
- umbilicated c.
- vascular c.
- Vogt's c.
- zonular c.

cataracta
- c. accreta
- c. adiposa
- c. aridosiliquata
- c. brunescens
- c. caerulea
- c. centralis pulverulenta
- c. complicata
- c. congenita membranacea
- c. coronaria
- c. dermatogenes
- c. electrica
- c. fibrosa

cataracta *(continued)*
- c. membranacea accreta
- c. neurodermatica
- c. nigra
- c. nodiformis
- c. ossea

cataractogenic
cataractous
catarase
catarrh
- sinus c.
- spring c.
- vernal c.

catarrhal
- c. conjunctivitis
- c. corneal ulcer

catheter
- Lincoff's balloon c.

catheterization
- c. of lacrimal duct
- c. of lacrimonasal duct

cations
catoptroscope
cautery
- Alcon hand c.
- Berkley Bioengineering bipolar c.
- bipolar c.
- Bovie wet field c.
- Concept disposable c.
- Concept hand-held c.
- disposable c.
- Fine's micropoint c.
- Geiger's c.
- Gonin's c.
- Hildreth's c.
- Mentor's wet field c.
- Mira c.
- Mueller's c.
- NeoKnife c.
- ophthalmic c.
- Op-Temp c.
- Parker-Heath c.

cautery *(continued)*
- Prince's c.
- Rommel's c.
- Rommel-Hildreth c.
- Scheie's c.
- Todd's c.
- Valilab c.
- von Graefe's c.
- Wadsworth-Todd c.
- wet field c.
- Ziegler's c.

cavern
- Schnabel's c.

cavernous
- c. hemangioma
- c. sinus fistula
- c. sinus syndrome
- c. sinus thrombosis

cavitation
Cavitron Irrigation/Aspiration System
Cavitron-Kelman Irrigation/Aspiration System
cavity
- optic papilla c.
- orbital c.

CCT — computerized corneal tomography
CD5 needle
cecal
cecocentral scotoma
cell
- giant c.
- sickle c. disease

cellophane retinopathy
cellophane-like band
cells
- air c.
- amacrine c.
- c. and flare
- bipolar retinal c.
- clump c.
- cone c.

cells *(continued)*
- corneal c.
- ganglion c.
- giant c.
- goblet c.
- horizontal c.
- Langerhans c.
- lipid c.
- mast c.
- membrane lipid c.
- multinucleated giant c.
- neural crest c.
- c. of Müller
- photoreceptor c.
- radial c. of Müller
- retinoblastoma c.
- rod c.
- visual c.
- wing c.

cellula
cellulae lentis
cellular debris
cellularity
cellulitis
- orbital c.
- periorbital c.

Celsus'
- lid
- operation
- spasmodic entropion operation

Celsus-Holtz entropion
center
- c. of rotation
- optic c.

centering ring
centigray — cGy
centistoke
centrad
centrage
central
- c. amaurosis
- c. angiospastic retinitis
- c. artery
- c. canal
- c. cataract
- c. choroiditis
- c. cloudy dystrophy of Francois
- c. disk-shaped retinopathy
- c. fields
- c. fixation
- c. fovea of retina
- c. fusion
- c. iridectomy
- c. island of vision
- c. keyhole of vision
- c. nervous system
- c. posterior curve
- c. reflex stripe
- c. retinal artery occlusion
- c. retinal vein
- c. retinal vein occlusion
- c. scotoma
- c. serous retinitis
- c. serous retinochoroidopathy
- c. stellate laceration
- c. suppression
- c. vision
- c. visual acuity
- c. yellow point

centrally fixing eye
centraphose
centration
centripetally
centrocecal scotoma
centroperipheral
cephalo-orbital
ceratectomy
cerclage
cerebellar
- c. hemisphere
- c. hemorrhage

cerebellar *(continued)*
c. notch
c. tonsil
c. vermis
cerebellomedullary
cerebellopontine
cerebelloretinal
cerebellospinal
cerebellotegmental
cerebellothalamic
cerebellum
cerebral
c. angiography
c. arteriography
c. arteriosclerosis
c. atrophy
c. cortex
c. dyschromatopsia
c. infarction
c. palsy
c. radionuclide angiography
c. ventricle
cerebritis
cerebrohepatorenal syndrome
cerebrospinal fluid
cerebrovascular accident
cerebrovasculature
cerebro-ocular
cerebro-ophthalmic
cerebrum
ceroid
cerulean cataract
cervical ganglion
Cestan's syndrome
Cestan-Chenais syndrome
CF — counting fingers
cGy — centigray
chalazia
chalazion
c. clamp
c. curet
c. forceps
chalazion
c. trephine
chalcitis
chalcosis
cornea c.
c. lentis
chalkitis
Challenger Digital Applanation Tonometer
chamber
anterior c.
aqueous c.
eye c.
flat c.
posterior c.
reformation of c.
shallow c.
vitreous c.
Chamber's sterile adhesive bubble
Chan's wrist rest
Chandler's
iridectomy
forceps
syndrome
Chandler-Verhoeff lens extraction
channel
scleral c.
chaotic
Charcot's triad
Charles'
anterior chamber sleeve
infusion sleeve
intraocular lens
lensectomy
vacuuming needle
chart
Amsler's c.
astigmatic dial c.
Bailey-Lovie Log MAR c.
Donder's c.
Ferris' c.

chart *(continued)*
- Guibor's c.
- Kindergarten eye c.
- Lancaster-Regan dial 1 c.
- Lancaster-Regan dial 2 c.
- Landolt's broken ring c.
- Lebensohn's c.
- Randot's c.
- reading c.
- Reuss' color c.
- Snellen's c.
- sunburst dial c.
- University of Waterloo c.
- ventograph c.

check ligaments
Chédiak-Higashi syndrome
cheese wire
cheiroscope
chelating agent
chemical conjunctivitis
chemokinesis
chemosis
chemotatic
chemotaxis
chemotherapy
chemotic
cherry red spot
Cheyne's nystagmus
chiasm
- optic c.

chiasma opticum
chiasmal
- c. arachnoiditis
- c. compression
- c. glioma
- c. syndrome

chiasmatic
- c. field defects
- c. syndrome

chiastometer
Chievitz fiber layer
chisel
- lacrimal sac c.

Chlamydia trachomatis
chloasma
chlorolabe
chloroma
chlorophane
chloropia
chloropsia
chocolate agar
choked disk
cholesterol emboli of retina
cholesterosis bulbi
cholinergic
chondroitin sulfate
chord
- c. incision
- c. length

chordoma
choriocapillaris
choriocele
chorioid
chorioidea
choriopapillaris
chorioretinal
- c. atrophy
- c. degeneration

chorioretinitis
- central c.
- leutic c.
- peripheral c.
- sclerosing panencephalitis c.
- senile c.
- syphilitic c.
- toxoplasmosis c.

chorioretinopathy
choristoma tumor
choroid
- crescent c.

choroidal
- c. detachment
- c. dystrophy
- c. flush
- c. folds

choroidal *(continued)*
c. gyrate atrophy
c. hemorrhage
c. hyperfluorescence
c. infiltration
c. ischemia
c. lesion
c. myopic atrophy
c. neoplasm
c. nevus
c. primary sclerosis
c. scan
c. sclerosis
c. secondary atrophy
c. tap
c. tubercles
c. vessels
choroidea
choroideremia
choroiditis
acute diffuse serous c.
anterior c.
areolar c.
areolar central c.
central c.
diffuse c.
disseminated c.
Doyne's familial honeycombed c.
exudative c.
focal c.
Förster's c.
c. guttata senilis
Jensen's juxtapapillaris c.
macular c.
metastatic c.
c. myopia
nongranulomatous c.
senile macular exudative c.
c. serosa
serpiginous c.
suppurative c.

choroiditis *(continued)*
syphilitic c.
Tay's c.
toxoplasmic c.
traumatic c.
choroidocyclitis
choroidoiritis
choroidopathy
choroidoretinitis
Choyce's implant
Choyce-Mark VIII implant
chromatic
c. aberration
c. dispersion
c. perimetry
c. vision
chromaticities
chromatin
chromatometer
chromatopsia
chromatoptometer
chromatoptometry
chromatoskiameter
chromic
c. catgut suture
c. collagen suture
c. myopia
chromodacryorrhea
chromometer
chromophane
chromophobe adenoma
chromoretinopathy
chromoscope
chromoscopy
chromostereopsis
chronic
c. angle-closure glaucoma
c. conjunctivitis
c. open-angle glaucoma
c. progressive external ophthalmoplegia
chrysiasis

Ciaccio's glands
Cibis
  conjunctivitis
  ectropion
  electrode
  entropion
  liquid silicone procedure
  needle
  pemphigoid
  ski needle
cibisotome
cicatricial
  c. ectropion
  c. entropion
  c. mass
  c. pemphigoid
  c. retrolental fibroplasia
  c. strabismus
cicatrix
  filtering c.
cicatrization
cicatrizing
CILCO
  argon laser
  Frigitronics
  Hoffer Laseridge
  krypton laser
  Lasertek A/K laser
  Sonometric A-SCAN
  Ultrasound Unit
cilectomy
cilia
  c. base
ciliaris muscle
ciliariscope
ciliarotomy
ciliary
  c. arteries
  c. block
  c. body
  c. body band
  c. disk
  c. epithelium
ciliary *(continued)*
  c. flush
  c. folds
  c. ganglion
  c. glands
  c. hyperemia
  c. injection
  c. ligaments
  c. margin
  c. muscle
  c. nerves
  c. processes
  c. reflex
  c. ring
  c. spasm
  c. staphyloma
  c. sulcus
  c. vein
  c. zonule
ciliate
ciliated
ciliectomy
ciliochoroidal effusion
cilioequatorial fibers
ciliogenesis
cilioposterocapsular fibers
cilioretinal artery
cilioscleral
ciliosis
ciliospinal
  c. center of Budge
  c. reflex
ciliotomy
ciliovitreal block
ciliovitrectomy
cilium
cillo
cillosis
cinch
cinching
cinctured
Cine-Microscope
circadian heterotropia

circinate
- c. exudate
- c. retinitis
- c. retinopathy

circle
- arterial c. of greater iris
- arterial c. of lesser iris
- Berry's c.
- c. of confusion
- c. diffusion
- c. of dispersion
- c. dissipation
- c. of greater iris
- c. of Haller
- Hovius c.
- c. of least confusion
- c. of lesser iris
- Minsky's c.
- vascular c. of optic nerve
- Vieth-Muller c.
- c. of Willis'
- Zinn's c.

circling band

circular
- c. ciliary muscle
- c. fibers
- c. synechiae

circulus
- c. arteriosus halleri
- c. arteriosus iridis major
- c. arteriosus iridis minor
- c. vasculosus nervi optici
- c. zinnii

circumbulbar

circumcorneal

circumduction

circumferential

circumlental

circumocular

circumorbital

circumpapillary

circumscribe

circumscribed episcleritis

circus senilis

cirsophthalmia

cirsophthalmus

cis retinal

cisterna
- chiasmatic c.

cisternography

Citelli's rongeur

clamp
- Berke's c.
- bulldog c.
- Castroviejo's lid c.
- cheek c.
- cross-action c.
- Erhard's c.
- Gladstone-Putterman entropion c.
- muscle c.
- Prince's muscle c.
- Putterman's levator resection c.
- Putterman's ptosis c.
- Putterman-Müller blepharoptosis c.
- Robin's chalazion c.
- Schaedel's cross-action towel c.
- serrefine c.

Clark's eye speculum

Clayman's intraocular lens

clear windows

Cleasby's
- iridectomy operation
- spatulated needle

cleavage

cleft
- congenital c. of iris
- corneal c.

Clerf's needle holder

Clinitex Charles endophotocoagulator probe

Clinometer

Clinoscope
clip
    double tantalum c.
    holding c.
    tantalum c.
clip-applying forceps
clivus
clock dial
clock-mechanism esotropia
C-loop posterior chamber lens
Cloquet's canal
closed-angle glaucoma
closed-funnel vitreoretinopathy
closed-system pars plana vitrectomy
cloud
cloudy cornea
clumped
    c. cells
    c. pigmentation
    c. retinal pigment
clumping
cluster headaches
clusters
    c. of pigmented spots
    c. of retinoblastoma cells
CME — cystoid macular edema
CMI — cell mediated immunity
CMI — cytomegalic inclusion
CNS — central nervous system
COAG — chronic open-angle glaucoma
coagulate
coagulating electrode
coagulation
coagulum
coalesce
coalesced
coalescing
coal-mining lensectomy
coarctate retina
coarse punctate staining
coat
coat *(continued)*
    fibrous c. of eye
    sclerotic c.
    uveal c.
    vascular c. of eyeball
coated vicryl suture
Coats'
    disease
    retinitis
    white ring
coaxial
cobblestone
    c. appearance
    c. papillae
    c. retinal degeneration
Coburn's
    camera
    irrigation/aspiration unit
    lensometer
    refractor
Coburn-Meditec
Coburn-Rodenstock lamp
cocaine test
Coccidioides immitis
coccidioidomycosis
Cockayne's syndrome
Codman/Micra
Cogan's
    apraxia
    congenital oculomotor apraxia
    dystrophy
    sign
    syndrome
Cogan-Boberg-Ans lens implant
cogwheeling
Cohan's
    corneal forceps
    needle holder
Cohan-Barraquer microscope
Cohan-Vannas iris scissors
Cohan-Westcott scissors
Coherent Radiation

Coherent Radiation *(continued)*
- argon/krypton laser
- Fluorotron

Coleman's retractor
Colibri's forceps
collagen
- c. disease
- c. fibers
- c. lamellae
- c. shield
- c. vascular disease

collagenolytic trabecular ring
collar
collarette
colliculus
Collier's sign
collimated
collimator
Collin's 140 color adaptometer
Collin-Beard operation
colliquative
collodion dressing
colloid
- c. bodies
- c. deposits

collyria
collyrium
coloboma
- atypical c.
- bridge c.
- chorioretinal c.
- choroid c.
- ciliary body c.
- complete c.
- fissure c.
- Fuchs's c.
- c. iridis
- c. lentis
- c. lobuli
- c. of fundus
- c. of iris
- c. of lens
- c. of optic nerve

coloboma *(continued)*
- c. of retina
- c. of vitreous
- c. palpebrale
- peripapillary c.
- c. retinae
- retinochoroidal c.
- typical c.

colobomata
colobomatous
- c. cyst
- c. microphthalmia

color
- c. blindness
- complementary c.
- c. confusion
- c. contrast
- c. disk
- end-point c.
- incidental c.
- metameric c.
- Munsell's c.
- c. perimetry
- primary c.
- pseudoisochromatic c. plates
- pure c.
- c. saturation
- c. sense
- c. vision
- c. washout

Color Vision Test
colossal agenesis
colposcope
columnar layer
coma aberration
Comberg's
- foreign body operation
- lens
- localization

Combiline System
comedo pattern
comet scotoma

comitant
 c. exodeviations
 c. exophoria
 c. exotropia
 c. heterotropia
 c. strabismus
 c. vertical deviations
comminuted orbital fracture
commissura
 c. palpebrarum lateralis
 c. palpebrarum medialis
 c. palpebrarum nasalis
 c. palpebrarum temporalis
 superior c. of Meynert
commissurae opticae
commissure
 arcuate c.
 interthalamic c.
 lateral c. of eyelids
 medial c. of eyelids
 c. of Gudden
 optic c.
 palpebral c.
 posterior chiasmatic c.
 supraoptic c.
common canaliculus
commotio retinae
complementary
 c. after-image
 c. chromaticities
 c. colors
complexus basalis choroideae
component
 quick left/right c.
compound
 c. astigmatism
 c. eye
 c. hyperopic astigmatism
 c. myopic astigmatism
 c. spectacles
compression
compressor
compressor *(continued)*
 Anthony's orbital c.
 Berens' orbital c.
computed tomography
Computon Microtonometer
concave
 c. cylinder
 c. lens
concavoconcave
concavoconvex
concentric
 c. constriction
 c. folds
 c. lesion
 c. stria
concentrically
Concept
 disposable cautery
 hand-held cautery
concha bullosa
conclination
concomitant
concretions
concussion of the retina
condensate
condensing lens
cone
 c. dysfunction
 c. dystrophy
 c. monochromacy
 monochromatic c.
 ocular c.
 c. photopigments
 retinal c.
 twin c's
 visual c.
configuration
confluent
conformer
 Fox's c.
 McGuire's c.
 silicone c.
 Universal c.

confrontation fields
Confrontation Visual Field Test
confrontational
confusion
  color c.
congenital
  c. abducens nerve palsy
  c. amaurosis
  c. anomaly
  c. astigmatism
  c. bulbar paralysis
  c. cataract
  c. cleft of iris
  c. conus
  c. crescents
  c. dacryocele
  c. dacryocystitis
  c. dystropic ptosis
  c. dysversion
  c. ectropion
  c. entropion
  c. esotropia
  c. facial diplegia
  c. fibrous syndrome
  c. glaucoma
  c. hemianopia
  c. hereditary corneal dystrophy
  c. heterochromia
  c. ichthyosis
  c. impatency
  Leber's c. amaurosis
  c. lens dislocation
  c. lens opacities
  c. limbal corneal dermoid tumors
  c. medullated optic nerve fibers
  c. melanosis oculi
  c. nasolacrimal duct obstruction
  c. nystagmus

congenital *(continued)*
  c. oculodermal melanocytosis
  c. oculomotor apraxia
  c. oculomotor nerve palsy
  c. optic nerve coloboma
  c. optic nerve pits
  c. optical atrophy
  c. ptosis
  c. retinal folds
  c. retinoschisis
  c. rubella syndrome
  c. syphilis
  c. toxoplasmosis
congested vessels
congestion
  deep c.
  superficial c.
  transient c.
Congo red
congruity
congruous
  c. field defects
  c. homonymous hemianopic scotoma
conical
  c. cornea
  c. implant
  c. protrusion
conjugate
  c. deviation
  c. focus
  c. gaze
  c. movements
  c. ocular movements
  c. paralysis
  c. point
conjugately
conjunctiva
  bulbar c.
  c. forceps
  palpebral c.

conjunctiva *(continued)*
- c. retractor
- c. scissors
- c. spreader

conjunctivae

conjunctival
- c. arteries
- c. bleb
- c. brachium
- c. break
- c. calcifications
- c. concretions
- c. contusions
- c. cul-de-sac
- c. deposits
- c. dermoids
- c. discharge
- c. edema
- c. epithelial cells
- c. exudate
- c. flap
- c. fold
- c. follicles
- c. glands
- c. goblet cell
- c. goblet cell densities
- c. graft
- c. hemorrhage
- c. hyperemia
- c. injection
- c. lacerations
- c. lipodermoids
- c. lithiasis
- c. lymphangioma
- c. lymphoid tumors
- c. melanoma
- c. melanotic lesions
- c. necrosis
- c. nevus
- c. papilloma
- c. patch graft
- c. phlyctenulosis
- c. reaction

conjunctival *(continued)*
- c. reflex
- c. ring
- c. sac
- c. scarring
- c. scrapings
- c. slough
- c. staining
- c. tear
- c. ulcer
- c. veins
- c. xerosis

conjunctive movement

conjunctiviplasty

conjunctivitis
- acne rosacea c.
- actinic c.
- actinomyces c.
- acute catarrhal c.
- acute contagious c.
- acute epidemic c.
- acute hemorrhagic c.
- adenovirus c.
- allergic c.
- anaphylactic c.
- angular c.
- arc-flash c.
- atopic c.
- atropine c.
- bacterial c.
- Beal's c.
- blenorrheal c.
- blepharitis c.
- calcareous c.
- candidiasis c.
- catarrhal c.
- chemical c.
- chronic catarrhal c.
- cicatricial c.
- congenital syphilitic c.
- croupous c.
- diphtheritic c.
- diplobacillary c.

conjunctivitis *(continued)*
- eczematous c.
- Egyptian c.
- Elschnig's c.
- epidemic c.
- erythema multiforme c.
- follicular c.
- giant papillary c.
- gonococcal c.
- gonorrheal c.
- gout c.
- granular c.
- hay fever c.
- inclusion c.
- infantile purulent c.
- infectious c.
- Koch-Weeks c.
- lagophthalmos c.
- larval c.
- c. ligneous
- lithiasis c.
- c. medicamentosa
- membranous c.
- meningococcus c.
- c. molluscum
- Morax-Axenfeld c.
- mucopurulent c.
- necrotic infectious c.
- c. necroticans infectiosus
- neonatal c.
- newborn c.
- c. nodosa
- nodular c.
- ocular vaccinia c.
- papillary c.
- Parinaud's oculoglandular c.
- Pascheff's c.
- c. petrificans
- phlyctenular c.
- pinkeye c.
- pneumococcal c.
- prairie c.

conjunctivitis *(continued)*
- pseudomembranous c.
- purulent c.
- Reiter's disease c.
- rubeola c.
- Sanyal's c.
- scrofular c.
- shipyard c.
- simple c.
- simple acute c.
- spring c.
- squirrel plague c.
- swimming pool c.
- toxic c.
- trachomatous c.
- tuberculosis c.
- tularenic c.
- c. tularensis
- uratic c.
- vernal c.
- viral c.
- Wegener's granulomatosis c.
- welder's c.
- Widmark's c.
- Wucherer's c.
- c. xeroderma pigmentosum

conjunctivodacryocystostomy
conjunctivoma
conjunctivoplasty
conjunctivorhinostomy
conjunctivotarsal
conjunctivo-Tenon's flap
conoid
- c. lens
- c. of Sturm

conophthalmus
Conrad's operation
Conradi's syndrome
consecutive
- c. esotropia
- c. exotropia

consecutive
- c. optic atrophy

consensual
- c. light reflex
- c. light response

constant
- c. monocular tropia
- c. nystagmus
- c. strabismus

constricted pupil

constriction

constructional apraxia

Contact A & B Scan

contact
- c. arc
- c. bandage lens
- c. burns of globe
- c. conjunctivitis
- c. dermatitis
- c. glasses
- hard c. lens
- c. lens
- c. lens overwearing syndrome
- long-wearing c. lens
- c. method
- soft c. lens

contactologist

contactology

contactoscope

contiguity

contiguous
- c. fibers
- c. pattern

Contino's
- epithelioma
- glaucoma

continuous wave argon laser

contracted socket

contraction
- c. and liquefaction
- anisocoria c.
- c. of cyclitic membrane

contraction *(continued)*
- c. of pupil
- pupillary c.

contralateral
- c. antagonist
- c. eye
- c. synergists

contrast material
- cyanographic c. m.
- cyanographin c. m.
- gallium citrate c. m.

contrecoup

contusion
- c. cataract
- c. of the choroid
- c. of the eye
- c. of the globe
- c. of the orbit
- corneal c.
- vitreoretinal c.

conular

conus
- congenital c.
- c. distraction
- inferior c.
- lateral oblique c.
- myopic c.
- c. of optic disk
- c. shell type eye implant
- c. supertraction
- underlying c.

converge

convergence
- accommodative c.
- c. amplitudes
- excess esotropia c
- far-point c.
- fusional c.
- c. insufficiency
- near-point c.
- negative c.
- positive c.
- proximal c.

convergence *(continued)*
relative c.
c. retraction nystagmus
c. spasm
tonic c.
voluntary c.
convergent
c. deviation
c. exercises
c. squint
c. strabismus
converging
c. lens
c. rays
convergiometer
convex lens
convexity
convexoconcave
convexoconvex
Conway's lid retractor
Cook's speculum
Cooper's
I & A Unit
implant
laser
operation
Surgeon-Plus Ultra Thin blades
Cooper Vision
camera
imaging perimeter
irrigating/aspirating unit
laser
microscope
refractive photokeratoscope
ultrasonography
Copeland's
implant
intraocular lens
pan chamber lens
streak retinoscope
copiopia
copper foreign bodies
copper-wire
c. arteries
c. arterioles
c. reflex
copper-wiring
Coquille plano lens
coralliform cataract
Corbett's spud
Corboy's
hemostat
needle holder
cordless monocular indirect ophthalmoscope
core
nerve c.
c. vitrectomy
coreclisis
corectasis
corectome
corectomedialysis
corectomy
corectopia
coredialysis
corediastasis
corelysis
coremorphosis
corenclisis
coreometer
coreometry
coreoplasty
coreoretinal
corestenoma congenitum
coretomedialysis
coretomy
corkscrew visual field defects
cornea
c. abrader
c. abrasion
c. anesthesia
c. arcus
artificial c.
Black's c.

cornea *(continued)*
- Burr's c.
- c. button
- c. chisel
- cloudy c.
- conical c.
- c. farinata
- flat c.
- c. globosa
- c. guttata
- c. guttate lesions
- c. holding forceps
- Kayser-Fleischer c. ring
- c. opaca
- opalescent c.
- oval c.
- c. plana
- c. scar
- c. sensitivity
- c. spot
- sugar-loaf c.
- Terrier's degeneration of c.
- c. urica
- c. verticillata
- Vogt's c.

corneal
- c. abrasion
- c. apex
- c. astigmatism
- c. bedewing
- c. bur
- c. burn
- c. button
- c. cap
- c. clouding
- c. contusion
- c. corpuscles
- c. crystals
- c. curet
- c. debrider
- c. deep opacity
- c. degeneration

corneal *(continued)*
- c. dehydration
- c. dellen
- c. dendrite
- c. deposits
- c. dissector
- c. distortion
- c. dysplasia
- c. edema
- c. endothelium
- c. enlargement
- c. epithelium
- c. erosion
- c. erysiphake
- c. fascia lata spatula
- c. fixation forceps
- c. foreign body bur
- c. full-thickness
- c. furrow degeneration
- c. graft
- c. guttata
- c. guttate dystrophy
- c. guttering
- c. implant
- c. inferior limbal infiltrates
- c. infiltrate
- c. inlays
- c. knife dissector
- c. lacerations
- c. lamellar groove
- c. leakage
- c. lens
- c. luster
- c. marginal furrow
- c. melting
- c. mushroom
- c. nebula
- c. needle
- c. onlays
- c. opacification
- c. opacity
- c. optical density

corneal *(continued)*
- c. pachometer
- c. pellucid
- c. perforation
- c. phlyctenulosis
- c. prosthesis forceps
- c. prosthesis trephine
- c. protrusion
- c. punctate infiltrates
- c. punctate lesion
- c. reflex
- c. scarring
- c. scissors
- c. spatulated scissors
- c. spot
- c. staining test
- c. staphyloma
- c. stria
- c. stroma
- c. stromal dystrophy
- c. thinning
- c. transplant marker
- c. trephine
- c. tube
- c. velum
- c. xerosis

corneal dystrophy
- Biber-Haab-Dimmer c.d.
- Buckler III c.d.
- central cloudy c.d.
- central speckled c.d.
- Cogan's microcystic epithelial c.d.
- congenital hereditary endothelial c.d.
- crystalline c.d.
- ectatic c.d.
- fingerprint c.d.
- fleck c.d.
- Fuchs' combined c.d.
- Fuchs' endothelial c.d.
- Fuchs' epithelial c.d.
- granular c.d.

corneal dystrophy *(continued)*
- Grayson-Wilbrant c.d.
- Groenouw–type I c.d.
- Groenouw–type II c.d.
- c. holding forceps
- lattice c.d.
- macular c.d.
- map-dot c.d.
- Meesman's epithelial c.d.
- Melsman's c.d.
- microcystic c.d.
- c.d. of Waardenburg-Jonkers
- parenchymatous c.d.
- posterior polymorphous c.d.
- Reis-Bücklers superficial c.d.
- Schnyder's crystalline c.d.
- vortex c.d.

corneal graft
- crescent c.g.
- full-thickness c.g.
- lamellar c.g.
- mushroom c.g.
- penetrating c.g.

corneal ulcer
- acne rosacea c.u.
- bacterial c.u.
- central c.u.
- fungal c.u.
- geographic herpes simplex c.u.
- herpes simplex c.u.
- marginal c.u.
- Mooren's c.u.

Corneascope

corneitis

corneoblepharon

corneoiritis

corneosclera

corneoscleral

corneoscleral *(continued)*
- c. button
- c. forceps
- c. groove
- c. lacerations
- c. lamellae
- c. melting
- c. punch
- c. right/left-hand scissors
- c. scissors
- c. sulcus

corona
- c. ciliaris
- Zinn's c.

coronal

coroparelcysis

coroplasty

coroscopy

corotomy

corpus
- c. adiposum orbitae
- c. callosum
- c. ciliare
- c. ciliaris
- c. vitreum

corpuscle
- corneal c.
- Toynbee's c.
- Virchow's c.

correctable

correspondence
- anomalous retinal c.
- harmonious retinal c.
- normal retinal c.
- c. points
- retinal c.

corrugator

cortex
- cerebellar c.
- c. lentis

cortical
- c. blindness
- c. cataract

cortical *(continued)*
- c. cleft
- c. clefting
- c. opacification
- c. psychic blindness
- c. spokes
- c. stripping
- c. vacuoles

cortices

corticonuclear fibers

corticosteroids

coruscation

coryza

cosmesis

cosmetic contact shell implant

Costen-Trent iris retractor

Costenbader's incision spreader

cotton-wool
- c. exudates
- c. spots

couching

count
- finger c.

counterpressor
- Amenabar's c.
- Gills' c.

counting fingers

Cover/Uncover Test

cranial
- c. arteritis
- c. foramen
- c. foramina
- c. nerve palsy

craniofacial
- c. dysostosis
- c. syndrome

craniometaphyseal dysplasia

craniopharyngioma

craniostenosis

craniosynostosis

craniotabes

Crawford's
- fascia

Crawford's *(continued)*
- forceps
- lacrimal set
- method
- needle
- sling operation
- stripper

creatinine clearance test

Crede's
- method
- prophylaxis

crenated

crepitance

crepitation

crepitus

crescent
- c. corneal graft
- c. graft
- myopic c.
- c. tonofilms

crescentic

crest
- lacrimal anterior c.
- lacrimal posterior c.
- orbital c.

cri-du-chat syndrome

cribra orbitalis of Welcker

cribral

cribrate

cribriform
- c. ligament
- c. plate
- c. spots

cribrosa

cribrum

Crile's needle holder

crisis
- glaucomatocyclitic c.
- ocular c.
- oculogyric c.
- Pel's c.

Critchett's operation

criterion-free measurement

Crock's encircling operation

crocodile
- c. lens
- c. shagreen
- c. tears

crofilcon A

Crookes' lens

cross cylinder
- Jackson's c.c.

cross-polarization photography

crossed
- c. amblyopia
- c. diplopia
- c. hemianopia
- c. parallax
- c. reflex

crossings
- arteriovenous c.

cross-action
- c. capsule forceps
- c. towel clamp

cross-eye

cross-fixation

cross-vector A scan

croupous conjunctivitis

Crouzon's disease

crowding phenomenon

crown
- ciliary c.

crow-foot closure

crusting lids

CRVO — central retinal vein occlusion

Cryo-Barrages vitreous implant

cryoablation

cryoapplication

cryocoagulation

cryoedema

cryoextraction

cryoextractor
- Alcon's c.
- Amoils' c.
- Bellows' c.

cryoextractor *(continued)*
- Kelman's c.
- Keeler's c.
- Rubinstein's c.
- Thomas' c.

cryofreeze
cryogenic
cryopencil
cryopexy
cryophake
- Alcon's c.
- Amoils' c.
- Bellows' c.
- Keeler's c.
- Kelman's c.
- Rubinstein's c.

cryopreservation
cryoprobe
- Amoils' c.
- Rubinstein's c.

cryoptor
- Thomas' c.

cryoretinopexy
cryostat
Cryostylet 2000
cryosurgery
cryosurgical
- Alcon's c. unit
- Frigitronics c. unit
- Keeler's c. unit
- Kelman's c. unit
- N20 c. unit

cryotherapy
crypt
- Fuchs' c.
- iris c.

Cryptococcus
cryptoglioma
cryptophthalmia
cryptophthalmos
cryptophthalmus
cryptosporidiosis
crystalline

crystalline *(continued)*
- c. deposits
- c. humor
- c. infiltrates
- c. keratopathy
- c. lens

crystallitis
Csapody's orbital repair operation
CT scan
CT — cover test
CUA needle
cuboidal
cuff
- Watzke's c.

Cuignet's
- method
- test

Culler's
- iris spatula
- lens spoon
- muscle hook

cul-de-sac
- conjunctival c.
- glaucomatous c.
- c. irrigating vectis
- c. irrigation T-tube
- c. irrigator
- ocular c.
- ophthalmic c.
- optic c.

cup
- Galin's bleb c.
- glaucomatous c.
- ocular c.
- ophthalmic c.
- optic c.
- physiologic c.

cupped disk
Cupper-Faden operation
cupping
- glaucomatous c.
- c. of disk

cupping *(continued)*
    c. of optic nerve
    pathologic c.
cupuliform cataract
cup-to-disk ratio
curb tenotomy
Curdy's
    blade
    sclerotome
Curdy-Hebra blade
curet
    Alvis' c.
    chalazion c.
    Fink's c.
    Gifford's c.
    Gill-Welch c.
    Green's c.
    Heath's chalazion c.
    Hebra's c.
    Kraff's capsule polisher c.
    Meyhoeffer's c.
    Skeele's c.
curettage
curette. *See curet*
curetted
curl backshell implant
curling of the capsule
Curran's knife needle
curvature
    c. ametropia
    c. hyperopia
    c. myopia
    c. of lens
curve
    visibility c.
curvilinear
Cushing's syndrome
cushingoid
Cusick's
    goniotomy knife
    operation
Cusick-Sarrail ptosis operation
Custodis'
    nondraining procedure
    operation
    procedure
    scleral buckling
    sponge
    suture
cutaneous
    c. horn
    c. myiasis
    c. tissue
cutdown incision
cuticular
Cutler-Beard operation
Cutler's
    implant
    lens spoon
cutter
    Buettner-Parel c.
    Douvas' c.
    Kloti's c.
    Machemer's c.
    Maguire-Harvey c.
    O'Malley-Heintz c.
    Parel-Crock c.
    Tolentino's c.
cutting bur
cyanoacrylate
    c. adhesive
    c. retinopexy
    c. tissue adhesive
cyanographic contrast material
cyanographin contrast material
cyanolabe
cyanopsia
cyanopsin
cyanosis
    bulbar c.
    c. bulbi
    retina c.
cyclectomy
cyclic
    c. esotropia

cyclic *(continued)*
- c. ocular motor spasm
- c. strabismus

cyclicotomy
cyclitic
- c. membrane

cyclitis
- chronic c.
- heterochromic Fuchs' c.
- c. in pars planitis
- plastic c.
- pure c.
- purulent c.
- serous c.

cycloanemization
cycloceratitis
cyclochoroiditis
cyclocryopexy
cyclocryotherapy
cyclodamia
cyclodeviation
cyclodialysis
- c. clefts
- c. spatula

cyclodiathermy
- c. electrode
- c. operation

cycloduction
cycloelectrolysis
cyclofusion
cyclogram
cyclokeratitis
cyclophoria
- accommodative c.
- c. minus
- c. negative
- c. plus
- c. positive

cyclophorometer
cyclopia
cycloplegia
cycloplegic
cyclops
cycloscope
cyclospasm
cyclotome
cyclotomy
cyclotropia
- c. minus
- c. negative
- c. plus
- c. positive

cyclovergence
cycloversions
Cyl. — cylindric lens or cylinder
cylicotomy
cylinder
cylindric
cylindrical lens
cyst
- bilateral c.
- Blessig-Iwanoff c's
- Blessig's c's
- corneal c.
- Dandy-Walker c.
- c. degeneration
- c. fibrosis
- inclusion c.
- intraepithelial c.
- iris c.
- Iwanoff's c's
- meibomian c.
- orbital c.
- pearl c.
- proteinaceous c.
- pupillary c.
- retinal c.
- scleral c.
- subconjunctival c.
- tarsal c.

cystic
- c. cataract
- c. eye
- c. fibrosis
- c. microphthalmia

cysticerci

cysticercoid
cysticercosis
cysticercus
cystine crystal
cystinosis
cystitome
cystitomy
cystoid
    c. bodies
    c. cicatrix of limbus
    c. macular edema
    c. macular hole
    c. maculopathy
    c. retinal degeneration
cystoplasmic organelles
cystotome
    Graefe's c.
    Kelman's c.
    Lewicky's formed c.
    Nevyas' double sharp c.
    von Graefe's c.
    Wheeler's c.
    Wilder's c.
cytomegalic inclusion disease
cytomegalovirus retinitis
Czermak's
    keratome
    pterygium operation

d

D — diopter
D trisomy syndrome
D&N — distance and near
Dacron suture
dacryadenalgia
dacryadenoscirrhus
dacryagogatresia
dacryagogic
dacryagogue
dacrycystalgia
dacrycystitis
dacryelcosis
dacryoadenalgia
dacryoadenectomy
dacryoadenitis
dacryoblennorrhea
dacryocanaliculitis
dacryocele
dacryocyst
dacryocystalgia
dacryocystectasia
dacryocystectomy
dacryocystis
    phlegmonous d.
    syphilitic d.
    trachomatous d.
    tuberculous d.
dacryocystitis
    acute d.
    chronic d.
    phlegmonous d.
    syphilitic d.
    trachomatous d.
    tuberculous d.
dacryocystoblennorrhea
dacryocystocele
dacryocystogram
dacryocystography
dacryocystoptosis
dacryocystorhinostenosis
dacryocystorhinostomy
    Moria-France d. clamp
dacryocystorhinotomy
dacryocystotome
dacryocystotomy
dacryogenic
dacryohelcosis
dacryohemorrhea
dacryolin
dacryolith
    Desmarres' d.
dacryolithiasis

dacryoma
dacryon
dacryops
dacryopyorrhea
dacryopyosis
dacryorhinocystotomy
dacryorrhea
dacryosinusitis
dacryosolenitis
dacryostenosis
dacryostomy
dacryosyrinx
Dailey's
  cataract needle
  operation
Dalen-Fuchs nodules
Dalgleish's operation
Dalrymple's
  disease
  sign
Danberg's forceps
Dannheim's eye implant
Darin's lens
dark
  d. adaptation
  d. adaptometry
  d. disk
  d. field examination
Darling's
  capsulotome
  capsulotomy
DaSilva's dermatome
Daviel's
  lens spoon
  operation
  scoop
Davis'
  knife needle
  spud
  trephine
Davis-Geck
  blepharoplasty
  suture
day
  d. blindness
  d. sight
  d. vision
Dean's
  iris knife
  knife holder
  needle
debrider
  Sauer's d.
debris-laden tear film
decenter
decentered
decentration of lenses
decimate
declination
decompression
  orbital d.
decreasing vision
decussate
decussation
deep
  d. blunt rake retractor
  d. corneal stromal opacities
  d. keratitis
defatted
defect
  altitudinal d.
  bitemporal field d.
  corkscrew visual field d.
  homonymous field d.
  inferior altitudinal d.
  superior homonymous quadrantic d.
deformity angle
degeneration
  Best's d.
  Biber-Haab-Dimmer d.
  congenital macular d.
  cystoid d.
  disciform macular d.

degeneration *(continued)*
- Doyne's familial colloid d.
- Doyne's honeycomb d.
- equatorial d.
- familial colloid d.
- hepatolenticular d.
- hyaline d.
- Kozlowski's d.
- lattice d. of retina
- lenticular d.
- macular d.
- macular disciform d.
- pellucid marginal corneal d.
- pellucid marginal retinal d.
- peripheral tapetochoroidal d.
- retinal lattice d.
- senile disciform d.
- senile exudative macular d.
- striatal nigral d.
- vitelliform macular d.
- vitelline macular d.
- Vogt's d.
- Wilson's d.

degenerative
de Grandmont's operation
degree
- prism d.

DeGrouchy's syndrome
dehisced
dehiscence
dehiscent
dehiscing
dehydroretinal
deinsertion
Deiters' operation
Dejean's syndrome
De Klair's operation
DeKnatel's silk suture
delacrimation
de Lapersonne's operation
DeLavega's vitreous aspirating cannula
delicate serrated straight dressing forceps
delimiting keratotomy
deliver
delivery
dellen
Deller's modification
Del Toro's operation
demarcation
de Mosier's syndrome
Demours' membrane
demyelinate
demyelinating plaque
demyelination
demyelinization
dendritic
- d. ghosts
- d. herpes simplex corneal ulcers
- d. herpes zoster keratitis
- d. keratitis
- d. lesions
- d. ulcer

denervate
denervated
denervation
dense
- d. brunescent nucleus
- d. opacities

denser
densities
density
- arciform d.

dentate
dentation
denudation
denude
denuding
deorsumduction

deorsumvergence
deorsumversion
depigmented spot
depressed fracture
depression of orbital floor
depressor
    Schepen's scleral d.
    Schocket's scleral d.
deprimens oculi
deprivation amblyopia
depth
    focal d.
    d. perception
Derby's operation
Derf's needle holder
Dermalon suture
dermatochalasis
dermatoconjunctivitis
dermatolysis palpebrarum
dermatome
    DaSilva's d.
dermatomyositis
dermato-ophthalmitis
dermoid
    congenital limbal corneal d.
    d. cyst
    orbital d.
    d. tumor
dermolipoma
Descartes' law
Descemet's
    folds
    membrane
    membrane detachment
    membrane punch
descemetitis
descemetocele
desiccant
desiccate
desiccation keratitis
Desmarres'
    chalazion
Desmarres' *(continued)*
    corneal dissector
    dacryolith
    forceps
    knife
    law
    lid clamp
    lid elevator
    lid retractor
    marker
    refractor
    retractor
    operation
    scarifier
desmosomal cellular attachment
desmosomes
desquamated epithelial debris
desquamation
dessicated
detached
    d. retina
    d. vitreous
detachment
    choroidal d.
    macular d.
    retinal d.
    rhegmatogenous d.
    vitreal d.
detectable foci
deturgescence
deutan
deuteranoma
deuteranomalopia
deuteranomalous
deuteranomaly
deuteranope
deuteranopia
deuteranopic
deuteranopsia
deuton color blindness
Deutschman's cataract knife
devascularization
developmental cataract

deviant color
deviation
- conjugate d.
- convergent d.
- Hering-Hellebrand d.
- heterotropic d.
- horizontal d.
- latent d.
- manifest d.
- minimum d.
- primary d.
- secondary d.
- skew d.
- squint d.
- strabismic d.
- supranuclear d.
- torsional d.
- tropic d.
- vertical d.

Devic's disease
DeVilbiss's irrigating/aspirating unit
deviometer
devitalized
DeWecker's
- anterior sclerotomy
- scissors

DeWecker-Pritikin scissors
dextroclination
dextrocular
dextrocularity
dextrocycloduction
dextrocycloversion
dextrodepression
dextroduction
dextrogyration
dextrotorsion
dextroversion
dextroverted
diabetes
- adult-onset d.
- d. albuminurinicus
- alloxan d.
- d. amaurosis

diabetes *(continued)*
- artificial d.
- brittle d.
- bronze d.
- bronzed d.
- chemical d.
- experimental d.
- gestational d.
- gouty d.
- growth-onset d.
- d. innocens
- d. inositus
- d. insipidus
- d. insipidus nephrogenic
- insulin-deficient d.
- insulin-dependent d.
- juvenile d.
- ketosis-prone d.
- ketosis-resistant d.
- Lancereaux's d.
- latent d.
- lipoatrophic d.
- lipoplethoric d.
- lipuric d.
- masked d.
- maturity-onset d.
- d. mellitus
- Mosler's d.
- non–insulin-dependent d.
- overflow d.
- overt d.
- pancreatic d.
- phlorhizin d.
- phosphate d.
- piqûre d.
- puncture d.
- renal d.
- skin d.
- steroid d.
- steroidogenic d.
- subclinical d.
- temporary d.
- toxic d.

diabetic
- d. Argyll-Robertson pupil
- d. cataract
- d. iritis
- d. melanosis
- d. optic atrophy
- d. retinopathy
- d. traction

diagnostic positions of gaze
dial
- astigmatic d.

dialyses
dialysis
- retinal d.

diamond
- d. blade knife
- d. bur
- d. dusted
- d. knife

Dianoux's operation
diaphanoscopy
diaphanous
diaphoresis
diaschisis
diastasis
- iris d.

diathermy
- d. applications
- Mira d.
- d. points
- d. puncture
- d. tip

diathesis
dichromasy
dichromat
dichromatic light
dichromatism
dichromatopsia
Dickey's operation
Dickey-Fox operation
Dickson Wright orbit decompression
Dieffenbach's operation
diffraction
diffuse
- d. angiokeratoma
- d. anterior scleritis
- d. inflammatory eyelid atrophy
- d. unilateral neuroretinitis

diffusion
Digilab tonometer
Digital B System
digital tonometry
digitalis toxicity
diktyoma
dilaceration
dilate
dilation
- d. lag
- d. of punctum
- d. of pupils

dilator
- Berens' d.
- Castroviejo's lacrimal d.
- Castroviejo-Galezowski d.
- French's lacrimal d.
- Heath's d.
- Hosford's d.
- House's lacrimal d.
- Jones' d.
- Muldoon's lacrimal d.
- muscle d.
- Nettleship-Wilder d.
- lacrimal d.
- punctal d.
- pupil d.
- Ruedeman's lacrimal d.
- Wilder's d.

dimefilcon A
Dimitry-Bell erysiphake
Dimitry's
- chalazion trephine
- erysiphake

Dimitry-Thomas erysiphake
Dimmer's keratitis

dimness of vision
dimple
Fuchs' d.
dimpling of eyeball
diopsimeter
diopter
prism d.
Dioptimum System
dioptometer
dioptometry
dioptoscopy
dioptre
dioptric
dioptrometer
dioptrometry
dioptroscopy
dioptry
diphtheroid
diplexia
diplopia
binocular d.
crossed d.
direct d.
heteronymous d.
homonymous d.
horizontal d.
monocular d.
paradoxical d.
pathological d.
physiological d.
stereoscopic d.
torsional d.
uncrossed d.
vertical d.
diplopiometer
diploscope
direct
d. astigmatism
d. diplopia
d. light reflex
d. method
d. ophthalmoscope
d. parallax
d. vision
director
grooved d.
disc. *See disk*
disci
disciform
d. chorioretinopathy
d. degeneration
d. herpes simplex keratitis
d. keratitis
d. macular degeneration
d. opacity
discission
discitis
disclination
disconjugate
d. gaze
discoria
discrete
d. colliquation
d. colliquative
discus
d. nevi optici
d. opticus
disease
Addison's d.
Albright's d.
Apert's d.
Arlt's d.
Ballet's d.
Basedow's d.
Batten's d.
Batten-Mayou d.
Behçet's d.
Behr's d.
Benson's d.
Berlin's d.
Best's d.
Bielschowsky's d.
Bourneville's d.
Bowen's d.
Bright's d.
carotid occlusive d.
Chédiak-Higashi d.

disease *(continued)*
- Coats' d.
- Cogan's d.
- collagen vascular d.
- Crouzon's d.
- cytomegalic inclusion d.
- Dalrymple's d.
- Devic's d.
- disseminated lupus erythematosus d.
- Eales' d.
- Englemann's d.
- Faber's d.
- Fabry's d.
- Farber's d.
- Favre's d.
- Flajani's d.
- Flatau-Schilder d.
- flecked retina d.
- Förster's d.
- Franceschetti's d.
- Francis' d.
- Gaucher's d.
- Gierke's d.
- gouty episcleritis d.
- Graefe's d.
- Graves' d.
- Hand-Schüller-Christian d.
- Harada's d.
- Heerfordt's d.
- Hippel's d.
- Hunter's d.
- Hutchinson's d.
- Jensen's d.
- Kimmelstiel-Wilson d.
- Koeppe's d.
- Krabbe's d.
- Krill's d.
- Kufs' d.
- Kuhnt-Junius d.
- Lauber's d.
- Leber's d.

disease *(continued)*
- Lindau's d.
- Lindau-von Hippel d.
- Masuda-Kitahara d.
- medullary optic d.
- Mikulicz's d.
- Möbius' d.
- Newcastle d.
- Niemann-Pick d.
- Norrie's d.
- Oguchi's d.
- Pompe's d.
- pulseless d.
- Purtscher's d.
- Recklinghausen's d.
- Reis-Bücklers d.
- Reiter's d.
- Sachs' d.
- Sanders' d.
- Sandhoff's d.
- Sanfilippo's d.
- Schilder's d.
- shipyard d.
- Sichel's d.
- Sjögren's d.
- Spielmeyer-Vogt d.
- Stargardt's d.
- Still's d.
- Takayasu's d.
- Tangier's d.
- Tay's d.
- Tay-Sachs d.
- Vogt's d.
- Vogt-Spielmeyer d.
- von Hippel's d.
- von Hippel-Lindau d.
- von Recklinghausen's d.
- Wagner's d.
- Weil's d.
- Westphal-Strümpell d.
- Wilson's d.

disinsertion of retina

disjugate movement

disjunctive movement

disk
- anangioid d.
- choked d.
- ciliary d.
- cupped d.
- d. drusen
- gelatin d.
- Krill's d.
- micrometer d.
- d. neovascularization
- d. neurovascular vessels
- Newton's d.
- d. new vessels
- optic d.
- d. pallor
- Placido's d.
- Rekoss' d.
- stenopeic d.
- stroboscopic d.
- Whipple's d.

dislocation of lens
disorganized globe
disparate retinal points
dispersion syndrome
disposable cautery
dissected half-thickness
dissecting scissors
dissector
- Barraquer's corneal d.
- Berens' corneal d.
- corneal d.
- Desmarres' corneal d.
- Green's corneal d.
- knife d.
- Martinez d.

disseminated
dissimilar
- d. image test
- d. target test

dissipation
dissociated
- d. hyperdeviation
- d. hypertropia

dissociated *(continued)*
- d. nystagmus
- d. vertigo deviation

dissociative state
distance
- d. and at near
- angular d.
- focal d.
- infinite d.
- interocular d.
- interpupillary d.

distichia
distichiasis
distometer
distortion
- barrel d.
- d. of lens
- d. of vision
- pin-cushion d.

distraction conus
diurnal intraocular pressure measurement
DIVA test
divergence
- d. amplitudes
- excess d.
- d. insufficiency
- negative vertical d.
- positive vertical d.
- d. reserves
- strabismus d.

divergent strabismus
diverticula of the lacrimal sac
Dix's spud
Dix-Hallpike test
DNCB - dinitrochlorobenzene
documentary photographs taken
Docustar fundus camera
Doherty's sphere implant
Dohlman's plug
doll's eye
- maneuver

doll's eye *(continued)*
reflex
sign
doll's head phenomenon
D'ombrain's operation
dome-shaped
dominance
ocular d.
dominant
d. eye
d. inheritance
Donaldson's eye patch
Donder's
chart
glaucoma
law
line
donor
d. cornea
d. eye
d. graft
d. tissue
Dorello's canal
dorsal midbrain syndrome
dorsolateral
dot
d. and blot hemorrhage
Gunn's d.
d. hemorrhage
Marcus Gunn d.
Mittendorf's d.
Trantas' d.
dot-like lens
double
d. arcuate scotoma
d. cutting sharp cystotome
d. cryopexy
d. dissociated hypertropia
d. elevator palsy
d. freeze-stalk cryopexy

double *(continued)*
d. freeze-thaw cryopexy
d. homonymous hemianopsia
d. hypertropia
d. irrigating/aspirating cannula
d. Maddox rod testing
d. refraction
d. row diathermy barrage
d. spatula
d. vision
Dougherty's irrigating/aspirating unit
doughnut-shaped
Douvas'
honeycombed choroiditis
rotoextractor
vitreous cutter
down to finger-counting
downbeat nystagmus
down-gaze
Down's syndrome
Doyne's
choroiditis
familial honeycombed choroiditis
iritis
Draeger's
high vacuum erysiphake
tonometer
dragged
d. disk
d. macula
d. retina
drainage
d. of lacrimal gland
d. of lacrimal sac
drape
3-M Steri-Drape d.
Alcon disposable d.
Barrier d.
Blair's head d.

drape *(continued)*
- Eye-Pak d.
- Hough's d.
- mini-ophthalmic d.
- Opraflex d.
- Steri-Drape d.
- Surgikos disposable d.
- VISIFLEX d.

dressing
- binocle d.
- binocular d.
- bolus d.
- Borsch's d.
- collodion d.
- compression d.
- crepe bandage d.
- Expo-Bubble d.
- eye pad d.
- fine moistened mesh gauze d.
- fluff d.
- fluffed-gauze d.
- lens d.
- monocular d.
- pressure d.
- pressure-patch d.
- ribbon-gauze d.
- sterile adhesive bubble d.
- Telfa plastic film d.
- tie-over Sellotape d.
- Tulle-gras d.
- wet d.
- wool saturated in saline d.

Drews'
- irrigating/aspirating unit
- lens

Drews-Rosenbaum
- iris retractor
- irrigation and aspiration

drooping upper eyelid

dropper
- Undine d.

droxifilcon A

drug abuse retinopathy

Drualt
- bundle of D.

drusen
- disk d.
- d. of optic disk
- d. of optic papilla

dry
- d. eye syndrome
- d. senile macular degeneration

dry-shelled cataract

DS-9 needle

Dualoop

Duane's
- accommodation chart
- classification
- retraction syndrome
- retractor
- syndrome

duct
- canalicular d.
- lacrimal d.
- lacrimonasal d.
- meibomian d.
- nasal d.
- nasolacrimal d.
- tear d.

duction test

ductions
- vertical d.
- d. and versions

ductional

ductule

ductulus

ductus
- d. lacrimales
- d. nasolacrimalis

Duddell's membrane
Duke-Elder
- lamp
- operation

Dulaney's lens
Dunnington's operation
duochrome test
Dupuy-Dutemps
- dacryocystorhinostomy dye test
- dacryostomy
- operation

dura
Duredge's knife
Durr's operation
dust-like opacities
Duverger and Velter operation
DVA — distance visual acuity
DVD — dissociated vertical divergence
dye test
dynamic
- d. refraction
- d. strabismus

Dyonics syringe injector
dysadaptation
dysaptation
dysautonomia
dyscephaly
- mandibulo-oculo-facial d.

dyschromasia
dyschromatopia
dyschromatopsia
dysconjugate gaze
dyscoria
dysgenesis
dyskeratosis
- d. congenita
- hereditary benign intraepithelial d.

dyslexia
dysmegalopsia
dysmetria
dysmetropsia
dysmorphic
dysmorphopsia
dysopia algera
dysopsia algera
dysostosis
dysphoric
dysplasia
- encephalo-ophthalmic d.
- oculoauricular d.
- oculoauriculovertebral d.
- oculodentodigital d.
- ophthalmomandibulomelic d.

dysplastic coloboma
dysthyroid optic neuropathy
dysthyroidism
dystonia
dystosis
- mandibulofacial d.

dystrophia
- d. adiposa corneae
- d. endothelialis corneae
- d. epithelialis corneae

dystrophy
- amorphous d.
- anterior membrane d.
- Best's vitelliform macular d.
- Biber-Haab-Dimmer d.
- Bietti's d.
- Buckler III d.
- butterfly macular d.
- central cloudy d. of Francois
- central cloudy parenchymatous d.
- central speckled d.
- choroidal d.

dystrophy *(continued)*
- choroidoretinal d.
- Cogan's microcystic corneal epithelial d.
- combined d. of Fuchs'
- cone d.
- congenital hereditary endothelial d.
- corneal endothelial guttate d.
- corneal stromal d.
- crystalline d.
- ectatic d.
- elastodystrophy
- endothelial d.
- epithelial d.
- epithelial d. of Fuchs'
- Fehr's macular d.
- fingerprint d.
- fleck d.
- Fleischer's d.
- Franceschetti's d.
- Fuchs' d.
- furrow d.
- granular d.
- Grayson-Wilbrandt d.
- Groenouw's type I d.
- Groenouw's type II d.
- hereditary epithelial d.
- hereditary vitelliform d.
- keratoconus d.
- lattice d.
- leukodystrophy
- macular corneal d.
- Maeder-Danis d.
- mandibulofacial d.
- map dot d.
- map dot fingerprint corneal epithelial d.
- marginal d.
- Meesman's d.
- Meesman's epithelial d.
- Melsman's d.

dystrophy *(continued)*
- microcystic d.
- muscular d.
- myotonic d.
- neonatal adrenoleukodystrophy
- d. of Waardenburg-Jonkers
- oculocerebrorenal d.
- Pillat's d.
- polymorphous d.
- posterior polymorphous d.
- progressive tapetochoroidal d.
- Reis-Bücklers superficial corneal d.
- retinal d.
- rod and cone d.
- Salzmann's nodular corneal d.
- Schlichting's d.
- Schnyder's crystalline corneal d.
- Stocker-Holt-Schneider d.
- tapetochoroidal d.
- vortex d.
- Wagner's vitreoretinal d.

e

Eales' disease

early
- e. lens opacities
- e. mature cataract

Easterman's visual function

ECCE — extracapsular cataract extraction

eccentric
- e. fixation

eccentric *(continued)*
e. limitation
e. viewing
eccentrically
ecchymoses
ecchymosis
ecchymotic
echinococcosis
echinophthalmia
echogram
echography
echo-ophthalmography
Echorule Ultrasonic Biometer
EchoScan by Nidek
echothiophate phospholine
eclipse
e. blindness
e. retinopathy
e. scotoma
ectasia
corneal e.
iris c.
scleral e.
ectatic corneal dystrophy
ectiris
ectochoroidea
ectocornea
ectoderm
ectodermatosis
ectodermosis
ectopia
cilia e.
e. iridis
e. lentis
macular e.
e. pupillae congenita
ectropion
atonic e.
e. cicatriceum
cicatricial e.
flaccid e.
e. luxurians
paralytic e.
ectropion *(continued)*
e. paralyticum
pigment layer e.
e. sarcomatosum
senile e.
e. senilis
spastic e.
e. spasticum
e. uveae
ectropionize
ectropium
eczematous
e. conjunctivitis
e. pannus
edema
Berlin's e.
boggy e.
brawny e.
cystoid macular e.
Iwanoff's retinal e.
microcystic e.
periretinal e.
Stellwag's brawny e.
edematous
Edinger-Westphal nucleus
edipism
edrophonium chloride test
Edwards' syndrome
effect
Braid's e.
Purkinje's e.
efferent
e. fibers
e. nerve
efficacy
effusion
egilops
egress
egressed
Egyptian
conjunctivitis
ophthalmia
Ehlers-Danlos syndrome

Ehrlich-Turck line
Ehrmann's test
eiconometer
eidoptometry
eight ball
  e.b. hemorrhage
  e.b. hyphema
eikonometer
elastic pseudoxanthoma
elastodysplasia
elastodystrophy
Elastoplast
  bandage
  dressing
  eye occlusor
elastosis
  e. dystrophica
  senile e.
Eldridge-Green lamp
electric shock cataract
electrocautery
electrocoagulation
electrode
  Gradle's e.
  Kronfeld's e
  Pischel's e.
  Weve's e.
electrodiaphake
electroencephalogram
electroencephalography
Electro-Keratome
electromagnetic removal of foreign body
electromagnetic spectrum
Electro-Mucotome
electron
  e. microscope
  e. microscopy
electron volt — eV
electronystagmogram
electronystagmograph
electronystagmography
electro-oculogram
electro-oculograph
electro-oculography
electroparacentesis
electrophysiology
electroretinogram
electroretinograph
electroretinography
electrospinogram
elephantiasis oculi
elevation
elevator
  Desmarres' lid e.
  Joseph's e.
Eliasoph's lid retractor
ELISA test — enzyme-linked immunosorbent assay
Elliott's
  corneal trephine
  operation
ellipse
ellipsoid
elliptical nystagmus
Ellis'
  foreign body spud
  needle holder
  needle probe
Elschnig's
  blepharorrhaphy
  bodies
  canthorrhaphy
  capsule forceps
  cataract knife
  central iridectomy
  conjunctivitis
  corneal knife
  cyclodialysis spatula
  fixation forceps
  iridectomy
  keratoplasty
  knife
  operation
  pearls
  pterygium knife

Elschnig's *(continued)*
 refractor
 retractor
 spatula
 spoon
 spots
 syndrome
Elschnig-O'Brien forceps
Ely's operation
embedded
embolism
 retinal e.
embryonal
 e. epithelial cyst of iris
 e. medulloepithelioma of ciliary body
 e. nuclear cataract
embryonic fixation syndrome
embryotoxon
emmetrope
emmetropia
emmetropic
Empac-Cavitron irrigation/aspiration unit
emphysema
 e. of conjunctiva
 e. of orbit
emplaced uveitis
en bloc ("ahn blok")
encanthis
encephalofacial angiomatosis
encephalomyelitis
encephalo-ophthalmic dysplasia
encephalopathy
 Wernicke's e.
encephalotrigeminal angiomatosis
encirclement
encircling
 e. band for scleral buckle
 e. element
 e. polyethylene tube

encircling *(continued)*
 e. silicone buckle
 e. tube
encroach
encroaching
encroachment
end-gaze nystagmus
endarteritis
endocapsular
endocarditis
endocrine
 e. exophthalmos
 e. lid retraction
 e. ophthalmopathy
endocryopexy
endocryophotocoagulation
endocryoretinopexy
endodiathermy
endogenous
 e. dyslexia
 e. uveitis
endoillumination
endoilluminator
endolaser probe tip
endophlebitis of retinal vein
endophotocoagulation
endophthalmitis
 bacterial e.
 fungal e.
 fusarium e.
 metastatic e.
 e. phacoallergica
 e. phacoanaphylactica
 e. phacogenetica
 systemic bacterial e.
 toxocariasis e.
endophthalmos
endophthalmus
endophytic
endoplasmic reticulum
endoretinal
Endo-Set by Haag-Streit
endothelial

endothelial *(continued)*
e. cell basement membrane
e. cell dystrophy
e. cell edema
e. cell side down
e. cell surface of cornea
corneal e. dystrophy
corneal e. pigmentary dispersion
endothelioma
Sidler-Huguenin e.
endothelium
e. camerae anterioris bulbi
corneal e.
e. oculi
endpoint nystagmus
en face ("ahn fahs")
ENG — electronystagmography
Englemann's disease
engorgement
enophthalmos
enophthalmus
enstrophe
entiris
entochoroidea
entocornea
entophthalmia
entoptic phenomenon
entoptoscope
entoptoscopy
entoretina
entropion
acquired e.
e. cicatriceum
cicatricial e.
congenital e.
Hotz's e.
senile e.
spastic e.
e. spasticum
e. uveae
uveal e.
entropionize
entropium
enucleate
enucleation
e. scissors
e. scoop
wire e. snare
enucleator
Banner snare e.
Botvin-Bradford e.
Bradford snare e.
Castroviejo's snare e.
Föerster's snare e.
Foster's snare e.
snare e.
enzymatic
e. cleaner
e. galactosemia
e. glaucoma
e. zonulolysis
enzyme-linked immunosorbent assay
EOG — electro-oculography
EOM — extraocular movement
eosinophil
ephelides
epiblepharon
epibulbar Fordyce nodules
epicanthal
e. fold
e. inversus
e. skin fold
epicanthic
epicanthine fold
epicanthus inversus
epicapsular lens stars
epicauma
epicenter
epidemic
e. blindness
e. conjunctivitis
e. keratoconjunctivitis
epidermidization
epidermoid carcinoma

epidermolysis bullosa
epikeratophakia
epilator
epilens
epinephrine
epiphora
epiphoria
epiretinal
episclera
episcleral
episcleritis
  gouty e.
  nodular e.
  e. partialis fugax
  simple e.
episclerotitis
epitarsus
epithelial
  e. barrier
  e. basement layer
  e. downgrowth
  e. dystrophy of Fuchs'
  e. edema
  e. implantation cyst
  e. inclusions
  e. ingrowth
  e. rolled edges
  e. scraping
  e. tumors
epithelioid
epithelioma
  Contino's e.
  intraepithelial e.
epitheliomata
epithelioplasty
epitheliosis desquamativa conjunctivae
epithelitis focal retinal pigment
epithelium
  e. anterius corneae
  corneal e.
  lens e.
  e. lentis
  pigmented e. of iris
epithelium *(continued)*
  e. pigmentosum iridis
  placoid pigmentation of e.
  posterior e. of cornea
  e. posterius corneae
  subcapsular e.
epizootic keratoconjunctivitis
epoch
Epstein's collar stud acrylic lens
equate
equator
  anatomic e.
  e. bulbi oculi
  crystalline lens e.
  eyeball e.
  lens e.
  e. lentis
equatorial
  e. degeneration
  e. drusen
  e. lentis
  e. meridian
  e. staphyloma
equilateral hemianopia
equilibrating operation
Erbakan's inferior fornix operation
erbium laser
ERG — electroretinogram
ergograph
Erhardt's lid forceps
erosion
  corneal e.
ERP — early receptor potential mottling
error
  astigmatic e.
eruptive keratoacanthoma
erysipelas
erysiphake
  Barraquer's e.
  Bell's e.
  Dimitry's e.

erysiphake *(continued)*
- Dimitry-Bell e.
- Dimitry-Thomas e.
- Draeger's high vacuum e.
- Esposito's e.
- Floyd-Grant e.
- Harrington's e.
- Johnson's e.
- Johnson-Bell e.
- Kara's e.
- L'Esperance's e.
- Maumenee's e.
- New York e.
- Nugent-Green-Dimitry e.
- Post-Harrington e.
- Sakler's e.
- Searcy's oval cup e.
- Storz-Bell e.
- Viers' e.
- Welch's rubber bulb e.
- Welsh's silastic e.

erythema multiforme
- e.m. bullosum
- e.m. exudativum

erythrogenic
erythrolabe
erythrometer
erythrometry
erythropia
erythropsia
Escapini's cataract operation
Eschenback's Optik
esocataphoria
esodeviation
esophoria
- accommodative e.
- nonaccommodative e.

esotropia
- accommodative e.
- acquired e.
- alternating e.
- congenital e.

esotropia *(continued)*
- consecutive e.
- constant e.
- cyclic e.
- infantile e.
- intermittent e.
- left e.
- nonaccommodative e.
- periodic e.
- right e.
- sensory e.
- V-pattern e.

esotropic
Esposito's erysiphake
essential
- e. hypotony
- e. iris atrophy

Esser's inlay operation
Esterman's scale
ET — esotropia
etafilcon A
ether guard
Ethicon
- Atraloc suture
- Micro-Point suture
- Sabreloc suture
- suture

Ethilon suture
ethmoid
- e. air cells
- e. bone
- e. canal
- e. sinuses

ethmoidal region
ethyl
- e. alcohol amblyopia
- e. cyanoacrylate

E trisomy
euchromatopsy
euploidic
euryopia
euthyphoria
euthyroid

euthyscope
eV — electron volt
evagination
    optic e.
evanescent
Evergreen Lasertek
    coagulator
    laser
Eversbusch's operation
eversion of punctum
everted
everter
    Berens's e.
    lid e.
    Roveda's e.
    Schachne-Desmarres e.
    Struble's e.
    Walker's e.
evisceration
    e. of eyeball
    e. spoon
evulsio nervi optici
evulsion
Ewald's law
Ewing's
    operation
    sarcoma
ex amblyopia
ex anopsia
exanthematous conjunctivitis
excavatio
    e. disci
    e. papillae nervi optici
excavation
    atrophic e.
    glaucomatous e.
    e. of optic disk
    physiologic e.
excessive
    e. cyclodialysis clefts
    e. lacrimation
Excimer laser
excretory duct
excursion
excycloduction
excyclophoria
excyclotropia
excyclovergence
exenteratio orbitae
exenteration
    orbital e.
exertional amblyopia
exfoliation
    e. of lens capsule
    e. syndrome
    true e.
exocataphoria
exodeviation
exogenous
exophoria
    alternating e.
    concomitant e.
    constant e.
exophoric
exophthalmic
exophthalmogenic
exophthalmometer
    Hertel's e.
    Luedde's e.
exophthalmometric
exophthalmometry
exophthalmos
    e. due to pressure
    e. due to tower skull
    endocrine e.
    malignant e.
    ophthalmoplegic e.
    pulsating e.
    thyrotoxic e.
    thyrotropic e.
exophthalmus
exophytic
exoplant
exorbitism
exotropia
    alternating e.

exotropia *(continued)*
- A-pattern e.
- basic e.
- comitant e.
- consecutive e.
- convergence insufficiency e.
- divergence excess e.
- flick e.
- intermittent e.
- left e.
- periodic e.
- right e.
- secondary e.
- sensory e.
- V-pattern e.

exotropic

experiment
- Mariotte's e.
- Scheiner's e.

Expo Bubble
- shield
- eye cover

exposure keratitis

expressor
- Arruga's e.
- Berens' e.
- Heath's e.
- hook e.
- Hosford's e.
- Kirby's hook e.
- lens e.
- e. loop
- McDonald's e.
- meibomian gland e.
- ring lens e.
- Rizzuti's e.
- Smith's e.
- Stahl's nucleus e.
- Verhoeff's e.

expulsive hemorrhage

extended round needle

external
- e. ankyloblepharon
- e. canthotomy
- e. geniculate body
- e. hordeolum
- e. limiting membrane
- e. ophthalmoplegia
- e. orbital fracture
- e. pterygoid-levator synkinesis
- e. strabismus

externus

extinction phenomenon

extirpation

extorsion

extracanthic

extracapsular cataract extraction

extracellular matrix

extraciliary

extraction
- e. flap
- e. of extracapsular cataract
- e. of intracapsular cataract

extractor
- Krwawicz's cataract e.
- roto e.

extramacular

extraocular
- e. movements
- e. muscles of Tillaux

extraocular muscles
- inferior oblique e.m.
- inferior rectus e.m.
- lateral rectus e.m.
- medial rectus e.m.
- superior oblique e.m.
- superior rectus e.m.

extrarectus

extraretinal

extrascleral

extravasated
extravasation
extrinsic muscles
extruded
extrusion
exudate
- hard e.
- soft e.

exudative
- e. retinitis
- e. senile maculopathy

eye
- aphakic e.
- artificial e.
- black e.
- blear e.
- Bright's e.
- cat's e.
- cinema e.
- crossed e.
- cystic e.
- dark-adapted e.
- deviating e.
- dominant e.
- e. epiphyseal
- exciting e.
- exudative e.
- fixating e.
- following e.
- Fox's e.
- hare's e.
- hop e.
- e. implant conformer
- e. infarction
- Klieg's e.
- lazy e.
- light-adapted e.
- monochromatic e.
- Nairobi's e.
- e. pad
- parietal e.
- pineal e.

eye *(continued)*
- primary e.
- pseudophakic e.
- racoon e.
- reduced e.
- e. removed in toto
- e. restored to normotensive pressure
- e. rotated inferiorly
- e. rotation
- schematic e.
- secondary e.
- shipyard e.
- Snellen's reform e.
- e. speculum
- squinting e.
- stony hard e.
- e. sweep
- sympathizing e.
- e. was quiet

EYE ANATOMY

- aqueous humor
- capsule
- choroid
- ciliary ligament
- ciliary muscle
- ciliary nerves
- cornea
- crystalline humor
- crystalline lens
- Descemet's membrane
- hyaloid membrane
- iris
- Jacob's membrane
- lamina cribrosa
- lamina fusca
- pupil
- retina
- sclera

EYE ANATOMY *(continued)*
- suspensory ligament
- uvea
- vitreous humor

eye bank
eye chart
Eye Con 5
eye contact
eye dropper
eye drops
eye/ear plane
eye lens
eye speculum
eyeball compression reflex
eyebrow
eyecup
eyed
eyedness
eyeglass
eyeground
eyehole
eyeing
eyelash
eyelid
- e. closure reflex
- e. coloboma
- e. contour
- e. crusting
- e. dermatochalasis
- e. ectropion
- e. entropion
- everted e.
- e. fissures
- e. flutter
- e. fold
- e. forceps
- e. fusion
- e. keratosis
- e. lymphangioma
- e. milia
- e. molluscum contagiosum infection
- e. myokymia

eyelid *(continued)*
- e. neurilemmoma
- e. neurofibroma
- e. nevi
- e. papilloma
- e. plaque
- e. ptosis
- e. retractor
- e. rhytids
- e. speculum
- e. strawberry hemangioma
- e. syringoma
- e. tumor
- e. vesiculation

EYELID ANATOMY

- aponeurosis
- canthus
- caruncula
- ciliary margins
- conjunctiva
- fibers of orbicularis oculi
- fornix
- inferior tarsus
- lacrimal ducts
- lacrimal sac
- lacus lacrimalis
- lamina
- lateral canthus
- levator palpebrae superioris
- medial palpebral ligament
- meibomian glands
- Müller's glands
- nasojugal
- nasolacrimal duct
- orbital margins
- orbital septum
- palpebral fissure

EYELID ANATOMY *(continued)*
- palpebral furrow
- palpebral raphe
- palpebrarum
- plica semilunaris
- posterior lamina
- Riolan's muscle
- superior fornix
- superior tarsus
- tarsal glands
- tarsal muscles
- tarsal plate
- tarsus
- tarsus orbital septum
- tunica conjunctiva

eyelids sutured closed

Eye-Pak II
- cover
- drape
- sheet

eyepatch
- oval e.

eyepiece
- comparison e.
- compensating e.
- demonstration e.
- huygenian e.
- negative e.
- positive e.
- Ramsden's e.
- wide field e.

eyepoint

eyeshield
- Barraquer's e.
- Buller's e.
- Cartella's e.
- Expo Bubble e.
- Fox's e.
- Green's e.
- Hessburg's e.
- Mueller's e.
- Paton's e.

eyeshield *(continued)*
- plastic e.
- ring cataract mask e.
- Universal e.
- Weck's e.

eyeshot

eyesight

eyespot

eyestrain

eyewash

EW — Edinger-Westphal

f

Faber's disease

Fabry's disease

face
- frog f.

facet

facetectomy

facetted
- f. avascular disciform opacity
- f. corneal scar

facial
- f. nerve
- f. palsy

facial block
- Nadbath's f.b.

facies
- f. anterior corneae
- f. anterior iridis
- f. anterior lentis
- f. anterior palpebrarum
- Hutchinson's f.
- f. orbitalis alae magnae
- f. orbitalis alae majoris
- f. orbitalis ossis frontalis
- f. orbitalis ossis zygomatici

facies *(continued)*
f. posterior corneae
f. posterior iridis
f. posterior lentis
f. posterior palpebrarum
facility of outflow
factor
diffusion f.
spreading f.
facultative
f. hyperopia
f. suppression
faculty fusion
Faden's
operation
sutures
faint flare
falciform fold of retina
false
f. image
f. macula
f. ptosis
f. vision
familial
f. autonomic dysfunction
f. colloid degeneration
f. dysautonomia
f. exudative vitreoretinopathy
f. lipoprotein deficiency
fan-like
Fanta's
cataract operation
speculum
fantascope
far point
f.p. accommodation
f.p. convergence
far sight
farinaceous epithelial keratitis
farinata
Farnsworth-Munsell 100 Hue Color Vision Test
farsighted
farsightedness
Fasanella-Servat ptosis operation
Fasanella's
lacrimal cannula
operation
retractor
fascia
bulbar f.
f. bulbi
f. lata
muscular f.
f. musculares bulbi
f. musculares oculi
orbital f.
palpebral f.
fasciae orbitales
fascia lata
f.l. musculares bulbi
f.l. musculares oculi
f.l. sling
f.l. stripper
Tenon's f.l.
fascicles
fascicular
f. keratitis
f. ophthalmoplegia
fasciculus maculary
fat
f. embolism of retina
f. graft
fatty exudate
Favre's disease
feathery clouding
Fechner's
intraocular lens
Federov's
4-loop iris clip lens implant
type I lens implant
type II lens implant
feeder-frond technique

feeder vessels
Fehr's macular dystrophy
Feldman's
    adaptometer
    RK optical center marker
fellow eye
fenestrae
fenestrated chain
fenretinide
Fenzel's
    angled manipulating hook
    manipulating hook
Fergus' operation
Ferree-Rand perimeter
Ferrein's canal
Ferris-Smith
    refractor
    retractor
Ferris-Smith-Sewall refractor
fetal
    f. alcohol syndrome
    f. fibrovascular sheath
    f. fissure
fiber
    accessory f.
    auxiliary f.
    Berneheimer's f.
    Brücke's f.
    chief f.
    cilioequatorial f.
    ciliposterocapsular f.
    circular f.
    circular ciliary muscle f.
    cone f.
    continuous f.
    corticonuclear f.
    Edinger's f's
    extraciliary f.
    Gratiolet's radiating f.
    interciliary f.
    f. layer of axon
    f. layer of Chevitz

fiber *(continued)*
    lens f.
    longitudinal f.
    main f.
    meridional ciliary muscle f.
    Müller's f.
    oblique f.
    optic nerve f.
    f. orbicularis oculi
    orbiculoanterocapsular f.
    orbiculociliary f.
    orbiculoposterocapsular f.
    principal f.
    radial f.
    Ritter's f.
    rod f.
    Sappey's f.
    sphincter f.
    sustentacular f.
    von Monakow's f.
    zonular f.
Fiberlite microscope
fiberoptic pick
fiberscope
Fibra Sonics phaco aspirator
fibrae
    f. circulares musculi ciliaris
    f. lentis
    f. longitudinales musculi ciliaris
    f. meridionales musculi ciliaris
    f. radiales musculi ciliaris
    f. zonulares
fibril
fibrillar material
fibrillation
fibrillogranuloma
fibrin
    f. dusting

fibrin *(continued)*
  f. platelet emboli
  f. thrombus
fibrinogen level
fibrinoid necrosis
fibroangioma
  nasopharyngeal f.
fibroblastic ingrowth
fibroblasts
fibrocytes
fibroglial
fibrogliotic
fibrogranular
fibroid cataract
fibroma
fibronectin
fibroplasia
  retrolental f.
fibroproliferative membrane
fibrosarcoma
fibrosis choroideae corrugans
fibrous
  f. dysplasia
  f. tunic of eyeball
fibrovascular
  f. fronds
  f. sheath
  f. tunic
Fick's
  axis
  halo
field
  binasal f.
  cribriform f.
  fixation f.
  Forel's f.
  f. of gaze
  f. loss
  spiral f.
  surplus f.
  f. of vision
  visual f.
field diaphragm setting
fifth cranial nerve
figure
  Purkinje's f.
  Stifel's f.
  Zollner's f.
fil d'Arion silicone tube
filament keratitis
filamentary
  f. keratitis
  f. keratome
filariasis
Filatov's keratoplasty
Filatov-Marzinkowsky operation
filter
  interference f.
  Millex f.
  Millipore f.
  neutral density f.
  red free f.
  UV blocking f.
  Whatman's f.
  Wrattan's f.
filtering
  f. bleb
  f. cicatrix
  f. operation
  f. wick
fimbriated
  f. edge
  f. margin
final threshold
fine
  f. iris processes
Fine's
  corneal carrying case
  dissecting forceps
  magnetic implant
  micropoint cautery
  toothed forceps
  tying forceps
Fine-Castroviejo forceps
fine-toothed forceps
finger-count

finger-counting
finger-like extensions
fingerprint dystrophy
finger vision
Fink's
  cataract aspirator
  cul-de-sac irrigator
  curet
  hook
  irrigator
  lacrimal retractor
  muscle hook
  muscle marker
  oblique muscle hook
  retractor
  tendon tucker
Fink-Jameson muscle forceps
Fink-Weinstein two-way syringe
Finnoff's transilluminator
first-grade fusion
fish eggs
Fisher's
  lid retractor
  needle
  spoon
  spud
  syndrome
Fisher-Arlt iris forceps
fishmouth tear
fishmouthing
Fison's indirect binocular ophthalmoscope
fissura
  f. orbitalis inferior
  f. orbitalis superior
fissure
  choroid f.
  corneal f.
  inferior orbital f.
  interpalpebral f.
  orbital f.
  palpebral f.
  sphenoccipital f.
fissure *(continued)*
  sphenoidal f.
  sphenomaxillary f.
  superior orbital f.
  f. zone
fistula
  corneal f.
  lacrimal f.
fistulae
fistulizing surgery
fixate
fixating eye
fixation
  axis f.
  binocular f.
  binocular f. forceps
  central f.
  f. forceps
  f. hook
  f. light
  f. object
  f. pick
  f. point
  f. reflex
  f. ring
  f. suture
fixed
  f. dilated pupil
  f. folds
  f. forceps
  f. point
  f. pupil
fixing eye
flaccid
Flajani's
  disease
  operation
flaky
flame hemorrhage
flame-shaped hemorrhage
flap
  conjunctival f.
  fornix-based f.

flap
 limbal-based f.
flare
 aqueous f.
flare and cells
flash
 f. blindness
 f. keratoconjunctivitis
flashes of light
flashing
flashlight examination
flat
 f. and shallow
 f. cornea
 f. cup
flecked
 f. corneal dystrophy
 f. retina disease
 f. retina of Kandori
Fleischer's
 dystrophy
 ring
Flexner-Winterstein rosette
flick
 f. exotropia
 f. hypertropia
flicker
flicker-fusion stimuli
Flieringa's
 fixation ring
 scleral ring
Flieringa-Kayser copper ring
Flieringa-Kayser fixation ring
Flieringa-LeGrand fixation ring
floaters
 vitreous f.
floccular
flocculent
floor fracture
floppy eyelid
Florentine's iris
florid
floriform cataract
Flouren's law
Floyd-Grant erysiphake
fluff dressing
fluffed gauze dressing
fluid cataract
fluid-gas exchange
fluorescein
 f. angiogram
 f. angiography
 f. dye and stain solution
 f. dye disappearance test
 f. fundus angioscopy
 f. test
fluorescence
fluorobiprofen
fluorophotometry
 vitreous f.
flush
 choroidal f.
flutter
 ocular f.
flux
 radiant and luminous f.
foam-appearing cytoplasm
foaming exudate
focal
 f. depth
 f. distance
 f. image point
 f. interval
 f. length
 f. point
 f. scotoma
foci
focimeter
focus
 aplanatic f.
 conjugate f.
 principal f.
 real f.
 virtual f.
focusing

Foerster's
- enucleation snare
- forceps

fogging system of refraction

foil sheet

Foix
- enucleation
- syndrome

folds
- ciliary f.
- congenital retinal f.
- conjunctival semilunar f.
- epicanthal f.
- epicanthine f.
- falciform f.
- fixed f.
- Hasner's f.
- iridial f.
- lacrimal f.
- palpebral f.
- palpebronasal f.
- retrotarsal f.
- semilunar f. of conjunctiva
- star f.
- stiff f.

follicle

follicles
- conjunctival f.

follicular
- f. conjunctivitis
- f. iritis
- f. plugging

folliculitis

Foltz's valve

Fontana's space

foot candle meter

foot plate

foramen
- Bozzi's f.
- inferior zygomatic f.
- infraorbital f.
- f. infraorbitale

foramen *(continued)*
- lacerate anterior f.
- lacerate middle f.
- lacerate posterior f.
- f. lacerum anterius
- f. of sclera
- f. of sphenoid bone
- optic f.
- f. opticus
- orbitomalar f.
- Soemmering's f.
- f. sphenoidalis
- supraorbital f.
- f. supraorbitale
- f. supraorbitalis
- rotundum f.
- zygomatic f.
- f. zygomatico-orbitale

foramina
- optic f.

forced
- f. duction test
- f. eye closure

forceps
- Adson's f.
- Alabama University utility f.
- Allen-Barker f.
- Allen-Braley f.
- Allis' f.
- Alvis' fixation f.
- Ambrose's suture f.
- Amenabar's capsule f.
- Arruga's f.
- Arruga-MacKool f.
- Asch's septal f.
- Ayer's chalazion f.
- B.B. shot f.
- Bailey's chalazion f.
- Baird's chalazion f.
- Ballen-Alexander f.
- Bangerter's muscle f.
- Banner's f.

forceps *(continued)*
- Bard-Parker f.
- Barkan's iris f.
- Barraquer's f.
- Barraquer's cilia f.
- Barraquer's conjunctival f.
- Barraquer's corneal f.
- Barraquer's hemostatic mosquito f.
- Barraquer-von Mondak capsule f.
- bayonet f.
- beaked f.
- Beaupre's cilia f.
- Bennett's cilia f.
- Berens' corneal transplant f.
- Berens' f.
- Berens' muscle f.
- Berens' ptosis f.
- Berens' suturing f.
- Berke's f.
- Berke's ptosis f.
- Berkley Bioengineering ptosis f.
- Bettman-Noyes fixation f.
- bipolar f.
- Birk-Mathelone micro f.
- Birks Mark II Colibri f.
- Birks Mark II f.
- Birks Mark II groove f.
- Birks Mark II micro needle holder f.
- Birks Mark II straight f.
- Birks Mark II suture tying f.
- Birks Mark II toothed f.
- Bishop-Harmon f.
- Blaydes' corneal f.
- blepharochalasis f.
- Bonaccolto's f.
- Bonaccolto's fragment f.

forceps *(continued)*
- Bonaccolto's jeweler f.
- Bonaccolto's magnet tip f.
- Bonaccolto's utility f.
- bone-biting f.
- Bonn's f.
- Boruchoff's f.
- Botvin's f.
- Botvin's iris f.
- Bracken's f.
- Bracken's fixation f.
- Bracken's iris f.
- Bronson-Magnion f.
- Callahan's lens loop fixation f.
- capsule f.
- capsule fragment f.
- Castroviejo's f.
- Castroviejo's capsule f.
- Castroviejo's clip applying f.
- Castroviejo's fixation f.
- Castroviejo's lid f.
- Castroviejo's scleral fold f.
- Castroviejo's suturing f.
- Castroviejo's wide grip handle f.
- Castroviejo-Arruga f.
- chalazion f.
- Chandler's f.
- cilia f.
- Clark's capsule fragment f.
- Clark-Verhoeff capsule f.
- Clayman's lens implant f.
- clip applying f.
- Cohan's corneal f.
- Coleman Taylor IOL f.
- Colibri's f.
- Colibri's micro f.
- corneal fixation f.

forceps *(continued)*
corneal holding f.
corneal prosthesis f.
corneal splinter f.
corneoscleral f.
Crawford's f.
cross-action capsule f.
Culler's fixation f.
Dallas lens inserting f.
Dan's chalazion f.
Danberg's iris f.
Dan-Gradle cilia f.
Davis' f.
Desmarres' f.
disk f.
Dixon-Thorpe vitreous foreign body f.
Douglas' cilia f.
dressing f.
Drews' cilia f.
Drews-Sato tying f.
Eber's needle holder f.
Ehrhardt's lid f.
Elschnig's f.
Elschnig's capsule f.
Elschnig's fixation f.
Elschnig-O'Brien f.
entropion f.
Erhardt's lid f.
Ewing's capsular f.
Fine's dissecting f.
Fine's tying f.
Fine-Castroviejo f.
Fink-Jameson muscle f.
Fisher-Arlt iris f.
fixation f.
fixation/anchor f.
fixed f.
Foerster's f.
fold f.
foreign body f.
Frances' spud chalazion f.

forceps *(continued)*
Francis' f.
Fuchs' capsule f.
Fuchs' iris f.
Furness' cornea holder f.
Gelfilm f.
Gifford's fixation f.
Gill-Arruga capsular f.
Gill-Hess iris f.
Girard's corneoscleral f.
Gradle's cilia f.
Graefe's fixation f.
Graefe's iris f.
Graefe's tissue f.
Grayson's corneal f.
Green's fixation f.
Grieshaber's diamond coated f.
Grieshaber's iris f.
Guist's fixation f.
Gunderson's muscle f.
Guyton-Clark fragment f.
Guyton-Noyes fixation f.
Halberg's contact lens f.
Halsted's curved mosquito f.
Halsted's mosquito hemostatic f.
Harms' corneal f.
Harms' tying f.
Harms-Tubingen tying f.
Hartman's f.
Hartman's mosquito hemostatic f.
Heath's chalazion f.
hemostatic f.
Hertel's stone f.
Hess' f.
Hess-Barraquer f.
Hess-Horwitz f.
Hirschman's lens f.
Holth's f.

forceps *(continued)*
- Hoskins' beaked Colibri f.
- Hoskins' fine straight f.
- Hoskins' fixation f.
- Hoskins' micro straight f.
- Hoskins' miniaturized micro straight f.
- Hoskins' straight micro iris f.
- Hoskins' suture f.
- Hoskins-Luntz f.
- Hoskins-Skeleton fine f.
- Hoskins-Skeleton micro grooved broad-tipped f.
- host tissue f.
- House's miniature f.
- Hubbard's corneoscleral f.
- Hunt's chalazion f.
- Hyde's double curved f.
- Ilg's capsule f.
- Ilg's curved micro tying f.
- Ilg's insertion f.
- intraocular f.
- Iowa State fixation f.
- iris f.
- Jacobs' capsule fragment f.
- Jameson's muscle f.
- Jansen's intraocular lens f.
- Jansen-Middleton septotomy f.
- Jervey's capsule fragment f.
- Jervey's iris f.
- jeweler's f.
- Jones' f.
- Judd's f.

forceps *(continued)*
- Kalt's f.
- Katena's f.
- Katzin-Barraquer f.
- Keeler's extended round tip f.
- Keeler's intraocular foreign body grasping f.
- Kelman's f.
- Kerrison's f.
- Kervorkian-Younge f.
- King-Prince muscle f.
- Kirby's capsule f.
- Kirby's corneoscleral f.
- Kirby's iris f.
- Kirby's tissue f.
- Knapp's f.
- Koby's cataract f.
- Kraff-Utrata capsulorrhexis f.
- Kraft's f.
- Kronfeld's f.
- Krukenberg's pigment spindle f.
- Kuhnt's fixation f.
- Kulvin-Kalt f.
- Lambert's chalazion f.
- large angled f.
- Leakey's chalazion f.
- Leigh's capsule f.
- lens threading f.
- Lester's fixation f.
- lid f.
- Linn-Graefe iris f.
- Lister's f.
- Littauer's cilia f.
- Llobera's fixation f.
- Lordan's chalazion f.
- Lucae's dressing f.
- Malis' f.
- Manhattan E & E suturing f.

forceps *(continued)*
marginal chalazion f.
Max Fine f.
McCullough's suturing f.
McGregor's conjunctiva f.
McGuire's marginal chalazion f.
McLean's capsule f.
McLean's muscle recession f.
McPherson's bent f.
McPherson's corneal f.
McPherson's micro iris f.
McPherson's micro suture f.
McPherson's tying f.
Mentor-Maumenee Suregrip f.
micro Colibri f.
miniature f.
Moehle's corneal f.
mosquito hemostatic f.
muscle f.
Neubauer's f.
New Orleans E & E fixation f.
Noble's f.
Noyes' f.
Nugent's rectus f.
O'Brien's fixation f.
O'Conner's sponge f.
O'Conner-Elschnig fixation f.
Ochsner's cartilage f.
Ochsner's tissue f.
Ogura's cartilage f.
Ogura's tissue f.
Osher's foreign body f.
Paton's anterior chamber lens implant f.
Paton's capsule f.

forceps *(continued)*
Paton's corneal transplant f.
Paton's suturing f.
Paton's tying/stitch removal f.
Paufique's suturing f.
Pavlo-Colibri corneal f.
Penn-Anderson scleral fixation f.
Perritt's f.
Peyman-Green vitreous f.
Phillips' fixation f.
Pierse's corneal f.
Pierse's fixation f.
Pley's extracapsular f.
Pollock's f.
Primbs' suturing f.
Prince's muscle f.
ptosis f.
Puntenny's f.
pupil spreader/retractor f.
Quevedo's fixation f.
Quevedo's suturing f.
Quire's mechanical finger f.
Reese's muscle f.
Reisenger's lens extracting f.
ring f.
Rizzuti's fixation f.
Rizzuti's rectus f.
Rizzuti-Furness cornea holding f.
Rolf's f.
Russian f.
Rycroft's tying f.
Sachs' tissue f.
Sanders-Castroviejo suturing f.
Sandt's f.
Sauer's f.

forceps *(continued)*
Schaaf's foreign body f.
Schaefer's fixation f.
Scheie-Graefe fixation f.
Schepens' f.
Schweigger's capsule f.
scleral twist grip f.
Scott's lens insertion f.
Shepard-Reinstein f.
silicone rod and sleeve f.
silicone sponge f.
Skeleton fine f.
sleeve spreading f.
Smart's f.
Smart-Leiske cross-action intraocular lens f.
Snellen's entropion f.
Snider's corneal spring f.
Spender's chalazion f.
Spero's f.
Starr's fixation f.
Stern-Castroviejo f.
Stevens' f.
stitch removal f.
Storz's capsule f.
Storz's cilia f.
Storz's corneal f.
Storz-Bonn suturing f.
Storz-Utrata f.
Strow's corneal f.
superior rectus f.
suturing f.
Takahashi iris retractor f.
Terson's capsule f.
Terson's extracapsular f.
Thomas' fixation f.
Thorpe's f.
Thorpe-Castroviejo corneal f.
Thorpe-Castroviejo fixation f.

forceps *(continued)*
Thorpe-Castroviejo vitreous foreign body f.
Thrasher's lens implant f.
three-toothed f.
Troutman's f.
tying/stitch removal f.
Verhoeff's f.
Vicker's f.
vitreous foreign body f.
von Graefe's f.
von Mondak's f.
Wadsworth's lid f.
Wainstock's suturing f.
Waldeau's f.
Wies' chalazion f.
Worth's strabismus f.
Wullstein-House cup f.
Ziegler's f.
Fordyce's nodules
forebrain dysplasia
foreign body
f.b. bur
Ellis' f.b. spud
f.b. extraction
f.b. forceps
Shoch's f.b. pickup
f.b. spud
vitreous f.b.
Foerster's enucleation snare
Forel field
Forker's retractor
fornices
fornix
f. approach
inferior conjunctiva f.
lacrimal f.
f. sacci lacrimalis
superior conjunctival f.
fornix-based flap
Forssman's carotid syndrome
Förster's
choroiditis

Förster's *(continued)*
conjunctiva
lacrimal sac
operation
sacci lacrimalis
uveitis
Förster-Fuchs black spot
fossa
f. glandulae lacrimalis
glandular f. of frontal bone
hyaloid f.
f. hydoidea
lacrimal gland f.
lacrimal sac f.
lenticular f.
lenticular f. of vitreous body
optical f.
patellar f.
f. sacci lacrimalis
trochlear f.
f. trochlearis
f. tumor
fossae
fossette
Foster-Kennedy syndrome
Foster's enucleation snare
Fould's entropion operation
four
f. base-out prism testing
f. loop iris fixated implant
Four Dot Test
fourth
f. cranial nerve
f. nerve palsy
fovea
central f.
f. centralis
trochlear f.
f. trochlearis
foveae
foveal
f. avascular zone
f. flicker fusion frequency
f. reflex
f. vision
foveate
foveation
foveola
foveolae
foveolar
foveomacular retinitis
Foville's syndrome
Foville-Wilson syndrome
Fox's
aluminum shield
conformer
implant
irrigator/aspirator unit
operation
shield
sphere implant
fracture
apex f.
blow-out f.
floor f.
orbital f.
orbital floor f.
roof f.
fragmatome
Gill-Hess f.
Girard's f.
fragmentation-aspiration handpiece
fragmentor
Lieberman's f.
Framatome flute syringe
frame
trial f.
framework
scleral f.
uveal f.
framing

Franceschetti's
- coreoplasty operation
- deviation operation
- disease
- dystrophy
- keratoplasty operation
- operation
- syndrome

Francis'
- disease
- forceps
- spud

Francisella tularensis

Francois'
- dystrophy
- syndrome

Frankfort's horizontal plane

Franklin's
- glasses
- spectacles

Fraunfelder's "no touch" technique

Fraunhofer's line

free
- f. margin of eyelid
- f. running mode
- f. tenotomy

Freeman's solution

Freer's
- chisel
- elevator

freeze-thaw cryotherapy

French's
- hook spatula
- lacrimal dilator
- lacrimal probe
- lacrimal spatula
- needle holder
- pattern spatula

frequency
- fusion f.

Fresnel's
- lens

Fresnel's *(continued)*
- principle
- prism

Frey's
- implant
- tunneled implant

Fricke's operation

Friede's operation

Friedenwald's
- funduscope
- operation
- ophthalmoscope
- syndrome

Friedenwald-Guyton operation

Friedman's
- clip
- hand-held Hruby lens
- tantalum clips

Frigitronics
- freeze-thaw cryopexy probe
- nitrous oxide cryosurgery apparatus

fringes
- Moire's f.

Fritz vitreous transplant needle

Frog cortex remover

fronds
- fibrous f.
- sea f.

frons
- f. cranii
- f. of cranium

frontal
- f. bone
- f. nerve
- f. triangle

frontalis
- f. muscle
- f. muscle sling

frontispiece

frontolacrimal suture

Frost's
- scissors
- suture

Frost-Lang operation
frozen globe
Fuchs'
- aphakic keratopathy
- atrophy
- blackspot
- canthorrhaphy operation
- capsule forceps
- coloboma
- crypts
- cyclitis
- dimples
- dystrophy
- forceps
- heterochromia
- heterochromic cyclitis
- heterochromic iridocyclitis
- iris bombe transfixation operation
- iris forceps
- keratitis
- lancet type keratome
- operation
- retinal detachment syringe
- spot
- spot coloboma
- syndrome
- two-way syringe

Fuchs-Kraupa syndrome
Fukala's operation
full versions and ductions
fulminant
- f. myasthenia gravis
- f. ocular toxoplasmosis

Ful-Vue
- ophthalmoscope
- spot retinoscope
- streak retinoscope

function
- cone f.
- rod f.

functional
- f. amblyopia
- f. blindness
- f. defects

fundal reflex
fundi
fundus
- albinotic f.
- f. albipunctalis
- f. albipunctatus
- f. camera
- f. diabeticus
- f. flavimaculatus
- leopard f.
- f. microscopy
- f. oculi
- f. of eye
- salt-and-pepper f.
- tessellated f.
- f. tigre
- tigroid f.

funduscope
funduscopic examination
funduscopy
fungal
fungating
funnel
- muscular f.
- vascular f.

funnel-shaped retinal detachment
Furness' cornea holding forceps
furrow
- f. degeneration
- f. dystrophy
- f. keratitis
- scleral f.

Fusarium
- F. solanae

- Fusarium
  - F. solani
- fuscin
- fusiform cataract
- fusion
  - f. with amplitude
  - binocular f.
  - central f.
  - f. faculty
  - f. grade
  - peripheral f.
  - f. reflex
  - f. tube
- fusional convergence
- fusion-free position
- Fyoderov's lens (Federov's)

g

- galactokinase
- galactosemia
- galactosyl ceramide lipidosis
- Galen's vein
- galeropia
- galeropsia
- Galezowsky's lacrimal dilator
- Galin's
  - bleb cup
  - intraocular implant lens
- gallium citrate contrast
- Galt's aspirating cannula
- Gamboscope
- ganglion
  - g. cell layer
  - ciliary g.
  - g. layer of optic nerve
  - g. layer of retina
  - ophthalmic g.
  - optic g.
  - orbital g.

ganglion *(continued)*
  - Schacher's g.
  - g. stratum of optic nerve
- ganglionic
- ganglionitis
- gangliosidosis
  - generalized g.
- gangliosus ciliaris
- Gans' cannula
- Ganzfeld's electroretinograph
- Garcia-Ibanez camera
- Garcia-Novito eye implant
- gargoylism
- gas
  - g. bubble
  - hexafluoride g.
  - octofluoropropane g.
  - perfluoropropane g.
  - g. permeable contact lens
  - sulfur g.
- gas-fluid exchange
- Gass'
  - cannula
  - dye applicator
  - retinal detachment hook
  - scleral marker
  - scleral punch
  - vitreous aspirating cannula
- Gaucher's disease
- Gaule's spots
- Gault's reflex
- Gayet's operation
- gaze
  - conjugate g.
  - distant g.
  - disconjugate g.
  - dysconjugate g.
  - eccentric g.
  - evoked nystagmus
  - g. evoked tinnitus
  - g. movement

gaze *(continued)*
near g.
g. nystagmus
g. palsy
g. paretic nystagmus
Geiger's cautery
gelatinous material
gelatinous-appearing limbal hypertrophy
Gelfilm
cap
forceps
retinal implant
general anesthesia
geniculate
g. external body
g. lateral body
g. nucleus
geniculocalcarine tract
geographic
g. herpes simplex corneal ulcer
g. lesions
g. peripapillary choroiditis
geometric
g. axis
g. equator
g. perspective
Georgariou's cyclodialysis operation
German measles
gerontopia
gerontoxon lentis
Gerstmann's syndrome
gestational diabetes mellitus
Geuder's keratoplasty needle
ghost
g. cells
g. cell glaucoma
g. vessels
giant
g. cell arteritis

giant *(continued)*
g. papillae
g. papillary conjunctivitis
g. retinal break
g. tear
Giardet's corneal transplant scissors
Gibralter's headrest
Gibson's irrigating/aspirating unit
Giemsa stain
Gierke's disease
Gifford's
applicator
corneal curet
delimiting keratotomy operation
fixation forceps
iris forceps
needle holder
operation
reflex
sign
Gifford-Galassi reflex
Gill's
blade
corneal knife
counterpressor
double Luer Lok cannula
intraocular implant lens
iris forceps
knife
scissors
Gill-Fine corneal knife
Gill-Hess
blade
fragmatome
iris forceps
knife
scissors
Gill-Welch
curet
guillotine port

Gill-Welch *(continued)*
- knife
- scissors

Gillies' scar correction operation

Gilmore's intraocular implant lens

Girard's
- anterior chamber needle
- cataract aspirating needle
- corneoscleral forceps
- fragmatome
- keratoprosthesis operation
- phakofragmatome
- procedure
- scleral expander ring

Girard-Teulon law

girdle
- limbus g.
- white limbal g. of Vogt

Gish's micro YAG laser

Givner's lid retractor

glabella

glabellar

glabellum

Gladstone-Putterman transmarginal rotation entropion clamp

gland
- Baumgarten's g.
- Bruch's g.
- Ciaccio's g.
- ciliary g.
- conjunctival g.
- Harder's g.
- harderian g.
- Henle's g.
- inferior lacrimal g.
- Krause's g.
- lacrimal g.
- Manz's g.
- meibomian g.

gland *(continued)*
- Moll's g.
- Müller's g.
- palpebral g.
- Rosenmüller's g.
- sebaceous g's of conjunctiva
- superior lacrimal g.
- tarsal g.
- tarsoconjunctival g.
- trachoma g.
- Waldeyer's g.
- g. of Wolfring
- g. of Zeis
- zeisian g.

glanders

glandula lacrimalis
- g.l. inferior
- g.l. superior

glandulae
- g. ciliares conjunctivales
- g. conjunctivales
- g. lacrimales accessoriae
- g. mucosae conjunctivae
- g. sebaceae conjunctivales
- g. tarsales

glare
- direct g.
- peripheral g.
- g. test

glarometer

glass
- g. lens
- optical g.
- g. sphere implant

glassblower's cataract

glasses
- bifocal g.
- contact g.
- crutch g.
- executive bifocal g.
- Franklin's g.

glasses *(continued)*
Hallauer's g.
Masselon's g.
safety g.
sun g.
trifocal g.
glassine strands
glassy sheets
glaucoma
g. absolatum
absolute g.
acute g.
acute angle-closure g.
acute chronic g.
acute congestive g.
air-block g.
alpha-chymotrypsin–induced g.
angle-closure g.
angle-recession g.
aphakic g.
apoplectic g.
auricular g.
capsular g.
chronic g.
chronic angle-closure g.
chronic narrow-angle g.
chronic open-angle g.
chronic simple g.
ciliary block g.
closed-angle g.
combined g.
compensated g.
congenital g.
congestive g.
g. consummatum
Contino's g.
contusion g.
contusion angle g.
corticosteroid-induced g.
Donder's g.
enzyme g.
erythroclastic g.

glaucoma *(continued)*
fleken g.
g. fulminans
fulminant g.
ghost cell g.
hemolytic g.
hemorrhagic g.
hypersecretion g.
g. imminens
infantile g.
inflammatory g
intermittent angle-closure g.
juvenile g.
latent angle-closure g.
lens exfoliation g.
lenticular g.
low tension g.
malignant g.
monocular g.
melanomalytic g.
narrow-angle g.
neovascular g.
noncongestive g.
obstructive g.
ocular hypertension g.
open-angle g.
g. pencil
phacogenic g.
phacolytic g.
phacomorphic g.
phakogenic g.
phakolytic g.
phakomorphic g.
pigmentary g.
pigmentary dispersion g.
primary g.
primary angle-closure g.
primary open-angle g.
prodromal g.
pseudoexfoliative capsular g.
pseudoglaucoma g.

glaucoma *(continued)*
- pupillary block g.
- recessed-angle g.
- retrobulbar hemorrhage g.
- scleral shell g.
- secondary g.
- simple g.
- simplex g.
- steroid g.
- trabeculitis g.
- traumatic g.
- vitreous block g.
- wide-angle g.

glaucomatocyclitic crisis
glaucomatous
- g. cataract
- g. cup
- g. cupping
- g. excavation
- g. habit
- g. halo
- g. ring

glaucosis
glaukomflecken
glia
glial
- g. cells
- g. proliferation

gliocyte
- retinal g.

glioma
- astrocytic g.
- chiasmal g.
- g. endophytum
- g. exophytum
- optic g.
- peripheral g.
- retinal g.
- g. sarcomatosum
- telangiectatic g.

gliomatosis
gliomatous
gliosarcoma
- retinal g.

gliosis
- neonatal g.
- traumatic g.

gliotic
- g. membrane
- g. strip

glissade
glissadic
global
globe
globoid cell leukodystrophy
globule
- Morgagni's g.

globuli
glue
- butyl cyanoacrylate g.
- ethyl cyanoacrylate g.
- histoacryl g.
- methyl cyanoacrylate g.
- g. patch
- wicking g. patch

glued-on hard contact lenses
glutaraldehyde
glycogenesis
- hepatorenal g.

glycohemoglobin
glycolipid
goblet cells
goiter
- exophthalmic g.

Gold's
- sphere implant

Goldenhar's syndrome
Goldmann's
- Applanation Tonometer
- Coherent Radiation
- contact lens prism
- device
- goniolens
- kinetic technique
- multi-mirrored lens

Goldmann's *(continued)*
- perimeter
- perimetry
- serrated knife
- static technique
- three-mirror lens

Goldmann-Favre
- dystrophy
- syndrome

Goldmann-Larsson foreign body operation

Goldmann-Weeker Dark Adaptometer

Goldstein's
- anterior chamber syringe
- cannula
- golf club spud
- lacrimal sac retractor
- lacrimal syringe
- retractor

golf club spud

Golgi's
- complex
- neurons

Goltz-Gorein syndrome

Gomez-Marquez lacrimal operation

gonia

gonial

Gonin's
- cautery
- operation

goniofocalizing lens

goniogram
- Becker's g.

goniolens
- 4-mirror g.
- Allen-Thorpe g.
- Goldmann's g.
- Koeppe's g.
- single-mirror g.
- Thorpe-Castroviejo g.

goniophotocoagulation

goniophotography

gonioplasty

gonioprism

goniopuncture knife

gonioscope
- Lovac's g.
- Sussman's 4 mirror g.
- Zeiss' g.

gonioscopic
- g. lens
- g. prism

gonioscopy

goniosynechia

goniosynechiae

goniotomy
- g. knife
- g. needle holder

Gonnin's marker

Gonnin-Amsler marker

gonoblennorrhea

gonococcal conjunctivitis

gonorrheal conjunctivitis

Good's retractor

Gormley's double cannula

gossamer scarring

gouge
- lacrimal sac g.
- spud g.
- Todd's g.

Gould's intraocular implant lens

gouty
- g. episcleritis
- g. iritis

Gower's sign

GPC — giant papillary conjunctivitis

graceful swirling rods

Gradenigo's syndrome

Gradle's
- cilia forceps
- corneal trephine
- electrode
- forceps

Gradle's *(continued)*
keratoplasty operation
operation
retractor
Graefe's
cataract knife
cystotome
disease
forceps
iris forceps
knife
operation
sign
strabismus hook
syndrome
graft
g. carrier spoon
corneal g.
lamellar g.
mushroom g.
penetrating g.
g. preservation solution
Graither's
collar button
refractor
retractor
gram-negative bacteria
gram-positive bacteria
Gram stain
granular
g. corneal dystrophy
g. dystrophy
granularity
granule
cone g.
rod g.
granuloma
g. gangraenescens
g. iridis
granulomatous uveitis
Graves' disease
gravid retinitis
gray
g. cataract
g. line
g. plaque
Grayson's corneal forceps
Grayson-Wilbrandt anterior corneal dystrophy
gray-white corneal scar
greater
g. ring of iris
g. wing of the sphenoid
Greave's operation
Green's
blindness
caliper
capsule forceps
cataract
cataract knife
chalazion forceps
corneal knife
curet
dissector
double spatula
eyeshield
fixation forceps
forceps
hook
iris replacer
knife
muscle hook
muscle tucker
needle holder
refractor
replacer spatula
spatula
strabismus hook
strabismus tucker
trephine
Gregg's syndrome
Greig's syndrome
grid
Amsler's g.

Gridley's intraocular lens
Grieshaber's
- corneal trephine
- keratome
- needle
- needle holder
- ruby knife
- trephine
- ultrasharp microsurgery
- vertical cutting scissors
- vitreous scissors

Grimsdale's operation
Groenholm's
- refractor
- retractor

Groenouw's dystrophy
Grönblad-Strandberg syndrome
groove
- Blessig's g.
- infraorbital g.
- lacrimal g.
- lamellar g.
- nasolacrimal g.
- optic g.
- g. silicone implant
- g. sutures
- Verga's lacrimal g.

Gross'
- retractor
- stereopsis

Grossmann's operation
ground glass sheet
Gruning's magnet
GS-9 needle
gt - drop
gtt - drops
guard
- cataract knife g.
- forceps g.
- keratome g.
- knife g.
- scalpel g.

Gudden's commissure
Guibor's
- chart
- duct tube
- shield

Guillain-Barré syndrome
guillotine
- g. cutting tip
- g. vitrectomy instrument

Guist's
- enucleation hemostat
- enucleation scissors
- fixation forceps
- hemostat
- implant
- scissors
- speculum
- sphere implant

Guist-Bloch speculum
Gullstrand's
- law
- loupe
- ophthalmoscope
- reduced eye
- slit lamp

gumma
gummas
gummata
Gunderson's
- conjunctival flap
- muscle forceps

Gunn's
- dots
- pupil
- syndrome

gutta — gt. (drop)
gutta
- g. amaurosis
- g. serena

guttae — gtt. (drops)
Guttat. — guttatim
guttate (drop-shaped lesions)

guttatim (drop by drop)
guttation (exudation of liquid)
Gutzeit's dacryostomy operation
Guyton's
  corneal transplant trephine
  electrode
  operation
  ptosis operation
Guyton-Clark fragment forceps
Guyton-Friedenwald suture
Guyton-Lundsgaard
  cataract knife
  keratome
  scalpel
  sclerotome
Guyton-Maumenee speculum
Guyton-Minkowski Potential Acuity Meter
Guyton-Noyes fixation
Guyton-Park speculum
gymnastics
  ocular g.
gyrate atrophy

h

Haab's
  knife needle
  magnet
  reflex
  scleral resection knife
  striae
Haag-Streit slit lamp
habit
  glaucomatous h.
Haenig's irrigating scissors
Haemophilus
  H. aegyptius
  H. influenzae
Hagberg-Santavuori syndrome
Hague's
  cataract lamp
Haidinger's brush
Haik's implant
hair of eyebrow
halation
Halberg's trial clip occluder
Hallauer's
  glasses
  spectacles
Haller's layer
Hallermann-Streiff-Francois syndrome
Hallermann-Streiff syndrome
Hallpike's maneuver
hallucinations
halo
  h. demonstrator
  Fick's h.
  glaucomatous h.
  h. saturninus
  senile h.
  visual h.
halogen ophthalmoscope
halometer
halometry
halos
halothane
Halpin's operation
Halsey's needle holder
Halstead's curved mosquito forceps
hamartoblastoma
hamartoma
  orbit h.
  uveal tract h.
hamartomatosis
hammock pupil
hamulus
  h. lacrimalis
  trochlear h.
Hand-Schüller-Christian disease

handle
    Beaver's h.
hand-held
    h. eye magnet
    h. fundus camera
    h. Hruby's lens
    h. rotary prism
hand-motion visual acuity test
hand-movement visual acuity test
Hansel's stain
Hansen's keratome
Hanson's keratome guard
haplopia
haploscope
    mirror h.
haploscopic
hapten
haptic contact
Harada's
    disease
    syndrome
Harada-Ito procedure
hard
    h. contact lens
    h. exudates
Hardesty's tenotomy hook
Hardy's punch
Hardy-Rand-Littler screening plates
Harmon's forceps
harmonious abnormal retinal correspondence
Harms'
    corneal forceps
    trabeculotome
Harms-Dannheim trabeculotomy operation
Harms-Tubingen tying forceps
Harrington's
    erysiphake
    retractor
    tonometer
Harrison's
    retractor
    scissors
Hartman's
    forceps
    hemostatic forceps
Hartstein's
    irrigator
    refractor
    retractor
Hasner's
    lid forceps
    operation
    valve
Hassall-Henle
    bodies
    warts
HCL — hard contact lens
head-tilt test
Healon
Heath's
    chalazion curet
    curet
    dilator
    expressor
    forceps
heat-ray cataract
heavy ion irradiation
Hebra's
    blade
    curet
    hook
hedger cataract
Heerfordt's disease
hefilcon A
Heidenhaim's syndrome
Heine's
    cyclodialysis
    operation
helcoma
helicoid
heliotrope
helium

helium *(continued)*
- h. ion aiming laser
- h. neon aiming laser

hemangioma
- capillary h.
- cavernous h.
- strawberry h.
- uveal tract h.

hemangiomatosis
hemangiopericytomas
hematic cyst
hematocrit
hematogenous pigmentation
hematoma
hemeralope
hemeralopia
hemiamblyopia
hemianopia
- absolute h.
- altitudinal h.
- bilateral h.
- binasal h.
- binocular h.
- bitemporal fugax h.
- complete h.
- congruous h.
- crossed h.
- equilateral h.
- heteronymous h.
- homonymous h.
- horizontal h.
- incomplete h.
- incongruous h.
- lateral h.
- nasal h.
- quadrant h.
- quadrantic h.
- relative h.
- temporal h.
- true h.
- unilateral h.
- uniocular h.

hemianopia *(continued)*
- upper h.
- vertical h.

hemianopic
hemianopsia
hemianoptic
hemianosmia
hemichromatopsia
hemicrania
hemidecussate
hemifacial
- h. atrophy
- h. microsomia

hemiopalgia
hemiopia
hemiopic
hemiparesis
hemiplegia
- alternating oculomotor h.

hemiscotosis
hemisphere
- h. eye implant
- h. projection perimetry

hemispherical
hemochromatosis
hemoglobin
Hemophilus
- *H. aegyptius*
- *H. influenzae*

hemophthalmia
hemophthalmos
hemophthalmus
hemorrhage
- choroidal h.
- disk drusen h.
- dot and blot h.
- "eight ball" h.
- expulsive h.
- flame h.
- nasal h.
- retinal h.
- retinopathy h.

hemorrhage *(continued)*
- round h.
- splinter h.
- subhyaloid h.
- subretinal h.
- vitreal h.
- vitreous break-through h.
- white centered h.
- yellow ochre h.

hemorrhagic
- h. conjunctivitis
- h. glaucoma
- h. retinopathy

hemostat
Hemovac
Henle's
- fiber layer
- glands
- layer

hepatolenticular degeneration
hepatorenal glycogenesis
HEPES buffer
heptachromic
Herbert's
- operation
- pits

hereditary
- h. benign intraepithelial dyskeratosis syndrome
- h. epithelial corneal dystrophy
- h. macular dystrophy
- h. progressive arthro-ophthalmopathy
- h. spherocytosis
- h. telangiectasia

heredofamilial optic atrophy
heredogenerative neurologic syndrome
Hering's
- after-image mechanism
- law of equal innervation

Hering's *(continued)*
- test
- theory

Hering-Bielschowsky after-image test
hernia of the iris
herpes
- h. corneae
- h. epithelial tropic ulceration
- h. follicular keratoconjunctivitis
- h. iridis
- h. iridocyclitis
- h. keratitis
- neonatal h.
- ocular h.
- h. ophthalmicus
- h. panuveitis
- h. simplex
- h. uveitis
- h. zoster ophthalmicus

herpesvirus
herpetic metakeratitis
herpetoid lesion
Hertel exophthalmometer
Hertwig-Magendie syndrome
Hertzog's
- lens spatula
- pliable probe

Hess'
- diplopia screen
- eyelid operation
- forceps
- operation
- ptosis operation
- screen test
- spoon

Hess-Barraquer forceps
Hess-Horowitz forceps
Hess-Lee screen

Hessberg's
- corneal shield
- intraocular lens glide
- subpalpebral lavage system

Hessberg-Barron vacuum trephine
heterochromia
- h. cataract
- h. cyclitis
- Fuchs' h.
- h. iridis
- h. uveitis

heterograft
heterokeratoplasty
heterometropia
heteronymous diplopia
heterophoralgia
heterophoria
heterophoric
heterophthalmia
heterophthalmos
heteropia
heteropsia
heteroptics
heteroscope
heteroscopy
heterotropia
- comitant h.
- concomitant h.
- paralytic h.

heterotropy
hexachromic
Heyer-Schulte microscope
Heyner's
- cannula
- curet
- dilator
- double cannula
- expressor
- forceps

Hg — mercury
HGH laser
Hiff's ptosis
high
- h. hyperopia
- h. intensity illuminator
- h. myopia
- h. tension suturing technique

Hildreth's cautery
Hill's
- procedure
- retractor

Hillis'
- refractor
- retractor

Hilton's
- self-retaining infusion cannula
- sutureless infusion cannula

Hippel's
- disease
- operation

Hippel-Lindau syndrome
hippus
Hirschberg's
- magnet
- method
- test

Hirschman's
- spatula
- speculum

histiocytosis
histo spots
histoacryl glue patch
histoplasma capsulatum
histoplasmosis syndrome
HM — hand motion
HM — hand movement
Hogan's operation
hole
- retinal h.

Hollenhorst's plaque
hollow sphere implant

hollowing and shadowing
Holmgren's
- color test
- wool skein test

Holofax
Holth's
- forceps
- iridencleisis
- operation
- punch
- scleral punch
- sclerectomy

homatropine dilatation
homeostasis
Homer-Wright rosettes
homocystinuria
homokeratoplasty
homolateral
homologous
homonymous
- h. crescent
- h. diplopia
- h. hemianopia
- h. hemianopsia
- h. quadrantopsia

Honan's
- cuff
- manometer

hook
- Amenabar discission h.
- anchor h.
- Berens' h.
- Birks Mark II h.
- boat h.
- corneal h.
- Culler's muscle h.
- discission h.
- Drews-Sato suture pickup h.
- expressor h.
- Fenzle's manipulating h.
- Fink's muscle h.
- fixation h.

hook *(continued)*
- flat h.
- Gass' retinal detachment h.
- Graefe's strabismus h.
- Green's muscle h.
- Green's strabismus h.
- Hardesty's tenotomy h.
- Hebra's h.
- Hunkeler's ballpoint h.
- iris h.
- Jameson's muscle h.
- Kirby's h.
- Knapp's h.
- Kuglein's h.
- Maumenee iris h.
- McReynolds' lid retracting h.
- muscle h.
- Nugent's h.
- O'Conner's flat h.
- O'Conner's sharp h.
- oblique muscle h.
- Ochsner's h.
- Osher's h.
- Praeger's iris h.
- retinal detachment h.
- scleral h.
- sharp h.
- Shepard's iris h.
- Shepard's reversed iris h.
- Sinskey's lens h.
- Smith's expressor h.
- spatula h.
- squint h.
- St. Martin-Franceshetti cataract h.
- Stevens' tenotomy h.
- strabismus h.
- suture pickup h.
- tenotomy h.
- Tomas' iris h.
- Tomas' suture h.

hook *(continued)*
- twist fixation h.
- Tyrell's iris h.
- von Graefe's h.
- Weiner's h.

Hoopes' corneal marker
Hopkins' Rod Lens Telescope
Horay's operation
hordeola
hordeolum
- external h.
- internal h.

horizontal
- h. band pallor
- h. cells
- h. gaze center
- h. meridian
- h. nystagmus
- h. prism bars
- h. raphe

Horner's
- law
- muscle
- ptosis
- pupil
- syndrome

Horner-Bernard syndrome
Horner-Trantas spots
horopter
- Vieth-Muller h.

horopteric
horror fusionis
horseshoe tear
Horvath's operation
Hosford's
- expressor
- lacrimal dilator
- spud

Hoskins' razor blade fragments
Hoskins-Castroviejo corneal scissors
Hoskins-Westcott tenotomy scissors
host tissue forceps
Hotz's entropion operation
Hotz-Anagnostakis operation
Hough's drape
House's
- knife
- lacrimal dilator
- miniature forceps
- myringotomy knife

House-Bellucci alligator scissors
House-Dieters nipper
House-Urban Pentax camera
Houser's cul-de-sac irrigation T tube
Hovius'
- canal
- circle
- membrane
- plexus

Howard's abrader
Hruby's
- contact lens
- lens

HSV — herpes simplex virus
Hubbard's forceps
Hudson's line
Hudson-Stahli line of corneal pigmentation
hue
Huey's scissors
Hughes'
- implant
- modification of Burch technique
- operation

Hummelsheim's procedure
humor
- aqueous h.
- h. aquosus
- h. cristallinus
- crystalline h.
- ocular h.
- plasmoid h.

humor *(continued)*
vitreous h.
h. vitreus
humoral
Humphrey's
automatic refractor
perimeter
Hunkeler's ball point hook
Hunt's chalazion scissors
Hunter's
disease
syndrome
Hunter-Hurler syndrome
Hurler's
disease
syndrome
Huschke's valve
Hutchinson's
disease
facies
pupil
syndrome
triad
huygenian eyepiece
hyaline
h. artery
h. cast
h. degeneration
h. masses
h. membrane
hyalinization
hyalitis
h. anterior membrane
h. artery
asteroid h.
h. punctata
punctate h.
h. suppurativa
suppurative h.
hyaloid
h. asteroid
h. canal
h. face
hyaloid *(continued)*
h. fossa
h. membrane
h. posterior membrane
h. system
hyaloidal
hyaloideocapsular ligament
hyaloiditis
hyaloidotomy
hyalomucoid
hyalonyxis
hyalosis
hyaluronidase
hydatoid
Hyde's
forceps
irrigator/aspirator unit
hydraulic retinal reattachment
hydroblepharic
hydroblepharon
hydrocephalus
hydrodiascope
Hydron lens
hydrophthalmia
hydrophthalmos
anterior h.
posterior h.
total h.
hydrophthalmus
hydrops of iris
hyfrecator
hyperacuity
hyperbaric oxygen
hyperbolic
hyperemia
hyperemic
hyperesophoria
hyperesthesia
optic h.
hypereuryopia
hyperexophoria
hyperfluorescence
hyperhidrosis

hyperkeratosis
hyperlipidemia
hyperlipoproteinemia
hypermaturation
hypermature cataract
hypermetrope
hypermetropia
hypermetropic astigmatism
hyperope
hyperophthalmophic syndrome
hyperopia
  absolute h.
  axial h.
  curvature h.
  facultative h.
  high h.
  index h.
  latent h.
  manifest h.
  refractive h.
  relative h.
  total h.
hyperopic astigmatism
hyperostosis
hyperparathyroidism
hyperphoria
  circumduction h.
  left h.
  right h.
hyperpresbyopia
hypersecretion
hypertelorism
  ocular h.
  orbital h.
hypertension
  ocular h.
hypertensive
  h. neuroretinopathy
  h. oculopathy
  h. retinitis
  h. retinopathy
hyperthyroidism
hypertonia oculi
hypertonic
hypertropia
  alternating h.
  constant h.
  dissociated h.
hypervitaminosis
  vitamin A h.
  vitamin D h.
hypha
hyphae
hyphal
hyphema
hyphemia
hypnagogic
hypochromic
hypocyclosis
hypoesophoria
hypoexophoria
hypofluorescence
hypometric
hypophoria
hypophysis
hypopituitarism
hypoplasia
hypoplastic disk
hypopyon
hyposcleral
hypotelorism
  ocular h.
  orbital h.
hypothalamus
hypothyroidism
hypotonia oculi
hypotonus
hypotony
hypotropia
  alternating h.
  constant h.
hypovitaminosis
hypsiconchous
hysteria
hysteric
  h. amaurosis

hysteric *(continued)*
  h. amblyopia
  h. field
hysterical
  h. blindness
  h. constricted field

i

Ialo photocoagulator
ianthinopsia
iatrogenic
  i. breaks
  i. retinal break
  i. retinal hole
  i. retinal tear
ICCE — intracapsular cataract extraction
ICD — intercanthal distance
ICE — iridocorneal epithelial syndrome
ice ball
ichthyosis
icteric
icterus
IDI corneoscope
idiopathic arteritis of Takayasu
idioretinal
IK — interstitial keratitis
Ilg
  lens loop
  micro needle holder
  needle
  probe
  push/pull
Iliff's
  exenteration
  lacrimal probe
  lacrimal trephine
  operation
Iliff-House sclerectomy
Iliff-Park speculum
Iliff-Wright fascia needle
illacrimation
illaqueation
Illiterate Eye Chart
illuminance
illuminated suction needle
illuminating
illumination
illumining
illusion
  Kuhnt's i.
  passive i.
image
  accidental i.
  i. degradation
  i. displacement
  false i.
  heteronymous i.
  homonymous i.
  incidental i.
  i. jump
  mirror i.
  negative i.
  ocular i.
  optical i.
  i. point
  Purkinje's i.
  Purkinje-Sanson i.
  real i.
  retinal i.
  Sanson's i.
  spectacular i.
  true i.
  virtual i.
  visual i.
  i. of mires
imbalance
  binocular i.
immature
  i. cataract
  i. neuroglia

immersion method
immunofluorescence
impending macular hole
impinge
impinged
impingement
impinging

IMPLANT MATERIALS

- glass
- gold
- plastic
- polyethylene
- Silastic
- silicone

implant
- 4-loop iris clip i.
- 4-loop iris fixated i.
- 45-degree bent re-form i.
- acorn-shaped i.
- acrylic i.
- Allen's orbital i.
- Allen-Braley i.
- Alpar's i.
- Arruga's i.
- Arruga-Moura-Brazil i.
- Berens' conical i.
- Berens' pyramidal i.
- Berens-Rosa scleral i.
- Binkhorst's i.
- Boberg- Ans i.
- Bonaccolto's orbital i.
- Boyd's orbital i.
- Brawner's i.
- Brown-Dohlman Silastic corneal i.
- build-up i.
- Bunker's i.
- Cardona's focalizing fundus i.

implant *(continued)*
- Cardona's gonio-focalizing i.
- Castroviejo's acrylic i.
- Choyce's i.
- Choyce Mark VIII i.
- Cogan-Boberg-Ans i.
- conical i.
- conventional shell i.
- Copeland's i.
- corneal i.
- cosmetic contact shell i.
- Cryo-Barrages vitreous i.
- Cutler's i.
- Dannheim's i.
- Dermostat i.
- Doherty's i.
- Epstein's collar stud acrylic i.
- Federov's type I i.
- Federov's type II i.
- Ferguson's i.
- Fox's sphere i.
- Frey's i.
- Frey's tunneled i.
- front build-up i.
- full dimpled Lucite i.
- Garcia-Novito i.
- Gelfilm i.
- glass sphere i.
- gold sphere i.
- Goldmann's 3 mirror i.
- Gold-Mules i.
- grooved silicone i.
- Guist's i.
- Haik's i.
- hemisphere i.
- hollow sphere i.
- hook type i.
- Hruby's i.
- Hughes' i.
- Iowa i.
- Ivalon's sponge i.
- Jordan's i.

implant *(continued)*
- King's i.
- Koeppe's gonioscopic i.
- Kryptok's i.
- Landegger's i.
- Lemoine's i.
- Levitt's i.
- Lincoff's scleral sponge i.
- Lovac 6-mirror i.
- Lucite sphere i.
- Lyda-Ivalon-Lucite i.
- magnetic i.
- McGhan's i.
- Melauskas' acrylic i.
- meridional i.
- methyl methacrylate i.
- motility i.
- Mulberger's i.
- Mules' i.
- Müller's i.
- Nocito's i.
- O'Malley's i.
- optic i.
- orbital floor i.
- peanut i.
- plastic sphere i.
- Plexiglass i.
- polyethylene i.
- Radin-Rosenthal i.
- Rayner-Choyce i.
- reverse-shape i.
- Ridley's i.
- Ridley Mark II i.
- Rodin's i.
- Rosa-Berens i.
- Ruedeman's i.
- Ruiz's plano fundus i.
- Schepens' hollow hemisphere i.
- scleral i.
- semishell i.
- Severin's i.
- shelf-type i.
- shell i.

implant *(continued)*
- Sichi's i.
- Silastic i.
- silicone mesh i.
- sleeve i.
- Smith's orbital floor i.
- Snellen's conventional reform i.
- solid silicone with Supramid mesh i.
- sphere i.
- spherical i.
- sponge i.
- Stampelli's i.
- Stone's i.
- subperiosteal i.
- Supramid i.
- Supramid Allen i.
- surface i.
- tantalum mesh i.
- Teflon i.
- Tennant's i.
- Tensilon i.
- tire i.
- Troncosco's gonioscopic i.
- Troutman's i.
- tunneled i.
- Ultex i.
- Uribe's i.
- VA magnetic i.
- Varigray i.
- Varilux i.
- Vitallium i.
- Volk's conoid i.
- Walter Reed i.
- Wheeler's eye sphere i.
- wire mesh i.

implantation

implantoptic

impression tonometer

Imre's
- keratoplasty
- lateral canthoplasty

Imre's *(continued)*
- operation
- sliding flap

in toto
in tumbling fashion
incident
- flux i.
- ray i.

incidental
- i. color
- i. image

incipient cataract
incision
- chord i.
- grooved i.
- relaxing i.
- i. spreader
- i. terminus
- von Noorden's i.

incisura
- i. ethmoidalis ossis frontalis
- i. frontalis
- i. lacrimalis
- i. maxillae
- i. supraorbitalis

incisurae
incisure
- ethmoidal i.
- frontal i.
- lacrimal i.
- supraorbital i.

inclinometer
inclusion bodies
incomitant vertical strabismus
incomplete hemianopia
incongruent
incongruous field defects
incontinentia pigmenti
increment
incrementally
incycloduction
incyclophoria
incyclotropia
incyclovergence
indentation
index
- hyperopia i.
- myopia i.
- i. of refraction
- refractive i.

indirect ophthalmoscope
indirect ophthalmoscopy
induced anisophoria
inelastic
infantile
- i. cataract
- i. esotropia
- i. glaucoma
- i. optic atrophy

infarct
infarction
infectious mononucleosis
inferior
- i. arcade
- i. canaliculus
- i. fasciculus
- i. fornix
- i. longitudinal fasciculus
- i. nasal artery
- i. nasal vein
- i. oblique
- i. ophthalmic vein
- i. orbital fissure
- i. orbital rim
- i. punctum
- i. rectus
- i. tarsus
- i. temporal arcade
- i. temporal artery
- i. temporal vein

inferonasal
inferonasally
inferotemporal
inferotemporally
infiltrates
infoldings
infraciliary

infraduct
infraduction
infraepitrochlear nerve
infranasal
infranasally
infranuclear pathway
infraorbital
    i. artery
    i. canal
    i. foramen
    i. groove
    i. margin
    i. nerve
infrapalpebral sulcus
infrared radiation
infrared slit lamp
infravergence
infraversion
ingrowth
    epithelial i.
inhibition palsy
injection
    circumcorneal i.
    Van Lint's i.
injector
    automatic twin
        syringe i.
inner
    i. canthus
    i. nuclear layer
    i. plexiform layer
    i. retina
    i. segment
innervate
innervation
InnoMed Corporation
INNOVA System 920
INO — internuclear ophthalmoplegia
input nerve
insertion
in situ
instilled
instillation
insufficiency
    i. of the externi
    i. of the eyelids
Insulin pump CPI90-100
intercanthal distance
intercanthic
intercellular space
interciliary fibers
intercilium
interface
interferometer
interlamellar
Intermedics Phaco & I/A Unit
intermittent
    i. esotropia
    i. exotropia
    i. strabismus
    i. tropia
intermuscular membrane
internal
    i. carotid artery
    i. limiting membrane
    i. ophthalmoplegia
    i. strabismus
internuclear ophthalmoplegia
interpalpebral
interpupillary
interstitial
    i. keratitis
    i. neovascularization
interval
    focal i.
    Sturm's i.
intima
intimal
intorsion
intorter
intra-axonal
intracameral
intracanicular
intracapsular
intracavernous
intracellular
intracorneal

intracranial
intracytoplasmic inclusion bodies
intraepithelial
  i. epithelioma
  i. plexus
intralesional
intramarginal sulcus
intranuclear
intraocular
  i. cataract extraction
  i. cysticerci
  i. fistula
  i. foreign bodies
  i. gas bubbles
  i. hemorrhage
  i. lens dialer
  i. lens dislocation
  i. melanoma
  i. muscles
  i. optic neuritis
  i. pressure
  i. silicone oil tamponade
IntraOptics lensometer
intraorbital
intrapapillary drusen
intraretinal
intrascleral nerve loop
intrasheath tenotomy
intrastromal
intrathecal
intravitreal fibrin
intravitreous
intrinsic ocular muscles
introducer
  Carter's sphere i.
  silicone i.
  sphere i.
intumescent cataract
invaginated
invagination
inversion
inverted posture
involution
involutional
  i. senile ectropion
  i. senile entropion
  i. senile ptosis
IO — inferior oblique
IOCARE titanium needle
IOL — intraocular lens
IOLAB I & A photocoagulator
IOLAB Titanium Instruments
IOM — intraocular muscles
ION — ischemic optic neuropathy
ion
  irradiation i.
  laser i.
ionizing radiation
iontophoresis
IOP — intraocular pressure
IOPTEX
ipsilateral antagonist
IR — inferior rectus
iridal
iridalgia
iridauxesis
iridectasis
iridectomesodialysis
iridectome
iridectomize
iridectomy
  basal i.
  complete i.
  optic i.
  patent i.
  peripheral i.
  preliminary i.
  preparatory i.
  preliminary i.
  preparatory i.
  scissors i.
  sector i.
  stenopeic i.
  therapeutic i.
iridectopia
iridectropium

iridemia
iridencleisis
iridentropium
irideremia
irides
iridescent
iridesis
iridiagnosis
iridial
iridian
iridic
iridis rubeosis
iridization
iridoavulsion
iridocapsulitis
iridocapsulotomy
iridocele
iridochoroiditis
iridocoloboma
iridoconstrictor
iridocorneal
 i. angle
 i. epithelial syndrome
iridocorneosclerectomy
iridocyclectomy
iridocyclitis
 Fuchs' heterochromic i.
 herpes simplex i.
 herpes zoster i.
 post-traumatic i.
 varicella i.
iridocyclochoroiditis
iridocycloretraction
iridocystectomy
iridodesis
iridodiagnosis
iridodialysis
iridodiastasis
iridodilator
iridodonesis
iridogoniocyclectomy
iridokeratitis
iridokinesia
iridokinesis
iridokinetic
iridoleptynsis
iridology
iridolysis
iridomalacia
iridomesodialysis
iridomotor
iridoncus
iridoparalysis
iridopathy
iridoperiphakitis
iridoplegia
 i. accommodation
 complete i.
 i. reflex
 sympathetic i.
iridoptosis
iridopupillary
iridorhexis
iridoschisis
iridosclerotomy
iridosteresis
iridotasis
iridotomy scissors
iridovitreosynechiae
iris
 i. bombé
 i. capture
 i. coloboma
 i. crypts
 i. cyst
 detached i.
 i. dilator
 i. epithelial hyperplasia
 Florentine i.
 i. hook cannula
 juvenile i. xanthogranuloma
 i. neurofibroma
 i. nodules
 i. pearls
 i. process
 i. prolapse
 i. repositor

iris *(continued)*
- i. ring
- i. roll
- i. root
- i. scissors
- i. spatula
- i. sphincter
- i. stroma
- i. sweep
- i. synechia
- tremulous i.
- umbrella i.

irisopsia
iritic
iritis
- i. blennorrhagique á rechutes
- i. catamenialis
- diabetic i.
- Doyne's i.
- i. fibrinitis
- follicular i.
- gouty i.
- i. papulosa
- plastic i.
- purulent i.
- i. nodosa
- i. recidivans staphylococcal allergica
- i. roseata
- serous i.
- spongy i.
- sympathetic i.
- syphilitic i.
- tuberculous i.
- uratic i.

iritoectomy
iritomy
IRMA — intraretinal microvascular abnormalities
IRMA shunt
irotomy
irradiance
irradiation
- heavy ion i.

irregular astigmatism
irreversible amblyopia
irrigating
- i. anterior chamber vectis
- i. cannula
- cul-de-sac i. vectis
- i. cystotome
- i. vectis

IRRIGATING/ASPIRATING UNITS

- Alcon
- Bishop-Harmon
- Bracken
- Cavitron
- Cavitron-Kelman
- Charles
- Cooper
- CooperVision
- DeVilbiss
- Dougherty
- Drews
- Drews-Rosenbaum
- Fink
- Fox
- Gass
- Gibson
- Hartstein
- Hyde
- IOLAB
- Irvine
- Kelman
- Kelman-Cavitron
- McIntyre
- Phaco Cavitron
- Rollet
- SITE TXR System
- Surg-E-Trol System
- Sylva
- Visitec 1624

Irvine's
irrigating/aspirating unit
probe pointed scissors
scissors
Irvine-Gass syndrome
ischemia
carotid i.
retinal i.
ischemic
i. atherosclerosis
i. choroidal atrophy
i. ocular syndrome
i. optic neuropathy
i. papillitis
i. papillopathy
i. retinae
i. retinopathy
iseiconic
iseikonia
Ishihara
Color Test
Pseudoisochromatic Plates
isocoria
isoiconia
isoiconic
isolated islands
isometropia
isophoria
isopia
isopter
isoscope
isotonic
I-Temp cautery
Ivalon sponge implant
IV slit lamp
Iwanoff's
cysts
retinal edema

j

J-shaped irrigating/aspirating cannula
jack-in-the-box phenomenon
Jacob's
membrane
ulcer
Jacob-Swann gonioscope
Jacobson's retinitis
Jaeger's
hook
keratome
lid plate
retractor
Visual Test
Jaesche-Arlt operation
Jaffee's
intraocular spatula
Jaffee-Bechert nucleus rotator
Jaffee-Givner lid retractor
Jaime's lacrimal operation
Jameson's
caliper
forceps
hook
muscle hook
operation
Jansky-Bielschowsky syndrome
jaundice
jaundiced
Javal's ophthalmometer
jaw claudication
jaw-winking syndrome
Jedmed A-scan
Jellinek's sign
Jenning's test
Jensen's
capsular scratcher
choroiditis juxtapapillaris
disease
intraocular lens forceps

Jensen's *(continued)*
jerk nystagmus
operation
procedure
retinitis
transposition procedure
jerk nystagmus
jeweler's tweezer
John Green caliper
Johnson's
double cannula
evisceration knife
operation
syndrome
Johnson-Bell erysiphake
Johnson-Tooke corneal knife
Jones'
dilator
keratome
operation
Pyrex tube
tear duct tube
test
Jordon's implant
Joseph's elevator
joule — J
joules — J
Judd's forceps
Judson-Smith manipulator
junction
corneoscleral j.
mucocutaneous j.
sclerocorneal j.
scotoma j.
junctional scotoma of Traquair
juvenile
j. arcus
j. cataract
j. corneal epithelial dystrophy
j. developmental cataract
j. GM_1 gangliosidosis
j. GM_2 gangliosidosis
j. glaucoma

juvenile *(continued)*
j. nevoxanthoendothelioma
j. optic atrophy
j. pilocytic astrocytoma
j. reflex
j. retinoschisis
j. rheumatoid arthritis
j. xanthogranuloma
juxtafoveal
juxtapapillaris
juxtapapillary nerve fiber layer
juxtaposition
JXG — juvenile xanthogranuloma

K

K readings
Kalt's
corneal needle
forceps
needle holder
spoon
Kamerling Capsular 90
kappa angle
Kara's
cataract needle
erysiphake
Karakashian-Barraquer scissors
Karickhoff's
double cannula
laser lens
Karl Ilg Instruments
Katena Products
katophoria
katotropia
Katzin's scissors
Katzin-Barraquer forceps
Kaufman's
media

Kaufman's *(continued)*
vitrector
Kayser-Fleischer ring
KCS — keratoconjunctivitis sicca
Kearney's side-notch IOL
Kearns-Sayre syndrome
Keeler's
Catford needle holder with micro jaws
cryophake
cryosurgical unit
extended round tip
Fison tissue retractor
intravitreal scissors
lancet tip
loupe
micro round tip
micro spear tip
micro tip
panoramic loupe
prism
Pulsair tonometer
puncture tip
razor tip
retractable blade
ruby knife
Specular Microscope
triple facet tip
ultrasonic cataract removal lancet
Keeler-Amoils
curved cataract probe
freeze
glaucoma probe
long shank retinal probe
Machemer retinal probe
micro curved cataract probe
Ophthalmic Cryosystem
retinal probe
straight cataract probe
vitreous probe
Keeler-Keislar lacrimal cannula
Keeler-Meyer diamond knife
Keeler-Pierse eye speculum
Keeler-Rodger iris retractor
Keith-Wagener
changes
retinopathy
Keith-Wagener-Barker classification
Keizer-Lancaster
eye speculum
lid retractor
Kelly's Descemet's membrane punch
Kelman's
cannula
cryoextractor
cyclodialysis cannula
cystotome
forceps
iris retractor
irrigating/aspirating unit
irrigating handpiece
knife
lens
operation
phacoemulsification unit
Kelman-Cavitron irrigating/aspirating unit
keloid
Kennedy's syndrome
KeraCorneoScope
Kerascan
keratalgia
keratectasia
keratectomy scissors
keratic
keratination
keratinous
keratitic precipitates
keratitis
acne rosacea k.
actinic k.
k. actinomyces
aerosol k.

keratitis *(continued)*
- alphabet k.
- annular k.
- arborescens k.
- artificial silk k.
- aspergillus k.
- bacterial k.
- band k.
- k. bandelette
- band-shaped k.
- bank k.
- k. bullosa
- catarrhal ulcerative k.
- deep k.
- deep punctate k.
- deep pustular k.
- dendriform k.
- dendritic k.
- desiccation k.
- Dimmer's nummular k.
- disciform k.
- k. disciformis
- epithelial diffuse k.
- epithelial punctate k.
- exfoliative k.
- exposure k.
- farinaceous k.
- farinaceous epithelial k.
- fascicular k.
- filamentary k.
- k. filamentosa
- Fuchs' k.
- fungal k.
- furrow k.
- herpes simplex k.
- herpes zoster k.
- herpetic k.
- hypopyon k.
- interstitial k.
- lagophthalmic k.
- lattice k.
- k. lesion
- Lyme disease k.

keratitis *(continued)*
- lymphogranuloma venereum k.
- marginal k.
- metaherpetic k.
- k. molluscum contagiosum
- mumps k.
- mycotic k.
- neuroparalytic k.
- neurotrophic k.
- k. nummularis
- oyster shuckers' k.
- padi k.
- parenchymatous k.
- k. petrificans
- phlyctenular k.
- k. post vaccinulosa
- k. precipitates
- k. profunda
- k. punctata leprosa
- k. punctata profunda
- k. punctata subepithelialis
- punctate k.
- purulent k.
- k. pustuliformis profunda
- pyknotic k.
- k. ramificata superficialis
- reaper's k.
- reticular k.
- ribbon-like k.
- rosacea k.
- Schmidt's k.
- sclerosing k.
- scrofulus k.
- secondary k.
- serpiginous k.
- k. sicca
- striate k.
- superficial k.
- superficial punctate k.
- suppurative k.

keratitis *(continued)*
- syphilitic k.
- Thygeson's k.
- trachomatous k.
- trophic k.
- tuberculous k.
- k. vaccinia
- varicella k.
- vascular k.
- vesicular k.
- xerotic k.
- zonular k.

keratoacanthoma
keratocele
keratocentesis
keratoconjunctivitis
- adenoviral k.
- atopic eczema k.
- epidemic k.
- epizootic k.
- flash k.
- herpes simplex k.
- herpes zoster k.
- phlyctenular k.
- shipyard k.
- k. sicca
- superior limbic k.
- viral k.
- welder's k.

keratoconus
keratocyte
keratoderma
keratodermatocele
keratoectasia
keratoglobus
keratohelcosis
keratohemia
keratoid
keratoiridocyclitis
keratoiridoscope
keratoiritis hypopyon
Kerato-Kontours Instruments
keratokyphosis
keratoleptynsis
keratoleukoma
Keratolux fixation device
keratolysis
keratoma
keratomalacia
keratomas
keratomata
keratome
- Agnew's k.
- Bard-Parker k.
- Beaver's k.
- Berens' partial k.
- Castroviejo's k.
- Czermak's k.
- Fuchs' lancet type k.
- Grieshaber's k.
- Guyton-Lundsgaard k.
- Hansen's k.
- Jaeger's k.
- Jones' k.
- Kirby's k.
- Lancaster's k.
- Martinez's k.
- McReynolds' k.
- Rowland's k.
- Storz's k.

keratometer mires
keratometric
keratometry
keratomileusis
keratomycosis
keratonosus
keratonyxis
keratopathy
- band k.
- bullous k.
- chloroquine k.
- climatic k.
- crystalline k.
- exposure k.
- filamentary k.
- idiopathic lipid k.

keratopathy *(continued)*
  indomethacin toxicity k.
  Labrador k.
  lipid k.
  phenothiazine k.
  striate k.
  vesicular k.
keratophakia
keratoplasty
  autogenous k.
  lamellar k.
  optic k.
  partial k.
  penetrating k.
  refractive k.
  k. scissors
  Sourdille's k.
  tectonic k.
  total k.
keratoprosthesis
keratorefractive
keratorhexis
keratoscleritis
keratoscope
keratoscopy
keratosis
  k. follicularis
  k. palmoplantaris
keratome
keratotomy
  delimiting k.
  radial k.
keratotorus
keratouveitis
kerectasis
kerectomy
keroid
Kerrison's
  forceps
  rongeur
Kestenbaum's
  capillary count
  procedure
  rule
Key's operation
keyhole
  k. pupil
  k. vision
Keystone test
Khodadoust line
kibisitome
Kiloh-Nevin syndrome
Kimmelstiel-Wilson syndrome
Kimura's platinum spatula
Kimwipes
Kindergarten Eye Chart
kinescope
kinetic
  k. perimeter
  k. perimetry
  k. strabismus
King's
  corneal trephine
  operation
  orbital implant
King-Prince knife
Kirby's
  angulated iris spatula
  cataract knife
  dislocator
  forceps
  hook
  intracapsular lens spoon
  intraocular lens scoop
  iris forceps
  iris spatula
  keratome
  knife
  lens dislocator
  lens loop
  operation
  refractor
  retractor
  scissors
  spoon
Kirby-Bauer disk sensitivity test
kissing choroidals
Kjer's dominant optic atrophy

Klebsiella pneumoniae
Klein's
- curved cannula
- keratoscope

Klieg eye
Klippel-Feil syndrome
Kloti's vitreous cutter
Knapp's
- cataract knife
- eye speculum
- forceps
- iris hook
- iris probe
- iris repositor
- iris scissors
- iris spatula
- knife
- knife needle
- lacrimal sac retractor
- law
- lens spoon
- operation
- procedure
- refractor
- retractor
- rule
- scissors
- spatula
- spoon
- streaks

Knapp-Imre operation
Knapp-Wheeler-Reese operation
Knie's sign
knife
- Agnew's canaliculus k.
- Alcon's surgical k.
- Bard-Parker k.
- Barkan's goniotomy k.
- Barraquer's k.
- Beaver's k.
- Beer's cataract k.
- Berens' cataract k.
- Berens' glaucoma k.
- Berens' keratoplasty k.

knife *(continued)*
- Berens' ptosis k.
- bladebreaker k.
- cannula k.
- Castroviejo's k.
- Castroviejo's twin k.
- corneal k.
- Cusick's goniotomy k.
- Desmarres' k.
- Deutschman's cataract k.
- diamond dusted k.
- discission k.
- dissector k.
- Duredge's k.
- Elschnig's k.
- Gill's k.
- Gill-Fine corneal k.
- Gill-Hess k.
- Gill-Welch k.
- Goldmann's serrated k.
- goniopuncture k.
- goniotomy k.
- Graefe's cataract k.
- Green's k.
- Grieshaber's ruby k.
- Guyton-Lundsgaard k.
- Haab's scleral resection k.
- House's myringotomy k.
- I-Knife microsurgical k.
- Johnson's evisceration k.
- Johnson-Tooke corneal k.
- Keeler's ruby k.
- Keeler-Meyer diamond k.
- Kelman's k.
- King-Prince k.
- Kirby's cataract k.
- Knapp's cataract k.
- KOI k.
- Lancaster's k.
- Lowell's glaucoma k.
- Lundsgaard's k.
- Martinez's k.

knife *(continued)*
McPherson-Wheeler k.
McPherson-Ziegler k.
McReynolds' pterygium k.
Meyer's Swiss Diamond lancet k.
Meyer's Swiss Diamond mini angled k.
Meyer's Swiss Diamond wedge k.
Microknife k.
Myocure k.
Parker's k.
Paton's corneal k.
Paufique's k.
ptosis k.
razor blade k.
Reese's ptosis k.
Rizzuti-Spizziri cannula k.
ruby k.
ruby diamond k.
Sato's corneal k.
Scheie's goniopuncture k.
scleral resection k.
Sharpoint k.
Sichel's k.
Smith's k.
Smith-Green cataract k.
Spizziri's cannula k.
Step-Knife diamond blade k.
stiletto k.
stitch removing k.
Storz's cataract k.
Storz Duredge steel cataract k.
Swan's discission k.
Tooke's k.
V-lancet k.
von Graefe's k.

knife *(continued)*
wave edge k.
Weber's k.
Wheeler's k.
Ziegler's k.
Knolle's capsule polisher
knuckle
k. of choroid
k. of loose vitreous
Koby's cataract
Koch-Weeks
bacillus
conjunctivitis
Kocher's sign
Koeppe's
disease
goniolens
lens
nodule
Koerber-Salus-Elschnig syndrome
Kofler's operation
KOI diamond knife
Kollmorgen's elements
Kollner's law
kopiopia
koroscope
koroscopy
KP — keratitic precipitates
KOWA
camera
Fluorescein System
fundus
Optimed slit lamp
Koyter's muscle
Krabbe's disease
Kraff's
capsule polisher curet
cortex cannula
polisher
Kraff-Utrata capsulorrhexis forceps
Krasnov's lens

- kratometer
- Kratz's
  - diamond dusted needle
  - lens needle
  - polisher
  - scratcher
- Kratz-Johnson lens
- Kraupa's operation
- Krause's
  - gland
  - syndrome
- Kreiger-Spitznas vibrating scissors
- Kreiker's
  - blepharochalasis
  - operation
- Kriebig's operation
- Krill's disease
- Krimsky's method
- Krimsky's test
- Krimsky-Prince Accommodation Rule
- Kronfeld's
  - electrode
  - forceps
  - refractor
  - retractor
- Kronlein's operation
- Kronlein-Berke operation
- Krukenberg's
  - corneal spindle
  - pigment spindle
  - sponge
- Krupin's valve
- Krwawicz's cataract extractor
- Kryospray II
- Kryptok lens
- krypton
  - k. laser
  - k. red/yellow
- Kufs's disease
- Kuglein's
  - hook
- Kuglein's *(continued)*
  - iris hook
  - irrigating lens manipulator
  - lens manipulator
  - push/pull
  - refractor
- Kuhnt's
  - dacryostomy
  - eyelid operation
  - forceps
  - illusion
  - operation
  - postcentral vein
  - tarsectomy
- Kuhnt-Helmbold operation
- Kuhnt-Junius
  - disease
  - maculopathy
  - repair
- Kuhnt-Szymanowski operation
- Kuhnt-Thorpe operation
- Kulvin-Kalt forceps
- Kurz's syndrome
- KW changes
- Kwitko's
  - conjunctival spreader
  - operation

L

- labyrinthine nystagmus
- Lacarrere's operation
- lacerate foramen
- laceration
  - corneoscleral l.
- lacertus musculi recti lateralis bulbi
- lacquer cracks
- lacrima

lacrimae
lacrimal
l. abscess
l. angleduct anomaly
l. apparatus
l. artery
l. awl
l. bay
l. bone
l. canal
l. canaliculi
l. cannula
l. caruncula
l. crest
l. duct
l. duct T-tube
l. fistula
l. fossa
l. gland acini
l. groove
l. intubation probe
l. irrigation test
l. lake
l. nerve
l. notch
l. papilla
l. point
l. probe
l. process
l. puncta
l. punctal stenosis
l. reflex
l. sac
l. sac chisel
l. sac gouge
l. sac retractor
l. sac rongeur
l. scintillography
l. sulcus of lacrimal bone
l. sulcus of maxilla
l. syringe
l. system
l. trephine

lacrimal *(continued)*
l. tubercle
l. vein
lacrimal gland
acinar l.g.
l.g. gallium uptake
Krause's l.g.
Wolfring's l.g.
lacrimalin
lacrimase
lacrimation
lacrimator
lacrimatory
lacrimoconchal suture
lacrimomaxillary suture
lacrimonasal duct
lacrimotome
lacrimotomy
lacrimoturbinal suture
lacteal cataract
Lactoplate
lacuna
Blessig's l.
lacunae
lacus lacrimalis
LaForce spud
lag dilation
Lagleyze's
needle
operation
Lagleyze-Trantas operation
lagophthalmic keratitis
lagophthalmos
lagophthalmus
Lagrange's
operation
scissors
Laird's spatula
laissez-faire lid operation
lake
lacrimal l.
Lambert's forceps
lamella of Fuchs'
lamellae

lamellar
- l. calcification
- l. cataract
- l. corneal graft
- l. developmental cataract
- l. graft
- l. groove
- l. keratoplasty
- l. separation of lens

lamellation

lamina
- anterior limiting l.
- basal l. of choroid
- basal l. of ciliary body
- basalis choroideae
- basalis corporis ciliaris
- Bowman's l.
- l. choriocapillaris
- l. choroidocapillaris
- l. cribrosa sclerae
- l. dots
- l. elastica anterior
- l. elastica posterior
- episcleral l.
- l. episcleralis
- l. fusca sclerae
- l. limitans anterior corneae
- l. limitans posterior corneae
- limiting l. anterior
- limiting l. posterior
- orbital l.
- l. orbitalis ossis ethmoidalis
- l. papyracea
- posterior limiting l.
- l. superficialis musculi
- suprachoroid l.
- l. suprachoroidea
- vascular l. of choroid
- l. vasculosa choroideae
- l. vitrea
- vitreal l.

lamina *(continued)*
- vitreous l.

laminar flow

laminated acellular mass

lamp
- Birch-Hirschfeld l.
- Duke-Elder l.
- Eldridge-Green l.
- Gullstrand slit l.
- Haag-Streit slit l.
- Hague cataract l.
- Rodenstock l.
- slit l.
- Zeiss l.

Lancaster's
- eye magnet
- eye speculum
- keratome
- knife
- lid speculum
- magnet
- operation
- Red-Green Test
- speculum

Lancaster-O'Connor speculum

Lancaster-Regan test

lance
- Rolfe's l.

lancet
- suture l.
- Swan's l.

Lanchner's operation

Landegger's orbital implant

Landers' vitrectomy ring

Landolt's
- bodies
- broken ring
- chart
- operation

Landström's muscle

Lane's needle

Lang's speculum

Langenbeck's operation

lantern test

Larcher's sign
large
  l. kappa angle
  l. physiologic cup
LASAG Microruptor
larva
  l. migrans
  ocular l.
larval conjunctivitis
laser
  Allergan Humphrey l.
  AMO YAG 100 l.
  argon blue l.
  argon green l.
  Biophysic Medical l.
  Britt BL-12 l.
  Britt argon l.
  Britt krypton l.
  Britt pulsed argon l.
  candela l.
  Carl Zeiss l.
  CILCO/Lasertek argon l.
  CILCO/Lasertek krypton l.
  CO_2 l.
  CO_2 Sharplan l.
  Coherent 7910 l.
  Coherent 920 argon l.
  Coherent dye l.
  Coherent krypton l.
  Cooper 2000 l.
  Cooper 2500 l.
  Cooper Laser Sonics l.
  CooperVision l.
  erbium l.
  Evergreen Lasertek l.
  Excimer l.
  Gish Micro YAG l.
  helium aiming ion l.
  helium neon aiming l.
  HGM l.
  ion l.
  l. iridotomy
  krypton l.
laser *(continued)*
  Lasertek l.
  liquid organic dye l.
  LPK-80 II argon l.
  Meditech l.
  Merrimac l.
  Microruptor II l.
  mode locked Nd:YAG l.
  molectron l.
  Nanolas Nd:YAG l.
  Nd:YAG l.
  NdiYAG l.
  neodymium YAG l.
  Nidek Laser System l.
  oculocutaneous l.
  Ophthalas argon l.
  Ophthalas krypton l.
  l. photocoagulation
  photodisrupting l.
  photovaporizing l.
  Q-switched neodymium YAG l.
  Q-switched ruby l.
  ruby l.
  Sharplan argon l.
  SITE l.
  Takata l.
  TE MOO mode beam l.
  l. trabeculoplasty
  tunable dye l.
  Visulas argon l.
  Visulas argon/YAG l.
  Visulas YAG C l.
  Visulas YAG E l.
  Visulas YAG S l.
lasered
Laserflex
  coagulator
  lens
Lasertek laser
lash margins
lastosis. *See elastosis*
latent
  l. congenital

latent *(continued)*
- l. hyperopia
- l. nystagmus
- l. squint
- l. strabismus

lateral
- l. angle
- l. canthus
- l. commissure of eyelid
- l. geniculate body
- l. geniculate nucleus
- l. hemianopia
- l. horn
- l. medullary syndrome
- l. orbital decompression
- l. orbital tubercle
- l. palpebral ligament
- l. palpebral tubercle
- l. phoria
- l. rectus muscle
- l. rectus palsy

lateroduction

laterotorsion

lattice
- l. corneal dystrophy
- l. degeneration
- l. dystrophy
- l. keratitis
- l. retinal degeneration

Lauber's disease

Laurence-Moon-Biedl syndrome

lavage

law
- Descartes' l.
- Desmarres' l.
- Donder's l.
- Ewald's l.
- Ferry-Porter l.
- Flouren's l.
- Giraud-Teulon l.
- Gullstrand's l.
- Hering's l.
- Horner's l.
- Knapp's l.

law *(continued)*
- Listing's l.
- Sherrington's l.
- Snell's l.
- Talbot's l.
- Wundt-Lamansky l.

Lawford's syndrome

Lawton's corneal scissors

layer
- bacillary l.
- basal l.
- Bowman's l.
- Bruch's l.
- cerebral l. of retina
- Chievitz's l.
- choriocapillary l.
- columnar l.
- ganglion cell l.
- ganglionic l. of optic nerve
- ganglionic l. of retina
- Haller's l.
- Henle's fiber l.
- limiting l.
- molecular external l.
- molecular inner l.
- molecular internal l.
- molecular outer l.
- nerve fiber l.
- nerve l. of retina
- neuroepithelial l. of retina
- nuclear external l.
- nuclear inner l.
- nuclear internal l.
- nuclear outer l.
- pigmented l. of ciliary body
- pigmented l. of eyeball
- pigmented l. of iris
- pigmented l. of retina
- plexiform external l.
- plexiform inner l.
- plexiform internal l.

layer *(continued)*
plexiform outer l.
l. of rods and cones
Sattler's l.
suprachoroid l.
lazy eye
LE — left eye
lead-filled mallet
lead incrustation of cornea
Leahey's operation
leak
glue patch l.
leaking
l. bleb
l. filtering bleb
leash
leaves of capsule
Lebensohn's Visual Acuity Chart
Leber's
amaurosis
congenital amaurosis
disease
miliary aneurysm
optic atrophy
Lederal Laboratories
left
l. deorsumvergence
l. gaze
l. hypertrophic
l. hypertropia
l. inferior oblique recession
l. inferior rectus muscle
l. sursumvergence
l. superior oblique tuck
l. superior rectus muscle
left-beating nystagmus
legal blindness
Leigh's encephalopathy
leiomyoma
l. of iris
l. of uveal tract
leiomyosarcoma
Leitz's microscope
Leland's refractor
lema
lemnici
lemnicus
Lemoine's
orbital implant
serrefine
Lemoine-Searcy fixation anchor loop
Lempert-Storz loupe
lens
3-mirror contact l.
3-mirror l.
4-mirror goniolens
Abraham peripheral button iridotomy l.
Accugel l.
achromatic l.
acrylic l.
adherent l.
Amenabar l.
American Medical Optics Baron l.
amnifocal l.
Amsoft l.
anastigmatic l.
Anis staple l.
aniseikonic l.
aplanatic l.
apochromatic l.
Appolionio l.
Aquaflex l.
Aquasight l.
Arlt l.
Arruga l.
aspheric cataract l.
astigmatic l.
auxilliary l.
Azar l.
Bagolini l.
bandage l.
Barkan gonioscopic l.
Baron l.
Barraquer l.

lens *(continued)*
- Bausch & Lomb Optima l.
- Bechert 7-mm l.
- Beebe l.
- biconcave l.
- biconvex l.
- bicylindrical l.
- Bietti l.
- bifocal l.
- Binkhorst l.
- Binkhorst-Fyodorov l.
- Bi-Soft l.
- bispherical l.
- Boys-Smith laser l.
- Brücke l.
- Carl Zeiss l.
- l. capsule
- cataract l.
- Centra-Flex l.
- Charles contact l.
- Choyce Mark VIII l.
- Cibasoft l.
- Cibathin l.
- CILCO-Simcoe II l.
- CILCO-Sonometrics l.
- Clayman l.
- clip l.
- Coburn l.
- concave l.
- concavoconcave l.
- concavoconvex l.
- condensing l.
- contact low-vacuum l.
- converging l.
- converging meniscus l.
- convex l.
- convexoconcave l.
- CooperVision PMMA-ACL Flex l.
- Copeland Radial panchamber UV l.
- Coquille plano l.
- corneal l.

lens *(continued)*
- corneal contact l.
- cortex l.
- Crookes l.
- crossed l.
- l. crystallina
- crystalline l.
- cylindrical l.
- decentered l.
- diagnostic fiberoptic l.
- direct gonioscopic l.
- dislocation l.
- dispersing l.
- diverging l.
- diverging meniscus l.
- Doubra l.
- Dura-T l.
- Emery l.
- ERG-Jet disposable contact l.
- Eschenback Optik l.
- Feister Dualens l.
- fiberoptic diagnostic l.
- flat l.
- Flexlens l.
- FormFlex l.
- Frelex l.
- Frenzel l.
- Friedman hand-held Hruby l.
- fundus contact l.
- fundus focalizing l.
- fused bifocal l.
- Galin l.
- gas permeable contact l.
- Genesis l.
- Gilmore l.
- glide l.
- Goldmann 3 mirror l.
- Goldmann macular contact l.
- goniofocalizing l.
- goniolens l.
- gonioscopic l.

lens *(continued)*
Gullstrand l.
hand-held Hruby l.
hard contact l.
Hessburg l.
Hoffer-Laseridge intraocular l.
honey bee l.
Hruby l.
Hunkeler l.
Hydracon l.
Hydrocurve l.
Hydron l.
Hydrosight l.
immersion l.
implant l.
infant 3-mirror laser l.
infant Karickhoff laser l.
Intermedics l.
Interspace YAG laser l.
intraocular l.
IOLAB 108 B l.
IOPTEX TabOptic l.
iridocapsular l.
iseikonic l.
iso-iconic l.
J-loop PC l.
Jaffee CILCO l.
Kamerling Capsular 90 l.
Karickhoff laser l.
Kearney side-notch l.
Kelman flexible tripod l.
Kelman Multiflex II l.
Kelman Omnifit l.
Kelman PC 27LB CapSul l.
Kirby l.
Koeppe l.
Krasnov l.
Kratz elliptical style l.
Kratz-Johnson l.
Krieger fundus l.
Kuler panoramic l.
Landers biconcave l.

lens *(continued)*
Landers contact l.
Landers-Foulks temporary keratoprosthesis l.
laser l.
Laseridge Optics l.
Layden infant l.
Leiske l.
l. loupe
l. meter
Lempert-Storz l.
lenticular l.
Lewis l.
Lieb-Guerry l.
Lindstrom Centrex l.
Liteflex l.
l. localizer
Lovac gonioscopic l.
Machemer flat l.
Machemer infusion contact l.
Machemer magnifying l.
macular contact l.
magnifying l.
Mainster retinal laser l.
March laser l.
Mark II magni-focuser l.
Mark IX l.
McGhan l.
McLean l.
Medallion l.
Meditec bandage contact l.
meniscus concave l.
meter l.
minus l.
Multi-Optics l.
negative meniscus l.
Neolens l.
New Orleans l.
Nova Aid l.
NOVACurve l.
Nova Soft II l.
nucleus l.

lens *(continued)*
Oculaid l.
Ocular Gamboscope l.
O'Malley-Pearce-Luma l.
omnifocal l.
Ophtec Co. l.
Optical Radiation l.
Optiflex l.
Opti-Vu l.
Opt-Visor l.
orthoscopic l.
O'Shea l.
Osher l.
panchamber UV l.
Pannu type II l.
PanoView Optics l.
PBII blue loop l.
pediatric Karickhoff laser l.
pediatric 3-mirror laser l.
periscopic l.
perioscopic concave l.
perioscopic convex l.
Permalens l.
Perspex CQ-Shearing-Simcoe-Sinskey l.
Petrus single-mirror laser l.
Peyman l.
Peyman-Tennant-Green l.
Peyman wide field l.
P.F. Lee pediatric goniolens l.
Pharmacia Visco J loop l.
photochromic l.
photosensitive l.
l. pits
l. plane
plano l.
planoconcave l.
planoconvex l.
Platina clip l.
plus l.

lens *(continued)*
positive meniscus l.
Posner diagnostic l.
Precision Cosmet l.
prismatic contact l.
prismatic gonioscopic l.
prismatic goniotomy l.
prosthetic l.
punctal l.
Rayner l.
Red Reflex Lens Systems l.
retroscopic l.
Ridley l.
Ritch trabeculoplasty laser l.
Rodenstock panfundus l.
rudiment l.
Ruiz fundus l.
safety l.
Sauflon PW l.
Schachar l.
Scharf l.
scleral contact l.
Severin l.
Shearing l.
Sheets l.
short C loop l.
Signet Optical l.
Silicone Elastomer l.
Silsoft contact l.
Simcoe II PC l.
Sinskey l.
l. size
Soflens l.
soft contact l.
spherical l.
spherocylindrical l.
star l.
stigmatic l.
Stokes l.
Strampelli l.
Style S2 clear loop l.
Surefit AC 85J l.

lens *(continued)*
- Surgidev l.
- Sutherland l.
- T l.
- Tennant Anchorflex AC l.
- Tolentino prism l.
- Topcon l.
- Toric-Optima series l.
- trial l.
- trifocal l.
- Trokel l.
- Trokel-Peyman laser l.
- Uniplanar style PC II l.
- Urrets-Zavalia retinal surgical l.
- UVEX l.
- Varilux l.
- l. vesicle
- Viscolens l.
- Vision Tech l.
- whorl l.
- Wild l.
- Wise iridotomy laser l.
- Wise iridotomy-sphincterotomy laser l.
- Woods Concept l.
- Yannuzzi fundus laser l.
- Yannuzzi l.
- Youens l.
- l. zonule

lensectomy
Lens-Eze inserter
lens-induced
- l. glaucoma
- l. uveitis

lensometer
- Allergen Humphrey l.
- A-O l.
- Carl Zeiss l.
- Coburn l.
- Marco l.
- Reichert l.
- Topcon l.

lentectomize
lentectomy
lenticonus
lenticula
lenticular
- l. astigmatism
- l. body
- l. cataract
- l. degeneration
- l. fossa
- l. ganglion
- l. glaucoma
- l. lens
- l. nucleus

lenticule
lenticulocapsular
lenticulo-optic
lenticulostriate
lenticulothalamic
lentiform
lentigines
lentiglobus
lentis articularis
Lenz's syndrome
leprosy
leptotrichosis conjunctiva
L'Esperance's erysiphake
lesser ring of iris
Lester lens manipulator
Lester-Burch speculum
Lester-Jones operation
letter blindness
letterbox technique
leucitis
leukemic
- l. cells
- l. infiltration
- l. retinitis
- l. retinopathy

leukocoria
leukocytic
leukodystrophy
leukokoria
leukoma

leukoma *(continued)*
l. adhaerens
adherent l.
leukomas
leukomata
leukomatous
leukoplakia
leukopsin
leukoscope
leukotomy
transorbital l.
levator
l. aponeurosis disinsertion
l. muscle
l. palpebrae superioris
l. resection
l. trochlear muscle
Levine's spud
Levitt's implant
levoclination
levocycloduction
levocycloversion
levoduction
levotorsion
levoversion
Lewicky's
formed cystotome
self-retaining chamber maintainer
Lewis'
lens loupe
scoop
Lewy's body
Lexer's operation
LGB — lateral geniculate body
LGN — lateral geniculate nucleus
LHT — left hypertropia
lichenified lids
Lichtenberg's corneal trephine
lid
l. agglutination

lid *(continued)*
l. crusting
l. eversion
l. everter
l. fissures
granular l.
l. lag
l. margin
l. notching
l. retraction
l. speculum
l. thrush
l. trephine
tucked l. of Collier
lid block
O'Brien l.b.
retrobulbar l.b.
Smith modification of Van Lint l.b.
lid everter
Berens' l.e.
Roveda's l.e.
Schachne-Desmarres l.e.
Struble's l.e.
Walker's l.e.
Lieberman's
fragmentor
phaco crusher
Liebreich's symptom
Life-Tech, Inc.
ligament
canthal l.
check l.
ciliary l.
cribriform l.
Hueck's l.
hyaloideocapsular l.
Lockwood's l.
medial palpebral l.
palpebral l.
pectinal l.
pectinate l.
suspensory l.
Zinn's l.

ligamenta
- l. anguli iridocornealis
- l. pectinatum anguli iridocornealis
- l. pectinatum iridis

light
- l. adaptation
- axial l.
- central l.
- l. coagulation
- l. difference
- l. discrimination
- idioretinal l.
- intrinsic l.
- minimum l.
- l. perception
- pipe l.
- l. projection test
- l. reflex
- l. response of pupil
- l. scatter

light-adapted eye
light-near dissociation
lightning cataract
Lignac-Fanconi syndrome
limbal
- l. approach
- l. girdle
- l. groove
- l. guttering
- l. incision
- l. neurofibroma
- l. parallel orientation
- l. palpebrales anteriores
- l. palpebrales posteriores
- l. luteus retinae

limbal-based flap
limbi
limbic
limbus
- conjunctival l.
- l. of cornea
- corneal l.

limbus *(continued)*
- l. guttering
- l. parallel orientation straddling tattoo mark
- l. of perception
- l. of sclera

limitation
- eccentric l.

limiting
- l. lamina
- l. membrane

limulus lysate test
Lincoff's
- balloon catheter
- implant
- operation
- sponge

Lindau-von Hippel disease
Linde's cryogenic probe
Lindner's
- operation
- sclerotomy
- spatula

line
- angular l.
- atropic l.
- blue l.
- l. of direction
- l. of fixation
- gray l.
- Helmholtz's l.
- Hudson's l.
- Hudson-Stähli l.
- Morgan's l.
- pigmented l. of the cornea
- primary l. of sight
- principal l. of direction
- pupillary l.
- Schwalbe's l.
- l. of sight
- Stähli's l.
- Stähli's pigment l.

line *(continued)*
- Stocker's l.
- superficial l. of the cornea
- triradiate l.
- visual l.
- Zöllner's l.

linea
- l. corneae senilis
- l. visus

linear
- l. echoes
- l. perspective
- l. visual acuity test

lipemia retinalis
lipemic retina
lipid degeneration
lipid-like inclusions
lipidoses
lipocytic lesion
lipodermoid
lipofuscinosis
lipogranuloma
lipoma
liposarcoma
lippa
lippitude
liquefaction
liquid
- l. organic dye laser
- l. vitreous aspirating cannula

liquefied vitreous
liquor
- l. corneae
- Morgagni's l.

Lister's
- forceps
- scissors

Lister-Burch speculum
Listing's
- law
- plane

lithiasis
- conjunctival l.

Littauer's cilia forceps
Littler's dissecting scissors
LKP — lamellar keratoplasty
lobe
- parietal l.
- temporal l.
- temporoparietal l.

lobulated
localization
- spatial l.

local tic
locator
- Berman's l.
- foreign body l.
- Roper-Hall l.
- Wildgren-Reck l.

loci
Lockwood's
- ligament
- light reflex
- tendon

locus
log
- l. rank
- l. units

logadectomy
Löhlein's operation
loiasis
Lombert's
- radiuscope
- tonometer

Londermann's
- corneal trephine
- operation

long
- l. ciliary nerve
- l. posterior ciliary arteries
- l. sight

longitudinal axis of Fick

long-scale contrast
longsightedness
Look
- I&A coaxial cannula
- capsule polisher
- cortex extractor
- cystotome
- irrigating lens loop
- irrigating vectis
- retrobulbar needle
- suture

loop
- angled nucleus removal l.
- intrascleral nerve l.
- Kirby's l.
- Lemoine-Searcy fixation anchor l.
- Meyer's l.
- nucleus delivery l.
- nucleus removal l.
- Pierse-Knoll irrigating lens l.
- Simcoe nucleus delivery l.
- two-angled polypropylene l.

loops of Axenfeld
Lopez-Enriquez
- operation
- scleral trephine

Lordan's chalazion forceps
Loring's ophthalmoscope
loss of vitreous
Lotman Visometer
Lo-Trau side-cutting needle
louchettes
Louis-Bar syndrome
loupe; see lens
Lovac's
- 6 mirror gonioscopic lens implant

Lovac's *(continued)*
- fundus contact lens implant
- gonioscopic lens

low
- l. contrast

low tension glaucoma
Lowe's
- ring
- syndrome

Lowe-Terrey-MacLachlan syndrome
Lowell's glaucoma knife
Löwenstein's operation
lower
- l. hemianopia
- l. punctum
- l. retina

Lowry's assay
LP — light perception
LPK-80 II argon laser
LR — lateral rectus
L.T. Jones tear duct tube
lucencies
lucency
Lucite implant
Luedde's
- exophthalmometer
- transparent rule

Luer's
- cannula lock
- connections
- tube

luetic
- l. chorioretinitis
- l. interstitial keratitis
- l. neuropathy

lumbar puncture
lumen
luminance
luminosity
Lumiwand light
Lundsgaard's

Lundsgaard's *(continued)*
knife
rasp
sclerotome
Lundsgaard-Burch
corneal rasp
sclerotome
lupus
l. erythematosus
l. oculopathy
lusterless
lustrous central yellow point
lux
luxated
luxation
l. of eyeball
l. of globe
l. of lens
Luxo Surgical Illuminator
Lyle's syndrome
Lyme disease
lymphangiectasis
lymphangioma
lymphedema
lymphocyte
lymphogranuloma
lymphoid tumor
lymphoma
anterior chamber l.
orbital l.
lymphomatosis
ocular l.
lymphoproliferative tumor
lymphosarcoma
Lyon hypothesis
lyophilized
lysed
lysis
lysozyme
lytic lesions

m

Machek's ptosis operation
Machek-Blaskovics operation
Machek-Gifford operation
Machemer's
caliper
cutter
vitreous cutter
Mack-Brunswick operation
MacKay-Marg tonometer
MacKool's capsule retractor
macroaneurysm
macroblepharia
macrocornea
macrophthalmia
macrophthalmic
macrophthalmos
macropia
macropic
macropsia
macula
cherry red m.
m. corneae
false m.
m. flava retinae
m. lutea retinae
m. retinae
maculae
macular
m. arteriole
m. corneal dystrophy
m. degeneration
m. displacement
m. heredodegeneration
m. hole
m. hypoplasia
m. leak
m. pucker
m. sparing
m. splitting

macular *(continued)*
m. star
m. stereopsis
m. surface wrinkling
m. suppression
m. venule
maculate
macule
maculocerebral
maculopapillary bundle
maculopapular
maculopathy
atrophic degenerative m.
bull's eye m.
cellophane m.
dry senile degenerative m.
Groenouw's type II m.
heredity m.
histoplasmosis m.
Kuhnt-Junius m.
pigment epithelial detachment m.
serous detachment m.
Sorsby's m.
Stargardt's m.
toxic m.
vitelliform m.
maculovesicular
MacVicar double-end strabismus retractor
Maddox
prism
rod test
wing test
Maeder-Danis dystrophy
mafilcon A
Magitot's keratoplasty operation
magnet
Bronson-Magnion m.
Gruning's m.
Haab's m.
hand-held m.

magnet *(continued)*
Hirschberg's m.
implant m.
Lancaster m.
original Sweet m.
rare earth m.
Schumann giant type m.
Storz-Atlas m.
magnetic
m. extraction
m. implant
m. operation
magnification
magnifying loupe
Magnus' operation
Maguire-Harvey vitreous cutter
Maier's sinus
main fibers
Mainster's retinal laser lens
Majewsky's operation
major
m. arcade
m. arterial circle of the iris
m. meridians
Maladie de Greffe's operation
malar eminence
Malbec's operation
Malbran's operation
malformation
Chiari's m.
malignant
m. exophthalmos
m. glaucoma
m. melanoma
m. myopia
m. pituitary lesion
malingerer
Malis Bipolar Coagulating/Cutting System
malleable
malprojection
mandible

mandibular
mandibulofacial
  m. dysostosis
  m. dystosis
  m. dystrophy
maneuver
  doll's eye m.
  Nylan-Baraney m.
Manhattan forceps
manifest
  m. deviation
  m. hyperopia
  m. refraction
  m. strabismus
manipulator
  Judson-Smith m.
Mann's sign
manner
  McLean's m.
manometer
  Honan's m.
  Tycos' m.
manoptoscope
Manz's gland
map dot corneal dystrophy
map dot fingerprint corneal epithelial dystrophy
marbelization
March's laser sclerostomy needle
Marchesani's syndrome
Marco's
  chart projector
  lensometer
  perimeter
  radiusgauge
  refractor
  slit lamp
  SurgiScope
Marcus Gunn
  afferent defect
  jaw-winking syndrome
  phenomenon
  pupil
  pupillary sign
  relative afferent defect
  sign
  syndrome
mare's hair lines
Marfan's syndrome
margin
  ciliary m. of iris
  free m. of eyelid
  infraorbital m. of maxilla
  intraorbital m. of orbit
  lateral m. of orbit
  orbital m.
  pupillary m. of iris
  supraorbital m. of frontal bone
  supraorbital m. of orbit
marginal
  m. blepharitis
  m. catarrhal ulcer
  m. keratitis
  m. melts
  m. myotomy
  m. tear strips
marginoplasty
margo
  m. ciliaris iridis
  m. infraorbitalis orbitae
  m. lacrimalis maxillae
  m. lateralis orbitae
  m. medialis orbitae
  m. orbitalis
  m. palpebrae
  m. pupillaris iridis
  m. supraorbitalis orbitae
  m. supraorbitalis ossis frontalis
Marinesco-Sjögren syndrome
Mariotte blind spot
marker
  Amsler's m.

marker *(continued)*
- bi-prong muscle m.
- Castroviejo's corneal transplant m.
- corneal transplant m.
- Desmarres' m.
- Feldman's RK optical center m.
- Fink's bi-prong m.
- Fink's muscle m.
- Gass' scleral m.
- Gonnin-Amsler m.
- O'Brien's m.
- radial keratotomy m.

Marlex mesh
Marlow's test
Maroteaux-Lamy syndrome
Marquez-Gomez conjunctival graft
Martin Surefit lens pusher
Martinez's
- corneal transplant centering ring
- corneal trephine blade
- disposable corneal trephine
- dissector
- keratome
- knife

mascara particle inclusions
maser
Massachusetts Vision Kit
Masselon's
- glasses
- spectacles

Master's two-step test
Masuda-Kitahara disease
matrix
Mattis' scissors
maturation
mature cataract
Mauksch's operation
Maumenee's
- erysiphake
- iris hook
- knife goniotomy cannula
- vitreous aspirating needle
- vitreous sweep spatula

Maumenee-Goldberg operation
Maumenee-Park speculum
Maunoir's iris scissors
Mauthner's test
Max Fine scissors
maxilla
maxillary
- m. bone
- m. nerve

Maxwell's
- ring
- spot

May's sign
Mayo's scissors
McCannell's ocular pressure reducer
McCarey-Kaufman transport medium
McCarthy's reflex
McClure's iris scissors
McCullough's forceps
McDonald's expressor
McGannon's
- refractor
- retractor

McGavic's operation
McGhan's
- 3M intraocular lens implant

McGuire's
- conformer
- corneal scissors
- forceps
- operation
- scissors

McIntyre's I/A System
McKinney's fixation ring
McLaughlin's operation
McLean's
- fashion
- forceps
- manner
- operation
- scissors
- suture
- tonometer

McNeill-Goldmann blepharostat
McPherson's
- forceps
- needle holder
- scissors
- spatula
- speculum

McPherson-Castroviejo scissors
McPherson-Vannas scissors
McPherson-Wheeler
- blade
- knife

McPherson-Ziegler knife
McReynolds'
- hook
- keratome
- knife
- operation
- pterygium transplant
- scissors
- technique

measles
meatus
- nasi inferior m.

mechanical
- m. ectropion
- m. ptosis
- m. strabismus

mechanism
- oculogyric m.
- pursuit m.

mechanized scissors
medallion lens
media
- chondroitin sulfate m.
- contrast m.
- dioptric m.
- K-Sol m.
- McCarey-Kaufman m.
- refracting m.

medial
- m. angle of eye
- m. arteriole of retina
- m. canthus
- m. commissure of eyelids
- m. horn
- m. longitudinal fasciculus
- m. palpebral ligament
- m. rectus
- m. venule of retina

mediaometer
median
medicamentosa conjunctivitis
Meditech laser
medium. See media
medullary
- m. cystic disease
- m. rays

medullated nerve fibers
medulloepithelioma
Meek's operation
Meesman's epithelial corneal dystrophy
megalocornea
megalopapilla
megalophthalmos
megalophthalmus
megalopia
megalopsia
megophthalmos
meibomian
- m. cyst
- m. gland

meibomian
m. sty
meibomianitis
meibomitis
melanin
melanocytes
melanocytic nevus
melanocytoma
melanokeratosis
melanoma
Cloudman mouse m.
ocular m.
melanomata
melanosis
m. bulbi
m. iridis
m. oculi
m. sclerae
melanotic
m. sarcoma
m. sarcomata
Melauskas' orbital implant
Melkersson's syndrome
Melkersson-Rosenthal syndrome
Meller's
operation
refractor
retractor
Mellinger's speculum
melting stromal
membrana
m. capsularis lentis posterior
m. choriocapillaris
m. epipapillaris
m. fusca
m. granulosa externa
m. granulosa interna
m. hyaloidea
m. limitans externa
m. limitans interna
m. nictitans
membrana *(continued)*
m. ruyschiana
m. vitrea
membrane
Bowman's m.
Bruch's m.
connective tissue m.
cyclitic m.
Demours' m.
Descemet's m.
Duddell's m.
epipapillary m.
external limiting m.
glassy m.
Haller's m.
Henle's m.
Hovius' m.
hyaloid m.
inner limiting m.
intermuscular m.
internal limiting m.
Jacob's m.
limiting m.
nictitating m.
outer limiting m.
periorbital m.
pupillary m.
purpurogenous m.
Reichert's m.
Ruysch's m.
ruyschian m.
stripping m.
tarsal m.
Tenon's m.
vitreous m.
Wackendorf's m.
wrinkling m.
Zinn's m.
membranectomy
membranous
m. cataract
m. conjunctivitis

mendelian
Mendez cystotome
meningioma
meningocele
meningococcus conjunctivitis
meniscus
  converging m.
  diverging m.
  Kuhnt's m.
  lens m.
  negative m.
  positive m.
Menkes' syndrome
Mentor's
  B-VAT II Video Acuity
  Exeter ophthalmoscope
  pre-cut drain
  wet field cautery
  wet field eraser
Mentor-Maumenee Suregrip forceps
mercury — Hg
mercury pressure — mmHg
meridian
  m. of cornea
  equatorial m.
  m. of eyeball
  horizontal m.
  vertical m.
meridiani bulbi oculi
meridianus
meridional
  m. amblyopia
  m. fibers of ciliary muscle
  m. implant
Merkel's cell neoplasm
Merocel Surgical Spears
meropia
Mersilene suture
Mesco
mesenchymal

mesenchymal *(continued)*
  m. cells
  m. ridge
mesh
  Marlex m.
  tantalum m.
meshwork
  trabecular m.
mesiris
mesochoroidea
mesocornea
mesodermal dysgenesis
mesophryon
mesopia
mesopic
mesoretina
mesoropter
metabolic-toxic
metachromic leukodystrophy
metaherpetic ulcer
metameric color
metamorphopsia varians
metaplastic epithelial cells
metarhodopsin
metastasis
metastatic
  m. choroiditis
  m. endophthalmitis
  m. retinitis
Metcher's speculum
method
  Barraquer's m.
  Credé's m.
  Cuignet's m.
  direct m.
  Hirschberg's m.
  modified band lid m.
  optical density m.
  Pfeiffer-Komberg m.
methulose
methylcellulose
methyl methacrylate

metric ophthalmoscopy
metronoscope
Meyer's
 Swiss diamond knife lancet
 Swiss diamond mini-angled knife
 Swiss diamond wedge knife
 temporal loupe
Meyer-Schwickerath light coagulation
Meyhoeffer's
 chalazion
 curet
Meynert's commissure
Meynerti
 superior commissura of M.
mica spectacles
micelles in vitreous
Michaelson's counter pressure
Michel's pick
microaneurysm
microaneurysmal leakage
microangiography
microblepharia
microblepharism
microblepharon
microblephary
microcoria
microcornea
microcytic
microgonioscope
microinfarction
Micro-Lite
micromegalopsia
micrometer
micronystagmus
micropannus
microphakia
microphotography
microphthalmia
microphthalmos
microphthalmoscope
microphthalmus
Micropigmentation System
micro-point
 m. needle
 m. suture
microproliferation
micropsia
microptic
micro-round tip needle
Microruptor II laser
microsaccades
microscope
 corneal m.
 slit lamp m.
 Wild M690 m.
 Zeiss m.
microscopy
 fundus m.
microspectroscope
microspherophakia
Microsponge
microstrabismus
microtremor
microtropia
microtropic syndrome
microvilli
microvillous
Microvit
 Probe System
 Vitrector
microwave radiation injury
midline position of gaze
midperiphery
migraine
 ophthalmic m.
 m. ophthalmoplegia
 ophthalmoplegic m.
Mikulicz's
 disease
 syndrome
milia

miliary aneurysm
milky cataract
Millard-Gubler syndrome
Miller's syndrome
Miller-Nadler glare tester
Millex filter
millijoules — mJ
millimicron
Millipore filter
mind blindness
miner's
  m. blindness
  m. nystagmus
mini ophthalmic drape
minimum
  m. cognoscibile
  m. deviation
  m. legibile
  m. light
  m. perceptible acuity
  m. separabile
  m. separable acuity
  m. visibile
  m. visual angle
Minsky's
  circles
  intramarginal splitting operation
minus
  m. cyclophoria
  m. cyclotropia
  m. lens
miosis
  irritative m.
  paralytic m.
  senile m.
  spastic m.
  spinal m.
  traumatic pupillary m.
  pupil m.
Mira
  AGL-400
  diathermy unit
Mira *(continued)*
  endovitreal cryopencil
  photocoagulator
mire
mires
mirror
  m. haploscope
  m. image
misdirected lashes
mitochondria
mitotic
Mittendorf's dot
mixed
  m. astigmatism
  m. cataract
MK IV ophthalmoscope
MLF — medial longitudinal fasciculus
mmHg — millimeters of mercury
Mobius'
  disease
  sign
  syndrome
modalities
mode-locked Nd:YAG laser
modified
  m. band lid method
  m. C-loop intraocular lens
  m. J-loop intraocular lens
Moehle's
  cannula
  forceps
Mohs' microsurgical resection
Moire's fringes
molecular layer
Moll's gland
Moller's microscope
molluscum conjunctivitis
Monakow's syndrome

Moncrieff's
- cannula
- discission
- operation

mongolism
mongoloid slant
monoblepsia
monochromasy
monochromat
monochromatic
- m. eye
- m. green

monochromatism
- cone m.
- rod m.

monocular
- m. confrontation visual field test
- m. depth perception
- m. diplopia
- m. dressing
- m. glaucoma
- m. oscillopsia
- m. patch
- m. strabismus
- m. temporal crescent
- m. vision

monoculus
monodiplopia
monofilament nylon suture
monofixation syndrome
monofixational
monolateral strabismus
mononuclear
mononucleosis
monopia
moon
- m. blindness
- m. circulated

Moore-Troutman corneal scissors
Mooren's ulcer
Moran's proptosis
Morax's
- keratoplasty
- operation

Morax-Axenfeld conjunctivitis
Moraxella lacunata
Morel-Fatio-Lalardie operation
Morgagni's liquor
morgagnian cataract
Morgan's line
Moria's
- obturator
- one-piece speculum
- trephine

Moria-France dacryocystorhinostomy clamp
morning glory
- m.g. anomaly
- m.g. optic atrophy
- m.g. retinal detachment

morning ptosis
Morquio's syndrome
Morquio-Brailsford syndrome
mosaic pattern
mosaicism
Mosher's operation
Mosher-Toti operation
Moss' traction
Motais' operation
motility
- m. implant
- ocular m. test

motion parallax
motor tic
Mot-R-Pak vitrectomy system
motor
- m. oculi
- m. fusion
- m. nerve
- m. root of ciliary ganglion
- m. tic

mottled
Moulton's lacrimal duct tube
movement
conjugate m.
conjunctive m.
gaze m.
saccadic m.
scissors m.
MP Video endoscopic lens attachment
MPC
automated intravitreal scissors
MR — medial rectus
MRI scan — magnetic resonance imaging scan
MTL trial frame
mucin
m. of tears
m. strands
mucinous
mucocele
mucocutaneous
mucoepidermoid
mucolipidoses
mucomycosis
mucopolysaccharide
mucopolysaccharidoses
mucopurulent
mucopyocele
mucotome
mucous
m. assay
m. membrane
m. threads
mucous-like strands
mucus
Mueller's
cautery
cell
electric corneal trephine
lacrimal sac retractor

Mueller's *(continued)*
muscle
refractor
retractor
shield
speculum
trephine
Mulberger's orbital implant
mulberry shaped mass
mulberry type papilloma
Muldoon lacrimal dilator
Mules'
implant
operation
scoop
sphere
vitreous sphere
Müller's
cells
fibers
glands
muscle
operation
shield
trigone
multicellular
multicentric
multifocal
m. lens
multilaminar
multilobar
Multilux
multimode
multiple
m. myeloma
m. sclerosis
m. vision
Munson's sign
mural cells
Murdock's speculum
Murdock-Wiener speculum
musca
muscae volitantes

muscegenetic
muscle
  m. belly
  Bowman's m.
  Brucke's m.
  ciliaris m.
  ciliary m.
  m. cone
  m. depressor
  dilator m. of pupil
  extraocular m's
  extrinsic m's
  m. of eye
  m. force
  Horner's m.
  inferior oblique m.
  inferior rectus m.
  inferior tarsal m.
  intraocular m's
  intrinsic m's
  iridic m.
  Koyter's m.
  Landström's m.
  lateral rectus m.
  levator m. of upper eyelid
  levator palpebrae superioris m.
  medial rectus m.
  Müller's m.
  ocular m.
  oculorotatory m.
  orbicular m. of eye
  orbicularis oculi m.
  orbicularis oris m.
  orbital m.
  palpebrae superioris m.
  pupillary sphincter m.
  rectus lateralis m.
  rectus medialis m.
  Riolan's m.
  Rouget's m.

muscle *(continued)*
  m. sheath
  sphincter m. of pupil
  superciliary m.
  superior oblique m.
  superior rectus m.
  superior tarsal m.
  yoked m.
muscle-paretic nystagmus
muscular
  m. asthenopia
  m. balance
  m. dystrophy
  m. fascia
  m. funnel
  m. strabismus
musculi
  m. bulbi
  m. ciliaris
  m. corrugator supercilii
  m. depressor supercilii
  m. dilator pupillae
  m. levator palpebrae superioris
  m. obliquus inferior bulbi
  m. obliquus inferior oculi
  m. obliquus superior bulbi
  m. obliquus superior oculi
  m. oculi
  m. orbicularis
  m. orbicularis oculi
  m. orbitalis
  m. procerus
  m. rectus inferior bulbi
  m. rectus inferior oculi
  m. rectus lateralis bulbi
  m. rectus lateralis oculi
  m. rectus medialis bulbi
  m. rectus medialis oculi

musculi *(continued)*
m. sphincter pupillae
m. tarsalis inferior
m. tarsalis superior
mushroom corneal graft
Mustarde's
awl
graft
mutton fat keratic precipitates
MVK — Massachusetts Vision Kit
MVR blade
MVS — Massachusetts XII Vitrectomy System
myasthenia gravis
mycelia
mycelial mass
Mycobacterium
mycotic
m. keratitis
m. snowball opacities
mydriasis
accidental m.
alternating m.
bounding m.
factitious m.
fixed m.
paralytic m.
spasmodic m.
spastic m.
spinal m.
springing m.
traumatic m.
mydriatic provocative test
myectomy
myelin
myelinated nerve fibers
myelinating
myelination
myelitis
myeloidin
myiocephalon
myiocephalum
myiodesopsia
myoclonal
myoclonus
myoculator
Myocure
blade
phaco blade
scalpel
myodesopsia
myodiopter
myofibromatosis
myogenic ptosis
myoid visual cell
myokymia
myoneural
myopathy
myope
myopia
axial m.
chromic m.
curvature m.
degenerative m.
high m.
m. index
malignant m.
pernicious m.
primary m.
prodromal m.
progressive m.
refractive m.
simple m.
myopic
m. astigmatism
m. choroidal atrophy
m. conus
m. crescent
m. degeneration
m. keratomileusis
m. reflex
myoscope
myosis

myositis
  orbital m.
myotomy
myotonic dystrophy
myringotomy blade
myxoid
myxoma

n

N. — cranial nerve
N — nasal
Nadbath's
  akinesia
  facial block
Naffziger's operation
Nagel's
  anomaloscope
  test
Nairobi eye
naked vision — Nv
Nanolas'
  Nd:YAG laser
  neodymium YAG laser
nanometer — nm
nanophthalmia
nanophthalmos
nanosecond — nsec
naphthalinic cataract
narrow
  n. slit illumination
  n.-angle glaucoma
nasal
  n. arteriole of retina
  n. border of optic disk
  n. canal
  n. duct
  n. hemianopia
  n. isopters
  n. periphery

nasal *(continued)*
  n. retina
  n. step
  n. venule of retina
nasalization
nasion
nasoantritis
nasociliary
  n. nerve
  n. neuralgia
nasojugal
nasolabial fold
nasolacrimal
  n. canal
  n. duct
  n. gland
  n. sac
nasoseptitis
nasosinusitis
Nd:YAG laser
Nd — neodymium
near
  n. fixation position of gaze
  n. point of accommodation
  n. point of convergence
  n. point of conversion
  n. reaction to light
  n. reflex spasm
  n. response
  n. sight
  n. vision
  n. visual acuity
nearsighted
nearsightedness
nebula
nebulae
necrosis
necrotizing scleritis
needle
  ACS n.
  Agnew's tattooing n.

needle *(continued)*
- Alcon's Surgical irrigating n.
- Alcon's Surgical reverse cutting n.
- Alcon's Surgical spatula n.
- Alcon's Surgical taper cut n.
- Alcon's Surgical taper point n.
- Amsler's aqueous transplant n.
- aqueous transplant n.
- Atkinson's retrobulbar n.
- Barraquer's n.
- Barraquer-Vogt n.
- bent blunt n.
- blunt n.
- Bowman's cataract n.
- Bowman's stop n.
- Burr's butterfly n.
- butterfly n.
- Calhoun's n.
- Calhoun-Hagler n.
- Calhoun-Merz n.
- cataract aspirating n.
- CD-5 n.
- Charles' n.
- Cibis' ski n.
- Cleasby's spatulated n.
- CooperVision irrigating n.
- CooperVision spatula n.
- corneal n.
- CUA n.
- Curran's knife n.
- Dailey's cataract n.
- Davis' knife n.
- Dean's knife n.
- discission n.
- Drews' cataract n.
- DS-9 n.

needle *(continued)*
- Ellis' foreign body n.
- Elschnig's extrusion n.
- extended round n.
- Fisher's n.
- flute n.
- Fritz's vitreous transplant n.
- Girard's cataract aspirating n.
- Girard's phacofragmatome n.
- Graefe's n.
- Grieshaber's n.
- Gueder's keratoplasty n.
- Haab's n.
- Heyner's n.
- Ilg's n.
- Iliff-Wright n.
- illuminated suction n.
- IOLAB n.
- Kalt's n.
- Kara's n.
- Knapp's n.
- knife n.
- Lagleyze's n.
- Lane's n.
- Lo-Trau n.
- March's n.
- Maumenee's n.
- micro-point n.
- micro-round tip n.
- Oaks' n.
- peribulbar n.
- probe n.
- puncture n.
- razor n.
- retrobulbar n.
- Reverdin's n.
- Riedel's n.
- Sabreloc n.
- Sato's n.
- Scheie's n.

needle *(continued)*
- sclerostomy n.
- side-cutting spatulated n.
- Simcoe's n.
- SITE n.
- spatulated n.
- spoon n.
- Stocker's n.
- Subco n.
- subconjunctival n.
- Swan's n.
- taper-cut n.
- titanium n.
- Ultrasonic lancet n.
- Viers' n.
- Vogt-Barraquer n.
- Weeks' n.
- Wergeland's n.
- Worst's n.
- Wright's n.
- Yale Luer-Lok n.
- Ziegler's n.

needle holder
- Alabama-Green n.h.
- Arruga's n.h.
- Barraquer's n.h.
- Birks' Mark II n.h.
- Boyce's n.h.
- Boynton's n.h.
- Castroviejo's n.h.
- Castroviejo-Kalt n.h.
- Clerf's n.h.
- Cohan's n.h.
- Crile's n.h.
- Derf's n.h.
- Gifford's n.h.
- Green's n.h.
- Grieshaber's n.h.
- Halsey's n.h.
- Ilg's n.h.
- Kalt's n.h.
- Keeler's Catford micro jaws n.h.

needle holder *(continued)*
- McPherson's n.h.
- Paton's n.h.
- Stephenson's n.h.
- Stevens' n.h.
- Tilderquist's n.h.
- Vicker's n.h.

negative
- n. scotoma
- n. vertical divergence
- n. vertical vergence

Neisseria
- *N. catarrhalis*
- *N. gonorrhoeae*
- *N. meningitidis*

neisserial conjunctivitis

neodymium — Nd

Neolens

neonatal
- n. adrenoleukodystrophy
- n. hypoglycemia
- n. inclusion blennorrhea

neovascular
- n. angle-closure glaucoma
- n. glaucoma
- n. net
- n. tufts

neovascularization

nephroblastoma

nephropathic
- n. cystine storage disease
- n. cystinosis

nephrotic syndrome

nerve
- abducens n.
- abducent n.
- afferent n.
- block n.
- ciliary n.
- n. core
- n. cross section
- n. fiber axons

nerve *(continued)*
  n. fiber bundle defect
  n. fiber bundle layer
  frontal n.
  n. head angioma
  n. head drusen
  infraorbital n.
  n. input
  intermedius n.
  intrascleral n. loops
  intratrochlear n.
  lacrimal n.
  motor n.
  nasociliary n.
  oculomotor n.
  ophthalmic n.
  optic n.
  n. palsy
  petrosal n.
  sensory n.
  n. sheath
  supraorbital n.
  supratrochlear n.
  tentorial n.
  trigeminal n.
  trochlear n.
  vidian n.
nervi
  n. ciliares breves
  n. ciliares longi
  n. infraorbitalis
  n. lacrimalis
  n. maxillaris
  n. nasociliaris
  n. oculomotorius
  n. ophthalmicus
  n. opticus
  n. supraorbitalis
  n. trigeminus
  n. trochlearis
  n. zygomaticus
nests and strands of cells
Nettleship iris repositor
Nettleship-Wilder dilator
network
  peritarsal n.
  vascular n.
Neubauer's forceps
neura
neural rim
neuralgia
  nasociliary n.
  supraorbital n.
neurectomy
  opticociliary n.
neurilemma
neurilemmitis
neurilemmoma
  ameloblastic n.
  malignant n.
neurilemmosarcoma
neurinoma
neurinomatosis
neurite
neuritic atrophy
neuritis
  atherosclerotic ischemic n.
  intraocular n.
  n. nodosa
  optic n.
  orbital n.
  postocular n.
  retrobulbar n.
neuroblast
neuroblastic
neuroblastoma
neurochorioretinitis
neurochoroiditis
neurodealgia
neurodeatrophia
neuroectoderm
neuroepithelial
neuroepithelioma
neurofibroma
neurofibromatosis

neurogenic
n. iris atrophy
n. ptosis
neurohumoral
neuromyelitis optica
neuromyotonia
neuron
Golgi I n.
Golgi II n.
neuronal
neuro-ophthalmology
neuroparalytic keratitis
neuroparalytic keratopathy
neuropathy
dysthyroid optic n.
neurophthalmology
neuroradiologic
neuroretinal rim
neuroretinitis
neuroretinopathy
neurospongium
neurosurgical
neurosyphilis
neurosyphilitic
neurotomy
opticociliary n.
neurotrophic keratitis
neurotropic
neutral density filter test
neutrality
neutralize
neutralizing
neutrophils
nevi
nevoid
nevoxanthoendothelioma
nevus
blue n.
compound n.
epithelial n.
junctional n.
n. of Ota
subepithelial n.
Nevyas' double sharp cystotome
Newcastle disease
New Orleans lens loupe
nicking
Nida's n. operation
n. of retinal vein
nictation
nictitating membrane
nictitation
Nida's nicking operation
Nidek laser
Niemann-Pick disease
night
n. blindness
n. sight
n. vision
nigroid body
Nikolsky's sign
niphablepsia
niphotyphlosis
nipper
Nizetic's operation
NLP — no light perception
no faci
no light perception
Noble's forceps
Nocardia
N. asteroides
N. brasiliensis
N. caviae
N. madurae
nocardiosis
Nocito's eye implant
nocturnal amblyopia
nodal point
node
Rosenmüller's n.
nodular
n. scleritis
n. episcleritis
nodule
Busacca's n.

nodule *(continued)*
  Dalen-Fuchs n.
  Koeppe's n.
  lentiform n.
nodules
  n. in actinomycosis
  n. in dirofilariasis
  n. in schistosomiasis
  n. in sparganosis
nodulus
  n. conjunctivales
  n. lymphatici
Nokrome bifocal lens
nonabsorbable suture
nonaccommodation
nonaccommodative
  n. esodeviations
  n. esotropia
nonarteritic
noncomitant
  n. heterotropia
  n. strabismus
nonconcomitant
noncongestive glaucoma
noncontact tonometer
  Reichert's n.t.
nondescript
nondisjunction
nonepithelial tumor
nonexudative
nongranulomatous
  n. choroiditis
  n. uveitis
noninfiltrative
noninvasive corneal redox fluorometry
nonleaking bleb
nonoptic reflex eye movements
nonorganic visual loss
nonparalytic strabismus
nonproliferative retinopathy
nonrhegmatogenous retinal detachment
nonsteroidal anti-inflammatory drugs
nonulcerative interstitial keratitis
normal retinal correspondence
Norman-Wood syndrome
normocytic hypochromic anemia
Norrie's disease
notch
  lacrimal n.
  n. of iris
notching
Noyes'
  forceps
  iridectomy scissors
  iris scissors
NPA — near point of accommodation
NPC — near point of convergence
NRC — normal retinal correspondence
NSAID — nonsteroidal anti-inflammatory drug
nubbin
nubecula
nuclear
  n. arc
  n. bronzing
  n. cataract
  n. changes
  n. cytoplasmic ratio
  n. developmental cataract
  n. inner layer
  n. ophthalmoplegia
  n. outer layer
  n. sclerosis of lens
nuclei
nucleocapsids
nucleolar
nucleoli
nucleoplasm

nucleus
accessory n.
n. delivery loop
Edinger-Westphal n.
n. of lens
lenticular n.
n. lentiform
n. lentis
Perlia's n.
pretectal n.
n. removal loop
Nugent's
forceps
hook
soft cataract aspirator
Nugent-Gradle scissors
Nugent-Green-Dimitry erysiphake
null point
nummular keratitis
Nurolon suture
nutritional amblyopia
Nv — naked vision
NVA — near visual acuity
nyctalope
nyctalopia
Nylan-Barany maneuver
nylon suture
nystagmic
nystagmiform
nystagmograph
nystagmoid-like oscillations
nystagmoid movements
nystagmus
acquired jerk n.
acquired pendular n.
ageotrophic n.
aural n.
Baer's n.
Bekhterev's n.
blockage n.
caloric n.
Cheyne's n.

nystagmus *(continued)*
congenital n.
convergence retraction n.
disjunctive n.
dissociated n.
downbeat n.
end-gaze n.
end-point n.
end-position n.
gaze-paretic n.
horizontal n.
jerk n.
labyrinthine n.
latent n.
left-beating n.
miner's n.
myoclonus n.
optokinetic n.
oscillating n.
periodic alternating n.
paretic n.
pendular n.
periodic alternating n.
rotary n.
rotational n.
torsional n.
undulatory n.
vestibular n.
vibratory n.

O

Oaks'
double needle
straight cannula
Oasis feather micro scalpel
obcecation
object
o. blindness
o. of regard

objective test
obligatory suppression
oblique
- o. astigmatism
- o. muscle hook
- o. palsy
- o. prism device

obliterated
O'Brien's
- akinesia
- block
- cataract
- forceps
- marker
- spud

obscuration
obscure
obstructive glaucoma
obturator
occipital cortex
occipitothalamic
occluder
occlusion
ochre
- o. hemorrhage
- o. mass
- ochre-colored whorls

ochronosis
- ocular o.

Ochsner's forceps
O'Conner's
- depressor
- flat hook
- forceps
- marker
- operation
- sharp hook

O'Conner-Peter operation
Octopus
- 500 EZ
- 201 perimeter
- test

ocufilcon
Oculab Tono-Pen
ocular
- o. albinism
- o. adnexa
- o. adnexal tumor
- o. angle
- o. ballottement
- o. bobbing
- o. cicatricial pemphigoid
- o. cone
- o. crisis
- o. cup
- o. dysmetria
- o. flutter
- o. histoplasmosis
- o. humor
- o. hypertelorism
- o. hypertension
- o. hypertensive glaucoma
- o. hypotony
- o. image
- o. ischemic syndrome
- o. lymphomatosis
- o. media
- o. melanoma
- o. meningioma
- o. motility test
- o. myoclonus
- o. myopathy
- o. neuromyotonia
- o. nocardiosis
- o. oscillations
- o. palsy
- o. paralysis
- o. pemphigus
- o. phthisis
- o. pressure reducer
- o. prosthesis
- o. refraction
- o. spectrum
- o. syphilis
- o. tension

ocular *(continued)*
  o. torticollis
  o. vesicle
Ocular Gamboscope loupe
oculentum
oculi uterque
oculist
oculistics
oculoauriculovertebral dysplasia
oculocalorie response
oculocardia
oculocardiac reflex
oculocephalic reflex
oculocephalogyric reflex
oculocerebral syndrome
oculocerebrorenal syndrome
oculocerebrovasculometer
oculocutaneous laser
oculodentodigital dysplasia
oculodermal
oculodigital reflex
oculofacial
oculoglandular syndrome
oculogyration
oculogyria
oculogyric
  o. crisis
  o. mechanism
oculomandibulodyscephaly
oculometroscope
oculomigraine
oculomotor
  o. apraxia
  o. decussation
  o. nerve
  o. palsy
  o. root of ciliary ganglion
oculomotorius
oculomycosis
oculonasal
oculopathy
  pituitarigenic o.
oculopharyngeal reflex
oculoplastic
oculoplasty corneal protector
oculopneumoplethysmography
oculopupillary
oculoreaction
oculorespiratory reflex
oculosensory cell reflex
oculospinal
oculosympathetic
  o. dysfunction
  o. paresis
oculotoxic
oculozygomatic
oculus
  o. dexter — OD (right eye)
  o. sinister — OS (left eye)
  o. unitas — OU (both eyes)
  o. uterque — OU (each eye)
Ocusan 400 Transducer
Ocusoft scrub
ocutome
Ocutome
  II Fragmentation System probe
OCVM System
OD — right eye
ODN — ophthalmodynamometry test
O'Donoghue's angled DCR probe
O'Gawa's cataract aspirating cannula
Ogston-Luc operation
Oguchi's disease
OHT — ocular hypertensive ointment
Oklahoma iris wire retractor

OKN — optokinetic nystagmus
old sight
Olivella-Garrigosa photocoagulator
Olk
  vitreoretinal pick
  vitreoretinal spatula
Olympus fundus camera
O'Malley-Heintz
  infusion cannula
  vitreous cutter
O'Malley self-adhering lens implant
OM
  4 ophthalmometer
  2000 operation microscope
OMNI Plus
omnifocal
OMS
  Empac Irrigation/Aspiration Unit
  Machemer/Parel VISC
Onchocerca
  O. caecutiens
  O. volvulus
onchocerciasis
onchercosis
one and one-half syndrome
one-snip punctum
onion skin–like membrane
onyx
opacification
opacified cuff
opacities
opacity
  Caspar's ring o.
opalescent cornea
opaque
  o. arcus
  o. media
open-angle glaucoma
open-funnel detachment
open-sky
  o. cryoextraction
  o. vitrectomy
opening of orbital cavity
operation
  Adams' o.
  Adler's o.
  Agnew's o.
  Agrikola's o.
  Allen's o.
  Allport's o.
  Alsus-Knapp o.
  Alvis' o.
  Ammon's o.
  Amsler's o.
  Anagnostakis' o.
  Anel's o.
  Angelucci's o.
  annular corneal graft o.
  Argyll-Robertson o.
  Arion's o.
  Arlt's o.
  Arlt-Jaesche o.
  Arrowhead's o.
  Arroyo's o.
  Arruga's o.
  Arruga-Berens o.
  Badal's o.
  Bangerter's pterygium o.
  Bardelli's lid ptosis o.
  Barkan's double cyclodialysis o.
  Barkan's goniotomy o.
  Barkan-Cordes linear cataract o.
  Barraquer's enzymatic zonulolysis o.
  Barraquer's keratomileusis o.
  Barrie-Jones canaliculodacryorhinostomy o.

operation *(continued)*
Barrio's o.
Basterra's o.
Beard's o.
Beard-Cutler o.
Beer's o.
Benedict's o.
Berens' pterygium transplant o.
Berens' sclerectomy o.
Berens-Smith o.
Berke's o.
Berke-Motais o.
Bethke's o.
Bielschowsky's o.
Birch-Hirschfeld entropion o.
Blair's o.
Blasius' lid flap o.
Blaskovics' canthoplasty o.
Blaskovics' dacryostomy o.
Blaskovics' inversion of tarsus o.
Blatt's o.
Bohm's o.
Bonaccolto-Flieringa scleral ring o.
Bonaccolto-Flieringa vitreous o.
Bonnett's o.
Bonzel's o.
Borthen's iridotasis o.
Bossalino's blepharoplasty o.
Bowman's o.
Boyd's o.
Brailey's o.
Bridge's o.
bridge pedicle flap o.
Briggs' strabismus o.

operation *(continued)*
Bromley's foreign body o.
Bronley's o.
Bronson's foreign body removal o.
Budinger's blepharoplasty o.
Burch's eye evisceration o.
Burow's flap o.
Buzzi's o.
Byron Smith's o.
Cairns' o.
Caldwell-Luc o.
Calhoun-Hagler o.
Callahan's o.
Campodonico's o.
Carter's o.
Casanellas' lacrimal o.
Casey's o.
Castroviejo's o.
Castroviejo-Scheie cyclodiathermy o.
cataract extraction o.
cautery o.
Celsus' spasmodic entropion o.
Celsus-Hotz o.
cerclage o.
Chandler's o.
Chandler-Verhoeff o.
Cibis' o.
cinching o.
Cleasby's o.
Collin-Beard o.
Comberg's foreign body o.
Conrad's orbital blowout fracture o.
Cooper's o.
corneal graft o.

operation *(continued)*
Crawford's sling o.
crescent o.
Critchett's o.
Crock's o.
cryoextraction o.
cryotherapy o.
Csapody's orbital repair o.
Cupper-Faden o.
Cusick-Sarrail ptosis o.
Custodis' o.
Cutler's o.
Cutler-Beard o.
cyclodiathermy o.
Czermak's pterygium o.
dacryoadenectomy o.
dacryocystectomy o.
dacryocystorhinotomy o.
dacryocystostomy o.
dacryocystotomy o.
Dailey's o.
Dalgleish's o.
Daviel's o.
decompression of orbit o.
Deiter's o.
de Grandmont's o.
De Klair's o.
de Lapersonne's o.
Del Toro's o.
Derby's o.
Desmarres' o.
de Wecker's o.
Dianoux's o.
diathermy o.
Dickey's o.
Dickey-Fox o.
Dickson-Wright o.
Dieffenbach's o.
dilation of punctum o.
discission of lens o.

operation *(continued)*
D'ombrain's o.
drainage of lacrimal gland o.
drainage of lacrimal sac o.
Duke-Elder o.
Dunnington's o.
Dupuy-Dutemps o.
Durr's o.
Duverger-Velter o.
Elliot's o.
Elschnig's canthorrhaphy o.
Ely's o.
encircling of globe o.
encircling of scleral buckle o.
enucleation of eyeball o.
equilibrating o.
Erbakan's inferior fornix o.
Escapini's cataract o.
Esser's inlay o.
Eversbusch's o.
evisceration o.
Ewing's o.
excision of lacrimal gland o.
excision of lacrimal sac o.
exenteration of orbital contents o.
extracapsular cataract extraction o.
Faden's o.
Fanta's cataract o.
Fasanella-Servat ptosis o.
fascia lata sling for ptosis o.
Fergus' o.
Filatov's o.

operation *(continued)*
- Filatov-Marzinkowsky o.
- filtering o.
- Fink's o.
- Flajani's o.
- Förster's o.
- Fould's entropion o.
- Fox's o.
- Franceschetti's corepraxy o.
- Franceschetti's keratoplasty o.
- Franceschetti's pupil deviation o.
- Fricke's o.
- Friede's o.
- Friedenwald's o.
- Friedenwald-Guyton o.
- Frost-Lang o.
- Fuchs' canthorrhaphy o.
- Fuchs' iris bombe transfixation o.
- Fukala's o.
- Gayet's o.
- Georgariou's cyclodialysis o.
- Gifford's delimiting keratotomy o.
- Gillies' o.
- Girard's keratoprosthesis o.
- Goldmann-Larsson foreign body o.
- Gomez-Marquez lacrimal o.
- Gonin's cautery o.
- goniotomy o.
- Gradle's keratoplasty o.
- Graefe's o.
- Greave's o.
- Grimsdale's o.
- Grossmann's o.
- Gutzeit's dacryostomy o.

operation *(continued)*
- Guyton's ptosis o.
- Halpin's o.
- Harman's o.
- Harms-Dannheim trabeculotomy o.
- Hasner's o.
- Heine's o.
- Heisrath's o.
- Herbert's o.
- Hess' ptosis o.
- Hiff's o.
- Hill's o.
- Hippel's o.
- Hogan's o.
- Holth's o.
- Holtz-Anagnostakis o
- Horay's o.
- Horvath's o.
- Hotz's entropion o.
- Hotz-Anagnostakis o.
- Hughes' o.
- Hunt-Transley o.
- Iliff's o.
- Iliff-Haus o.
- Imre's lateral canthoplasty o.
- indentation o.
- intracapsular cataract extraction o.
- iridectomy o.
- iridenclesis o.
- iridodialysis o.
- iridotasis o.
- iridotomy o.
- Irvine's o.
- Jaesche's o.
- Jaesche-Arlt o.
- Jaime's o.
- Jameson's o.
- Jensen's o.
- Johnson's o.
- Jones' o.

operation *(continued)*
Katzin's o.
Kelman's o.
keratectomy o.
keratocentesis o.
keratomileusis o.
keratoplasty o.
keratotomy
Key's o.
King's o.
Kirby's o.
Knapp's o.
Knapp-Imre o.
Knapp-Wheeler-Reese o.
Koffler's o.
Kraupa's o.
Kreiker's o.
Krieberg's o.
Krönlein's o.
Krönlein-Berke o.
Kuhnt's o.
Kuhnt's eyelid o.
Kuhnt-Helmbold o.
Kuhnt-Szymanowski o.
Kuhnt-Thorpe o.
Kwito's o.
Lacarrere's o.
Lagleyze's o.
Lagleyze-Trantas o.
Lagrange's o.
laissez-faire lid o.
Lancaster's o.
Lanchner's o.
Landolt's o.
Langenbeck's o.
Leahy's o.
Lester Jones o.
Lexer's o.
Lincoff's o.
Lindner's o.
Lindsay's o.
Löhlein's o.
Londermann's o.

operation *(continued)*
Lopez-Enriquez o.
Lowenstein's o.
Machek's o.
Machek-Blaskovics o.
Machek-Brunswick o.
Machek-Gifford o.
Magitot's o.
magnet o.
Magnus' o.
Majewsky's o.
Maladie de Graeffe's o.
Malbec's o.
Malbran's o.
Marquez-Gomez o.
Mauksch-Maumenee-Goldberg o.
McGavic's o.
McGuire's o.
McLaughlin's o.
McLean's o.
McReynolds' o.
Meek's o.
Meller's o.
Meyer-Schwickerath o.
Michaelson's o.
Minsky's o.
Moncrieff's o.
Moran's o.
Morax's o.
Morel-Fatio-Lalardie o.
Mosher-Toti o.
Moss' o.
Motais' o.
Mueller's o.
Mules' o.
Müller's o.
Mustarde's o.
myectomy o.
myotomy o.
Naffziger's o.
Neher's o.
Nehra-Mack o.

operation *(continued)*
- Nida's o.
- Nizetic's o.
- O'Conner's o.
- O'Conner-Peter o.
- Ogston-Luc o.
- one-snip punctum o.
- open-sky cryoextraction o.
- optical iridectomy o.
- orbital implant o.
- Pagenstecher's o.
- Panas' o.
- pars plana o.
- pattern cut corneal graft o.
- Paufique's o.
- peripheral iridectomy o.
- Peter's o.
- Physick's o.
- Pico's o.
- plombage o.
- pocket o.
- Polyak's o.
- Poulard's o.
- Power's o.
- Preziosi's o.
- probing lacrimonasal duct o.
- Putenney's o.
- Quaglino's o.
- Raverdino's o.
- Ray-Brunswick-Mack o.
- Ray-McLean o.
- reattachment of choroid o.
- reattachment of retina o.
- recession of ocular muscle o.
- Redmond-Smith o.
- Reese's o.
- Reese-Cleasby o.
- Reese-Jones-Cooper o.

operation *(continued)*
- removal of foreign body o.
- Richet's o.
- Rosenberg's o.
- Rosengren's o.
- Roveda's o.
- Rowbotham's o.
- Rowinski's o.
- Rubbrecht's o.
- Ruedemann's o.
- Rycroft's o.
- Saemisch's o.
- Safar's o.
- Sanders' o.
- Sato's o.
- Savin's o.
- Sayoc's o.
- Scheie's o.
- Schepens' o.
- Schimek's o.
- Schirmer's o.
- Schmalz's o.
- scleral fistulectomy o.
- scleral shortening o.
- scleroplasty o.
- sclerotomy o.
- sector iridectomy o.
- Selinger's o.
- Shaffer's o.
- Shugrue's o.
- Sichi's o.
- Silva-Costa o.
- Silver-Hildreth o.
- slant o.
- Smith's o.
- Smith-Kuhnt-Szymanowski o.
- Snellen's o.
- Soria's o.
- Soriano's o.
- Sourdille's keratoplasty o.

operation *(continued)*
- Sourdille's ptosis o.
- Spaeth's cystic bleb o.
- Spaeth's ptosis o.
- Speas' o.
- Spencer-Watson Z-plasty o.
- splitting lacrimal papilla o.
- Stallard's eyelid o.
- Stallard's flap o.
- Stallard-Liegard o.
- step graft o.
- Stock's o.
- Stocker's o.
- Straith's o.
- Strampelli-Valvo o.
- Streatfield's o.
- Streatfield-Fox o.
- Streatfield-Snellen o.
- Suarez-Villafranca o.
- Summerskill's o.
- suture of cornea o.
- suture of eyeball o.
- suture of iris o.
- suture of muscle o.
- suture of sclera o.
- Szymanowski's o.
- Szymanowski-Kuhnt o.
- Tansley's o.
- Tasia's o.
- tattoo of cornea o.
- Teale-Knapp o.
- tenotomy o.
- Terson's o.
- Tessier's o.
- Thomas's o.
- three-snip punctum o.
- Tillet's o.
- Toti's o.
- Toti-Mosher o.
- Townley-Paton o.
- trabeculectomy o.

operation *(continued)*
- Trainor's o.
- Trainor-Nida o.
- transfixion of iris o.
- transplantation of muscle o.
- Trantas' o.
- trapdoor scleral buckle o.
- Tripier's o.
- Troutman's o.
- Truc's o.
- Tudor-Thomas o.
- tumbling technique o.
- Ulloa's o.
- Uyemura's o.
- Van Milligen's o.
- Viers' o.
- Verhoeff's o.
- Verhoeff-Chandler o.
- Verwey's o.
- Vogt's o.
- Von Ammon's o.
- von Blaskovics-Doyen o.
- von Hippel's o.
- von Graefe's o.
- Waldhauer's o.
- Walter Reed o.
- Watzke's o.
- Weeker's o.
- Weeks' o.
- Weisinger's o.
- Wendell Hughes o.
- Werb's o.
- West's o.
- Weve's o.
- Wharton-Jones o.
- Wheeler's o.
- Wheeler-Reese o.
- Whitnall's o.
- Wicherkiewicz's o.
- Wiener's o.
- Wies' o.

operation *(continued)*
- Wilmer's o.
- Wolfe's ptosis o.
- Worst's o.
- Worth's o.
- Worth's ptosis o.
- Wright's o.
- Young's o.
- Ziegler's o.
- Z-plasty o.
- Zylik's o.

opercula
operculae
operculated
operculum
OPG — oculopneumoplethysmography
Ophthalas
- argon laser
- krypton laser

ophthalmagra
ophthalmalgia
ophthalmatrophia
ophthalmectomy
ophthalmencephalon
ophthalmia
- actinic ray o.
- catarrhal o.
- caterpillar o.
- o. eczematosa
- Egyptian o.
- electric o.
- o. electrica
- flash o.
- gonorrheal o.
- granular o.
- hivialis o.
- jequirity o.
- metastatic o.
- migratory o.
- mucous o.
- neonatorum o.
- neuroparalytic o.
- o. nodosa
- periodic o.
- phlyctenular o.
- purulent o.
- scrofulous o.
- spring o.
- strumous o.
- sympathetic o.
- transferred o.
- ultraviolet ray o.
- varicose o.

ophthalmiatrics
ophthalmic
- o. arteries
- o. artery
- o. cup
- o. ganglion
- o. migraine
- mini o. drape
- o. nerve
- o. plexus
- o. reaction
- o. solution
- o. vein

ophthalmitic
ophthalmitis
ophthalmoblennorrhea
ophthalmocarcinoma
ophthalmocele
ophthalmocopia
ophthalmodesmitis
ophthalmodiagnosis
ophthalmodiaphanoscope
ophthalmodiastimeter
ophthalmodonesis
ophthalmodynamometer
ophthalmodynamometry
ophthalmodynia
ophthalmodynomometry
ophthalmoeikonometer
ophthalmofunduscope
ophthalmograph

ophthalmogyric
ophthalmoleukoscope
ophthalmolith
ophthalmologic
ophthalmologist
ophthalmology
ophthalmomalacia
ophthalmomeningeal
ophthalmometer
ophthalmometroscope
ophthalmometry
ophthalmomycosis
ophthalmomyiasis
ophthalmomyitis
ophthalmomyositis
ophthalmomyotomy
ophthalmoneuritis
ophthalmoneuromyelitis
ophthalmopathy
- endocrine o.
- external o.
- internal o.

ophthalmophacometer
ophthalmophantom
ophthalmophlebotomy
ophthalmophthisis
ophthalmoplasty
ophthalmoplegia
- basal o.
- exophthalmic o.
- o. externa
- external o.
- fascicular o.
- infectious o.
- o. interna
- internal o.
- internuclear o.
- nuclear o.
- orbital o.
- Parinaud's o.
- partial o.
- o. partialis
- o. progressiva

ophthalmoplegia *(continued)*
- progressive o.
- Sauvineau's o.
- total o.
- o. totalis

ophthalmoplegic
- o. migraine
- o. muscular dystrophy

ophthalmoptosis
ophthalmoreaction
- Calmette's o.

ophthalmorrhagia
ophthalmorrhea
ophthalmorrhexis
ophthalmoscope
- binocular o.
- direct o.
- Friedenwald's o.
- ghost o.
- indirect o.
- Loring's o.
- Schepens's binocular indirect o.

ophthalmoscopy
- binocular indirect o.
- direct o.
- medical o.
- metric o.

ophthalmospectroscope
ophthalmospectroscopy
ophthalmostasis
ophthalmostat
ophthalmostatometer
ophthalmosteresis
ophthalmosynchysis
ophthalmothermometer
ophthalmotomy
ophthalmotonometer
ophthalmotonometry
ophthalmotoxin
ophthalmotrope
ophthalmotropometer
ophthalmotropometry

ophthalmovascular
ophthalmoxerosis
ophthalmoxyster
Ophthascan
OpMi microscope
Opraflex drape
opsin
opsinosis
opsiometer
opsoclonia
opsoclonus
Optacon
Op-Temp disposable cautery
optesthesia
optic
- o. angle
- o. aphasia
- o. atrophy
- o. axis
- o. canal
- o. chiasm
- o. coloboma
- o. cupping
- o. decussation
- o. demyelinating neuritis
- o. disk
- o. disk drusen
- o. evagination
- o. foramen
- o. foramina
- o. glioma
- o. hyperesthesia
- o. iridectomy
- o. keratoplasty
- o. lemniscus
- o. nerve
- o. nerve pits
- o. nerve sheath
- o. neuritis
- o. neuropathy
- o. papilla
- o. pits
- o. radiation

optic *(continued)*
- o. recess
- o. stalk
- o. sulcus
- o. thalamus
- o. tract
- o. vesicle

optic atrophy
- Behr's o.a.
- bow-tie o.a.
- congenital o.a.
- consecutive o.a.
- heredofamilial o.a.
- infantile o.a.
- ischemic o.a.
- juvenile o.a.
- Kjer's o.a.
- Leber's o.a.
- secondary o.a.
- simple o.a.
- tabetic o.a.

optical
- o. axis
- o. center
- o. nodal point
- o. zone

optician
opticianry
opticist
optic nerve
- o.n. coloboma
- o.n. disease
- o.n. drusen
- o.n. dysplasia
- o.n. fiber
- o.n. head
- o.n. hypoplasia
- o.n. lesion
- o.n. pit

opticochiasmatic
opticociliary
opticocinerea
opticokinetic

opticonasion
opticopupillary
optics
optimeter
optimum
Opti-Pure System
optist
optoblast
optociliary shunt vessels
optogram
optokinesis
optokinetic
optomeninx
optometer
optometrist
optometry
optomotor reflexes
optomyometer
optophone
optostriate
optotype
Opt-Visor loupe
ora
- o. globule
- o. serrata
- o. serrata retinae

orange punctate pigmentation
orbicularis
- o. ciliaris
- o. muscle
- o. reaction
- o. reflex
- o. sign

orbit
orbita
orbitae
orbital
- o. abscess
- o. akinesia
- o. aneurysm
- o. apex
- o. arch of frontal bone
- o. bone

orbital *(continued)*
- o. border of sphenoid bone
- o. canal
- o. cavity
- o. cellulitis
- o. compressor
- o. contents
- o. crest
- o. decompression
- o. emphysema
- o. enucleation compressor
- o. fascia
- o. fat pads
- o. fissure
- o. floor
- o. floor fracture
- o. floor prosthesis
- o. fracture
- o. hypertelorism
- o. hypotelorism
- o. implant
- o. inferior rim
- o. margin
- o. muscle
- o. opening
- o. ophthalmoplegia
- o. palsy
- o. periosteum
- o. periostitis
- o. pits
- o. plane
- o. plate of ethmoidal bone
- o. plate of frontal bone
- o. pseudotumor
- o. rim
- o. resilience
- o. roentgenogram
- o. roof
- o. section
- o. septum

orbital *(continued)*
- o. sulci of frontal bone
- o. sulcus
- o. superior fissure
- o. tomography
- o. wing of sphenoid bone

orbitale
orbitalis
orbitography
orbitomalar foramen
orbitonasal
orbitonometer
orbitonometry
orbitopathy
orbitostat
orbitotemporal
orbitotomy
organ
- accessory o. of eye
- o. of vision
- visual o.

organic amblyopia
organized vitreous
organum
- o. visuale
- o. visus

original Sweet's eye magnet
orthofusor
orthokeratology
Ortho-Lite
orthometer
orthophoria
orthophoric
orthopia
orthoposition
orthoptics
orthoptist
orthoptoscope
orthoscope
orthoscopic
orthoscopy
orthotrophic
os
- o. lacrimale
- o. orbiculare
- o. palatinum
- o. planum
- o. unguis

OS — left eye
OSCAR
oscillating vision
oscillopsia
Osher's hook
Osher-Fenzyl
osmolarity
osmotic
osseous
ossification
osteogenesis imperfecta
osteoma
Ota's nevus
otolith
OU — both eyes
OU — each eye
outer
- o. canthus
- o. nuclear layer
- o. plexiform layer
- o. retina
- o. segment

outpouching
output nerve
oval cornea
oval-shaped vernal ulcers
overaction
overcorrection
overlap
over-refraction
over-riding
over-ripe cataract
overwear syndrome
ovoid masses
OWS — overwear syndrome
oxyblepsia
oxygen flux

oxygen toxicity
oxyopia
oxyopter
ozena
ozenous

P

P & C — prism and cover test
P2 prolongation
Pach-Pen tonometer
pachometer
pachyblepharon
pachyblepharosis
pachymetry
Packo pars plana cannula
Packysonic II
paddy keratitis
padi keratitis
Paecilomyces lilacinus keratitis
Pagenstecher's operation
Paget's disease
pagetoid
pain reaction
painful ophthalmoplegia
palatine bone
palinopsia
pallor of disk
palpebra
  inferior p.
  superior p.
  tertius p.
palpebrae
palpebral
  p. adipose bags
  p. conjunctiva
  p. fascia
  p. fissure
  p. fold
  p. furrow

palpebral *(continued)*
  p. lobe
  p. opening
  p. raphe
palpebralis
palpebrarum
palpebrate
palpebration
palpebritis
palsy
  abducens p.
  Bell's p.
  cranial nerve p.
  cerebral p.
  gaze p.
  inhibitional p.
  lateral rectus p.
  nerve p.
PAM — Potential Acuity Meter
PAN — periarteritis nodosa
PAN — periodic alternating nystagmus
Panas' operation
panfundus
pannus
  allergic p.
  p. carnosus
  p. crassus
  degenerative p.
  p. degenerativus
  p. eczematosus
  glaucomatous p.
  phlyctenular p.
  p. siccus
  p. tenuis
  p. trachomatosus
panophthalmia
panophthalmitis
panoptic
panoramic loupe
panphotocoagulation
panretinal
  p. ablation

panretinal
p. photocoagulation
pansinuitis
pansinusitis
pantachromatic
pantankyloblepharon
pantoscope
Keeler's p.
pantoscopic
p. spectacles
p. tilt
panum area
panuveitis
papilla
Bergmeister's p.
lacrimal p.
optic p.
papillae
papillary
p. area
p. stasis
papilledema
papillitis
necrotizing p.
papilloma
papillomacular bundle
papilloretinitis
papillovitreal
parablepsia
paracentesis
paracentral
p. defects
p. nerve fiber bundle
p. scotoma
paracentric
parachromatism
parachromatopsia
paradoxical diplopia
parafovea
parafoveal
parafoveolar
parakinesis
parakinetic
parallactic
parallax
binocular p.
crossed p.
direct p.
heteronymous p.
homonymous p.
motion p.
stereoscopic p.
p. test
vertical p.
parallelism of gaze
paralysis
abducens p.
congenital abducens facial p.
congenital oculofacial p.
conjugate p.
internuclear p.
ocular p.
oculofacial p.
p. of accommodation
p. of gaze
Weber's p.
paralytic
p. ectropion
p. heterotropia
p. mydriasis
p. strabismus
paramacular
paramedian pontine reticular formation
parasellar syndrome
paraspinal
paraspinous
parastriate area
parasympathetic nerve system
parasympatholytic
parasympathomimetic
parathyroid
parathyroidism
paratrachoma
paravenous

paraxial lighting
Parel-Crock vitreous cutter
parenchyma
parenchymatous
  p. corneal dystrophy
  p. keratitis
paresis
paretic
parfocal
parietal lobe
paries
  p. interior orbitae
  p. lateralis orbitae
  p. medialis orbitae
  p. superior orbitae
Parinaud's
  conjunctivitis
  oculoglandular syndrome
  ophthalmoplegia
  syndrome
Park's speculum
Park-Guyton-Callahan speculum
Park-Guyton-Maumenee speculum
Parker's discission knife
Parker-Heath
  anterior chamber syringe
  cautery
  piggyback probe
Parks-Bielschowsky three-step head-tilt test
parophthalmia
parophthalmoncus
paropsis
paroxysm
paroxysmal
Parrot's sign
pars
  p. caeca oculi
  p. caeca retinae
  p. ciliaris retinae
  p. corneoscleralis
  p. iridica retinae

pars *(continued)*
  p. lacrimalis musculi orbicularis oculi
  p. marginalis musculi orbicularis oris
  p. nervosa retinae
  p. pigmentosa retinae
  p. optica hypothalami
  p. optica retinae
  p. orbitalis glandulae lacrimalis
  p. orbitalis gyri frontalis inferioris
  p. orbitalis musculi orbicularis oculi
  p. orbitalis ossis frontalis
  p. palpebralis glandulae lacrimalis
  p. palpebralis musculi orbicularis oculi
  p. plana approach
  p. plana corporis ciliaris
  p. plana vitrectomy
  p. planitis
  p. plicata
  p. plicata corporis ciliaris
  p. scleralis
  p. uvealis
partial
  p. cataract
  p. throw surgeon's knot
particulate matter
PAS — peripheral anterior synechia
Pascheff's conjunctivitis
passive
  p. forced duction test
  p. illusion
past-pointing
paster
PAT — prism adaptation test
Patau's syndrome

patch
Donaldson's eye p.
Hutchinson's p.
salmon p.
Scopolamine ear p.
Snugfit eye p.
venous sheath p.
wicking glue p.
patches
Bitot's p.
cotton-wool p.
patching
patchy window defects
pathogenesis
pathognomonic
pathologic diplopia
Paton's
corneal knife
corneal trephine
double spatula
eyeshield
knife
needle holder
single spatula
transplant spatula
pattern arborization
pattern-cut corneal graft
pattern-evoked electroretinogram
paucity
Paufique's
keratoplasty
knife
operation
synechiotomy
trephine
Paul's lacrimal sac retractor
paving stone degeneration
Payne's retractor
PC — posterior chamber
PCIOL — posterior chamber intraocular lens
PCLI — posterior chamber lens implant
PD — interpupillary distance prism diopter
PDR — proliferative diabetic retinopathy
peaking
Pierce's I/A
cannula
irrigating vectis
tripod implant
unit
pearl
p. cyst
p. white mounds
pearls
Elschnig's p.
peau de chagrin (shagreen skin)
pectinate
p. ligament of iris
p. villi
Peczon's I/A cannula
pediatric speculum
pedicle
flap p.
p. cone
pediculosis palpebrarum
pedunculated
PEK — punctate epithelial keratopathy
Pel's crises
pellucid
p. degeneration
p. marginal corneal degeneration
pemphigoid
pemphigus
ocular p.
p. vulgaris
pencil
cataract p.
glaucoma p.

pencil *(continued)*
retinal detachment p.
vitreous p.
pendular nystagmus
penetrating
p. full-thickness corneal graft
p. keratoplasty
penetration
pentachromic
pentagonal block excision
perception
color p.
depth p.
light p.
perfilcon A
perfluorodecalin
PERG — pattern-evoked electroretinogram
periarteritis nodosa
peribulbar needle
pericentral
perichiasmal
perichorioidal
perichoroidal
periconchitis
pericorneal plexus
peridectomy
perifovea
perifoveal
perifoveolar
perikeratic
perilenticular
perilimbal suction
Vactro p.s.
perimacular
perimeter
Allergan-Humphrey p.
Canon p.
CILCO p.
CooperVision p.
Digilab p.

perimeter *(continued)*
Ferree-Rand p.
Humphrey's p.
Marco's p.
Octopus 201 p.
Schweigger's p.
Topcon p.
Tubingen's p.
perimetry
perineuritis
perinuclear
periocular
periodic
p. alternating nystagmus
p. strabismus
periophthalmia
periophthalmic
periophthalmitis
perioptic sheath meningioma
perioptometry
periorbit
periorbital fat atrophy
periorbititis
periosteum
periostitis
peripapillary
periphacitis
periphakitis
peripheral
p. atrophy
p. anterior synechia
p. cataract
p. curve
p. fields
p. iridectomy
p. iris roll
p. retina
p. tapetochoroidal degeneration
p. uveitis
p. vision
peripherophose

periphery
periphlebitis retinae
periphoria
periretinal edema
periscleral space
perisclerotic
periscopic
peristriate
peritarsal network
peritectomy
peritomize
peritomy
perivascular sheathing
perivasculitis
PERK protocol
Perkins'
 applanation tonometer
 brailler
PERLA — pupils equal, reactive to light and accommodation.
Perlia nucleus
perpendicular
Perritt's forceps
PERRLA — pupils equal, round, reactive to light, accommodation.
persistent hyperplastic vitreous
perspective
 geometric p.
 linear p.
Peter's
 anomaly
 operation
Petit's canal
Petri dish
petrous
 p. bones
 p. ridges
Petzetakis-Takos syndrome
Peutz-Jeghers syndrome
Peyman's vitrector
Pfeiffer-Komberg method
phacitis
phacoanaphylactic endophthalmitis
phacoanaphylaxis
phacoantigenic
phacoblade
phacocele
phacocyst
phacocystectomy
phacocystitis
phacodonesis
Phaco Emulsifier Cavitron Unit
phacoemulsification
phacoerysis
phacoexcavation
phacoexcavator
phacofragmentation
phacoglaucoma
phacohymenitis
phacoiditis
phacoidoscope
phacolysin
phacolysis
phacolytic
phacoma
phacomalacia
phacomatoses
phacometachoresis
phacometecesis
phacometer
phacomorphic
phacopaligenesis
phacoplanesis
phacosclerosis
phacoscope
phacoscopy
phacoscotasmus
phacotoxic
phacozymase
phagocytized
phagocytosed cellular debris

phagocytosis
phagolysosomes
phakic eye
phakitis
phakoanaphylaxis
phakodonesis
phakolytic glaucoma
phakoma
phakomatoses
phakomatosis
phalangosis
Pharmacia Intermedics
pharmacological
pharmacological blockade
pharmacologically
pharyngoconjunctival fever
pharyngorhinitis
phemfilcon A
phengophobia
phenomenon
    aqueous-influx p.
    Ascher's glass-rod p.
    Aubert's p.
    autokinetic visible light p.
    Bell's p.
    blood-influx p.
    doll's head p.
    entoptic p.
    flicker p.
    Galassi's pupillary p.
    glass-rod negative p.
    glass-rod positive p.
    Hertwig-Magendie p.
    jack-in-the-box p.
    jaw-winking p.
    Le Grand-Geblewics p.
    Marcus Gunn p.
    orbicularis p.
    paradoxical pupillary p.
    phi p.
    Piltz-Westphal p.
phenomenon *(continued)*
    Purkinje's p.
    shot-silk p.
    Westphal's p.
    Westphal-Piltz p.
phenylephrine hydrochloride
phenylketonuria
phi phenomenon
pHisoHex
phlebophthalmotomy
phlycten
phlyctena
phlyctenae
phlyctenar
phlyctenoid
phlyctenosis
phlyctenula
phlyctenulae
phlyctenular
    p. conjunctivitis
    p. keratitis
    p. keratoconjunctivitis
    p. ophthalmia
    p. pannus
phlyctenule
phlyctenulosis
    allergic p.
    tuberculous p.
PHM — posterior hyaloid membrane
phoresis
phoria
phoriascope
phorometer
phorometry
phoro-optometer
phoropter retractor
phoroscope
phorotone
phosphene
photalgia
photerythrous

photoablative
photochromic lens
photocoagulation
 scatter p.
photocoagulator
 American Optical Co. p.
 Clinitex p.
 Mira p.
 Xenon p.
 Zeiss p.
photocoreoplasty
photodisrupting laser
photodisruption
photodynamic therapy
photodynia
photodysphoria
photoelectric vibration
photogene
photography
 fluorescence retinal p.
photogray lens
photokeratoscope
 Allergan Medical Optics p.
 CooperVision Refractive Surgery p.
photometer
 Forster's p.
photometry
photomydriasis
 Clinitex p.
photon
photons
photo-ophthalmia
photopapillometry
photophobia
photophthalmia
photopia
photopic
photopsia
photopsin
photopsy
photoptarmosis
photoptometer
photoptometry
photoreception
photoreceptive
photoreceptor
photoretinitis
photoscopy
photosun lens
Phototome System 2700
photovaporization
photovaporizing laser
PHPV — persistent hyperplastic primary vitreous
phthiriasis
phthisical eye
phthisis
 p. bulbi
 p. corneae
 essential p.
 ocular p.
phycomycosis
 cerebral p.
Physick's operation
physiologic
 p. blind spot
 p. excavation
 p. position of rest
physiological
 p. astigmatism
 p. retina
phytanic acid storage disease
PI — peripheral iridectomy
pial sheath
pick
 Burch's p.
 fixation/anchor p.
 Michel's p.
Pick's
 retinitis
 vision
Pickford-Nicholson anal-moscope
Pico's operation

"pie in the sky" defect
"pie on the floor" defect
Pierre-Robin syndrome
Pierse-Knoll irrigating lens loop
piezometer
piggyback
- p. contact lens
- p. probe

pigment
- p. cells
- p. clumping
- p. demarcation lines
- p. derangement
- p. dispersion
- p. dropout
- p. epithelitis
- p. epithelium
- p. granules
- p. placoid
- p. precipitates

pigmentary
- p. deposits on lens
- p. drop-out
- p. glaucoma
- p. halo
- p. migration
- p. rarefaction and clumping
- p. retinopathy

pigmentation rarefaction
pigmented
- p. layer of ciliary body
- p. layer of eyeball
- p. layer of iris
- p. layer of retina
- p. lesions
- p. stroma
- p. veils

pigmentum nigrum
pigtail
- p. fixation
- p. probe

Pillat's dystrophy
pilocarpine test
pilomatrixoma
pilot application
pimelopterygium
pin
- Pischel's p.
- Walker's p.

pince-ciseaux
pincushion distortion
pineal gland
pinealoma
pinguecula
pingueculae
pingueculum
Pinhole and Dominance Test
pinhole goggles
pinkeye disk
pinking
Pinky Ball
Pischel's
- electrode
- micropins
- pin
- scleral rule

pit(s)
- Gaul's p.
- Herbert's p.
- lens p.
- optic nerve p.

pituitarigenic
pituitary
- p. adenoma
- p. body
- p. gland
- p. tumor

PKP — penetrating keratoplasty
PKU — phenylketonuria
Placido's disk
placode lens
placoid pigment
pladarosis
plain catgut suture
plaited frill

plaiting
plane
    Broca's p.
    Daubenton's p.
    eye-ear p.
    Frankfort's horizontal p.
    horizontal p.
    Listing's p.
    orbital p. of frontal bone
    p. of regard
    vertical p.
    visual p.
planned extracapsular cataract extraction
plano
planoconcave
planoconvex
Plano T lens
planum orbitale
plaque
    Hollenhorst's p.
plaques
plasmoid
    p. agglutination
    p. aqueous humor
plastic
    p. disposable irrigating vectis
    p. lens
    p. prism
    p. shield
    p. sphere implant
plasticity
plate(s)
    Ishihara's p.
    isochromatic p.
    lid p.
    orbital p. of ethmoid bone
    orbital p. of frontal bone
    paper p.
    pseudoisochromatic p.
plate(s) *(continued)*
    reticular p.
    tarsal p.
plateau iris
Platina's
    clip
    lens
platinum
    p. probe spatula
    p. spatula
platycoria
platymorphia
platymorphic
platysmal reflex
pleomorphic adenoma
pleomorphism
pleoptic exercise
plesiopia
plethora
plethysmography
plexiform
    p. layer
    p. neuroma
Plexiglas implant
plexus
    annular p.
    ciliary ganglionic p.
    intraepithelial p.
    intrascleral p.
    ophthalmic p.
    pericorneal p.
    stroma p.
    subepithelial p.
Pley's forceps
plica
    p. lacrimalis
    p. lunata
    p. palpebronasalis
    p. semilunaris conjunctivae
plicae
    p. ciliares

plicae
- p. iridis

plombage

plug
- Berkley's Bioengineering brass scleral p.
- Dohlman's p.
- Eagle Vision-Freeman punctum p.

plus cyclophoria

PMMA lens — polymethyl methacrylate lens

Pneumococcus ulcer

pneumotonometer

pneumotonometry

p.o. — by mouth

pocket operation

pod

POHS — presumed ocular histoplasmosis syndrome

point
- cardinal p.
- conjugate p.
- convergence p.
- corresponding p.
- disparate p.
- eye p.
- far p.
- focal p.
- identical p.
- lacrimal p.
- near p.
- near p. absolute
- near p. relative
- nodal p.
- p. of dispersion
- p. of divergence
- p. of fixation
- principal p.
- p. of regard
- supraorbital p.
- stereoidentical p.

poisoning degenerative cataract

polar cataract

polarizing ophthalmoscope

pole
- anterior p.
- inferior p.
- posterior p.
- superior p.

poliosis

polisher
- Kraff's p.
- Kratz's p.

Polle pod attachment for ophthalmoscope

polus
- p. anterior bulbi oculi
- p. anterior lentis
- p. posterior bulbi oculi
- p. posterior lentis

Polyak's operation

polyarteritis nodosa

polychromatic lustre

polycoria
- p. spuria
- p. vera

polycythemia
- p. rubra vera
- p. vera

polyester suture

polyethylene
- p. implant
- p. T-tube
- p. tube

polyglactin suture

polyglycolic acid sutures

polygonal pigmented cells

polyhedral cells

polymacon

polymethyl methacrylate

polymorphonuclear

polyopia
binocular p.
p. monophthalmica
polyopsia
polyp
choanal p.
Hopmann's p.
nasal p.
presenile p.
polysinuitis
polysinusectomy
polysinusitis
polystichia
polystotic fibrous dysplasia
polytome x-ray
polytomography
polyvinyl alcohol
Pompe's disease
pons
pontes
pontile
pontine
p. gaze center
p. lesions
pontomesencephalic dysfunction
pooling
porcelain white end-point
porofocon
porus opticus
position
p. accommodation
p. ametropia
convergence p.
p. cyclophoria
dissociated p.
p. eyepiece
fusion-free p.
heterophoric p.
p. of rest
p. scotoma
position *(continued)*
sulcus fixated p.
vertical divergence p.
positive vertical divergence
Posner-Schlossman syndrome
post
p. cataract bleb
p. chamber
p. chiasmal
Post-Harrington erysiphake
post-placed
posterior
p. capsular polishing
p. capsular zonular barrier
p. capsular zonular disruption
p. chamber lens implant
p. ciliary arteries
p. discission
p. embryotoxon
p. fixation suture
p. hyaloid membrane
p. lamina
p. pole of eyeball
p. pole of lens
p. polymorphic dystrophy
p. scleritis
p. sclerotomy
p. staphyloma
p. subcapsular cataract
p. symblepharon
p. synechia
p. thermal sclerostomy
p. uveitis
p. veins
posteromedially
postganglionic
postkeratoplasty
postmarital amblyopia
postocular neuritis

postorbital
postvitrectomy fibrin
Potential Acuity Meter — PAM
Potter's syndrome
Potter-Bucky diaphragm
Poulard's
 entropion
 operation
Powell's wand
Power's operation
PPMD — posterior polymorphic dystrophy
PR — presbyopia
Prader-Willi syndrome
prairie conjunctivitis
PRAM Occluder
preauricular nodes
prechiasmal compression
precipitate(s)
 keratic p.
 mutton fat keratic p.
precipitating
precipitous
Precision Cosmet intraocular lens
precorneal
Preefer
prelacrimal
prelaminar
preliminary iridectomy
Prentice
 position
 rule
preparatory iridectomy
prephthisical
preplaced sutures
preproliferative
preretinal
 p. membrane
 p. neovascularization
 p. plaque
presage
presbycusis
presbyope
presbyopia
presbyopic
presbytia
presbytism
presenile melanosis
preseptal
 p. cellulitis
 p. orbicularis muscles
press-on Fresnel lens
press-on prism
pressure
 intraocular p.
 p. dressing
pretectal
 p. nucleus
 p. region
 p. syndrome
Prevost's sign
Preziosi's operation
primary
 p. cataract
 p. deviation
 p. dye test
 p. eye
 p. glaucoma
 p. line of sight
 p. mover
 p. open-angle glaucoma
 p. perivasculitis of the retina
 p. persistent hyperplastic vitreous
 p. position
 p. visual cortex
 p. vitreous
primordial
Prince's
 cautery
 clamp
 forceps

Prince's *(continued)*
- muscle clamp
- rule

principal
- p. axis
- p. foci
- p. line
- p. plane
- p. point
- p. visual direction

prism
- A-O rotary p.
- Allen-Thorpe gonioscopic p.
- apex p.
- ballast p.
- bar p.
- base-down p.
- base-in p.
- base-out p.
- base-up p.
- Becker's gonioscopic p.
- Berens's p.
- Fresnel's p.
- hand-held rotary p.
- Jacob-Swann gonioscopic p.
- Keeler's p.
- Maddox's p.
- oblique p.
- p. cover measurement
- p. cover test
- p. diopter
- p. spectacles
- press-on p
- right-angle p.
- Risley's rotary p.
- scanning p.
- square p.
- Wolff-Eisner p.

prismatic
- p. effect by lens

prismatic *(continued)*
- p. fundus
- p. gonioscopy lens

prismoid

prismoptometer

prismosphere

prisoptometer

Pritikin punch

p.r.n. — as needed

PRO CEM-4 microscope

proanomalopia

probe
- Alcon vitrectomy p.
- Anel's p.
- Bowman's p.
- Castroviejo's lacrimal sac p.
- Ellis' foreign body spud needle p.
- French's lacrimal p.
- Hertzog's pliable p.
- Iliff's p.
- Keeler-Amoils curved cataract p.
- Keeler-Amoils long shank p.
- Keeler-Amoils Machemer retinal p.
- Keeler-Amoils micro curved cataract p.
- Keeler-Amoils retinal p.
- Keeler-Amoils straight cataract p.
- Keeler-Amoils vitreous p.
- Knapp's iris p.
- lacrimal intubation p.
- Linde's cryogenic p.
- Manhattan E & E p.
- Mannis p.
- Microvit p.
- needle p.
- Ocutome p.

probe *(continued)*
Parker-Heath piggyback
pigtail p.
Quickert's lacrimal p.
Quickert-Dryden p.
Rolf's lacrimal p.
Rollet's lacrimal p.
Simpson's lacrimal p.
spatula p.
Theobald's p.
Vygantas-Wilder retinal drainage p.
Williams' p.
Worst's p.
Ziegler's p.
probing lacrimonasal duct
procedure
ciliary p.
Faden's p.
hamular p.
Hummelsheim's p.
Jensen's p.
Kestenbaum's p.
Krönlein's p.
PAM p.
Toti's p.
uncinate p.
process
zygomatico-orbital p.
processus
p. ciliares
p. frontosphenoidalis ossis zygomatici
p. orbitalis ossis palatini
p. zygomaticus maxillae
prodromal
progressive
p. addition lens
p. cataract
p. choroidal atrophy
p. external ophthalmoplegia
progressive *(continued)*
p. myopia
p. myopic degeneration
p. ophthalmoplegia
p. supranuclear palsy
p. tapetochoroidal dystrophy
projecting staphyloma
projection
erroneous p.
perimeter p.
Pro-Koester wide field SCM microscope
prolapse of iris
Prolene suture
proliferative
p. diabetic retinopathy
p. lupus retinopathy
p. vitreoretinopathy
prominence
Ammon's scleral p.
prominent
p. buckle
p. indentation
Pro-Ophtha
drape
dressing
eye pad
sponge
sticks
prophylactically
prophylaxis
Credé's p.
propionibacterium
proptometer
proptosis
proptotic
prosopantritis
prostheses
prosthesis
ocular p.
orbital p.

prosthesis
    socket p.
prosthokeratoplasty
protan color blindness
protanomal
protanomalous
protanomaly
protanope
protanopia
protanopic
protanopsia
protector
    Arruga's p.
protein electrophoresis
proteinaceous
    p. aqueous exudation
    p. coating
    p. cyst
protocol
protometer
proton beam
protruding eyes
protrusion
provocative test
Prowazek-Greeff bodies
Prowazek-Halberstaedter bodies
proximal convergence
PRP — panretinal photocoagulation
PRRE — pupils round, regular, and equal
PSC — posterior subcapsular cataract
pseudochiasmal
pseudocolomboma
pseudoesotropia
pseudoexfoliation
pseudoexophoria
pseudoexophthalmos
pseudoexotropia
pseudofluorescence
pseudogerontoxon
pseudo-Foster-Kennedy syndrome
pseudo-Graefe's sign
pseudoglandular
pseudoglioma
pseudoguttata
pseudoherpetic
pseudohypertropia
pseudohypoparathyroidism
pseudohypopyon
pseudoinflammatory macular dystrophy of Sorsby
pseudointernuclear ophthalmoplegia
pseudoisochromatic plates
pseudomembrane
pseudomembranous
Pseudomonas aeruginosa
Pseudomonas stutzeri
pseudomyopia
pseudoneuritis
pseudonystagmus
pseudopannus
pseudopapilledema
pseudopapillitis
pseudopemphigoid
pseudophacodonesis
pseudophakia
    p. adiposa
    p. fibrosa
pseudoproptosis
pseudopterygium
pseudoptosis
pseudoretinitis pigmentosa
pseudoscopic vision
pseudostrabismus
pseudotabes
    pupillotonic p.
pseudotrachoma
pseudotumor
    p. cerebri
    p. oculi
    orbital p.

pseudo–van Graefe's sign
pseudoxanthoma elasticum
psorophthalmia
PSP — progressive supranuclear palsy
psychic blindness
pterion
pterygia
pterygial tissue
pterygium
- congenital p.
- epitarsus p.
- p. scissors
- p. unguis

pterygoid levator synkinesis
ptilosis
ptosed
ptosis
- p. adiposa
- false p.
- Horner's p.
- p. lipomatosis
- morning p.
- p. scissors
- p. sympathica
- upside down p.
- waking p.

ptotic
puddler's cataract
puff of loose vitreous
pulley
pulsatile
pulse mode
pulseless disease
pulsers
pulsion
pulverization
pump-leak system
punch
- Berens' p.
- Castroviejo's p.
- corneoscleral p.
- Descemet's membrane p.

punch *(continued)*
- Gass' sclerotomy p.
- Holth's p.
- Kelly Descemet's membrane p.
- Klein's p.
- Pritikin's p.
- Rubin-Holth p.
- sclerectomy p.
- Storz's corneoscleral p.
- Walton's p.

punched-out lesion
puncta
punctae
punctal
- p. dilator
- p. openings
- p. stenosis

punctate
- p. cataract
- p. epithelial keratoplasty
- inner p. choroidopathy
- p. keratic precipitates
- p. keratitis
- p. retinitis

punctiform
punctograft
punctoplasty
punctum
- p. caecum
- inferior p.
- lacrimal p.
- p. lacrimale
- lower p.
- p. proximum of accommodation
- p. proximum of convergence
- p. remotum

punctumeter
puncture tip needle
pupil
- Adie's p.

pupil *(continued)*
  Argyll-Robertson p.
  artificial p.
  Behr's p.
  blown p.
  bounding p.
  Bumke's p.
  cat's eye p.
  cholinergic p.
  cornpicker's p.
  dilated p.
  fixed p.
  hammack p.
  Horner's p.
  Hutchinson's p.
  keyhole p.
  Marcus Gunn p.
  pear-shaped p.
  pinhole p.
  skew p.
  stiff p.
  tonic p.
  updrawn p.
pupilla
pupillae muscle of iris
pupillary
  p. aperture
  p. areflexia
  p. athetosis
  p. axis
  p. block
  p. capture
  p. distance
  p. margin of iris
  p. membrane
  p. miosis
  p. reflex
  p. paradoxic
  p. sphincter akinesis
  p. sphincter contractions
  p. zone
pupillatonia
pupilloconstrictor fibers
pupillograph
pupillometer
pupillometry
pupillomotor
pupilloplegia
pupilloscope
pupilloscopy
pupillostatometer
pupillotonia
pupil-to-root iridectomy
Purkinje's
  fibers
  image tracker
  images
  shift
Purkinje-Sanson mirror image
purpurogenous membrane
pursuit
  p. mechanism
  p. movements
Purtscher's
  angiopathic retinopathy
  disease
  retinopathy
purulent
  p. conjunctivitis
  p. iritis
  p. ophthalmia
push plus refraction technique
push/pull
  Birks Mark II Micro p.
  Ilg's p.
  Kuglein's p.
pusher
  Martin-Surefit lens p.
Putenney's operation
Putterman's ptosis clamp
Putterman-Chaflin ocular asymmetry measuring device
Putterman-Müller blepharoptosis clamp
PV Carpine

PVR — proliferative vitreoretinopathy
PXE — pseudoxanthoma elasticum
pyelonephritis
pyknotic nuclei
pyramidal cataract
Pyrex T-tube
pyrogenic granuloma
pyrophthalmia
pyrophthalmitis

q

q. — every
q.a.m. — every morning
q.d. — every day
q.h. — every hour
q.2h — every 2 hours
q.3h — every 3 hours
q.4h — every 4 hours
q.h.s. — at hour of sleep
q.i.d. — four times a day
q.l. — as much as desired
q.m. — every morning
q.n. — every night
q.o.d. — every other day
Q-switched
    neodymium YAG laser
    ruby laser
Quad's cutting tip
quadrant hemianopia
quadrantanopia
quadrantanopic
quadrantanopsia
quadrantic
    q. defect
    q. hemianopia
Quaglino's operation
quantitative
    q. static threshold
    q. threshold perimetry
Quevedo's
    fixation forceps
    suturing forceps
Quickert's
    lacrimal probe
    suture
Quickert-Dryden
    probe
    tube
quiescent
quiet chamber
quinine amblyopia

r

R&R — recess/resect
raccoon eyes
radial
    r. dilator muscles
    r. iridotomy scissors
    r. keratotomy marker
    r. vessel array
radially oriented
radian
radiance
radiant
    r. absorptance
    r. emittance
    r. energy
    r. flux
    r. intensity
    r. power
    r. reflectance
radiatio
    r. occipitothalamica
    r. optica

radiation
r. cataract
heavy ion r.
r. keratitis
occipitothalamic r.
optic r.
r. therapy
radices. *See radix*
radii
r. of lens
r. of lentis
Radin-Rosenthal eye implant
radioscope
radiotherapy
radius gauge
radix
r. lateralis tractus optici
r. medialis tractus optici
r. oculomotoria ganglii ciliaris
r. sympathica ganglii ciliaris
Raeder's syndrome
railroad nystagmus
rainbow
r. syndrome
r. vision
Raji cell assay
ramollitio retinae
Ramsden's eyepiece
ramus
Randolph's
cyclodialysis cannula
irrigator
Randot's Dot E Stereotest
range of accommodation
RAPD — relative afferent pupillary defect
raphe
horizontal r.
lateral palpebral r.
r. palpebralis lateralis
r. palpebrarum
raphe *(continued)*
r. plica semilunaris
posterior lamina r.
rapid eye movements
rarefaction
rasp
Lundsgaard-Burch corneal r.
Rathke's pouch tumor
ratio
Raverdino's operation
Ray-Brunswick-Mack operation
Ray-McLean operation
Raymond-Cestan syndrome
Rayner-Choyce implant
razor
r. blade knife
r. bladebreaker
r. tip needle
RD — retinal detachment
reaction
conjunctival r.
hemiopic pupillary r.
Loewi's r.
near-point r.
ophthalmic r.
orbicularis r.
pain r.
vestibular pupillary r.
Wernicke's r.
reading chart
reagent strips
real
r. focus
r. image
reaper's keratitis
reattachment
r. of choroid
r. of retina
receptor
r. amblyopia
visual r.
recess
optic r.

recess/resect — R&R
recession
    angle r.
    optic muscle r.
recessive
    r. dystrophic epidermolysis bullosa
    r. inheritance
    r. keratosis palmoplantaris
recessus opticus
reciprocal innervation
Recklinghausen's disease
reclination
recrudescence
recti
rectus muscle
red
    r. blindness
    r. blush
    r. desaturation
    r. eye
    r. glare test
    r. glass test
    r. reflex
    r. scaly plaques
red-green blindness
Redmond Smith operation
reduced eye
redundant
reduplication cataract
re-epithelialization
Reeh's scissors
reel aspiration cannula
Reese's
    forceps
    ptosis knife
    ptosis operation
    syndrome
Reese-Cleasby operation
Reese-Jones-Cooper operation
refined refraction
refixation
reflectance echo
reflected echo
reflection
reflectometry
reflex
    accommodation r.
    r. amaurosis
    r. amblyopia
    Aschner's r.
    attention r.
    auditory r.
    Bekhterev's r.
    Bell's r.
    blink r.
    cat's eye r.
    cerebral cortex r.
    choked r.
    ciliary r.
    ciliospinal r.
    cochleopapillary r.
    conjunctival r.
    consensual light r.
    convergency r.
    copper wire r.
    corneal r.
    corneomandibular r.
    corneomental r.
    corneopterygoid r.
    crossed r.
    cutaneous pupillary r.
    dazzle r.
    direct light r.
    doll's eye r.
    emergency light r.
    eyeball compression r.
    eyeball-heart r.
    eyelid closure r.
    fixation r.
    foveolar r.
    fundus r.
    fusion r.
    Gifford's r.
    Gifford-Galassi r.
    Haab's r.
    iridoplegia r.

reflex *(continued)*
- iris contraction r.
- juvenile r.
- lacrimal r.
- lacrimation r.
- lid r.
- light r.
- McCarthy's r.
- myopic r.
- oculocardiac r.
- oculocephalogyric r.
- oculopharyngeal r.
- oculopupillary r.
- oculosensory r.
- opticofacial winking r.
- orbicularis pupillary r.
- paradoxical pupillary r.
- platysmal r.
- Plitz's r.
- pupillary r.
- pupillary paradoxic r.
- red r.
- reversed pupillary r.
- Ruggeri's r.
- senile r.
- shot-silk r.
- skin-pupillary r.
- supraorbital r.
- tapetal light r.
- threat r.
- trigeminal r.
- r. trigeminus
- water-silk r.
- Weiss' r.
- Westphal's pupillary r.
- Westphal-Piltz r.
- white r.
- yellow r.

refract

refractile
- r. body
- r. crystals

refracting media

refraction
- direct light r.
- double r.
- dynamic r.
- homatropine r.
- manifest r.
- ocular r.
- static r.

refractionist

refractive
- r. amblyopia
- r. ametropia
- r. error
- r. index
- r. media

refractivity

refractometer

refractometry

refractor
- Agrikola's r.
- Allergan-Humphrey r.
- Amoils' r.
- Berens' r.
- Brawley's r.
- Bronson-Turz r.
- Campbell's r.
- Canon's r.
- Castallo's r.
- Castroviejo's r.
- Coburn's r.
- CooperVision Diagnostic Imaging r.
- Desmarres' r.
- Elschnig's r.
- Ferris-Smith-Sewall r.
- Fink's r.
- Goldstein's r.
- Gradle's r.
- Graither's r.
- Green's r.
- Groenholm's r.
- Hartstein's r.
- Hillis' r.

refractor *(continued)*
- Kirby's r.
- Knapp's r.
- Kronfeld's r.
- Kuglein's r.
- Marco's r.
- McGannon's r.
- Meller's r.
- Mueller's r.
- Reichert's r.
- Rizzuti's r.
- Rollet's r.
- Schepens' r.
- Stevenson's r.
- Topcon's r.

Refsum's disease
regeneration
region
- ciliary r.
- infraorbital r.
- ocular r.
- orbital r.

regress
regression
regular astigmatism
regurgitation test
Reichert's
- binocular indirect ophthalmoscope
- camera
- Ful-Vue ophthalmoscope
- Ful-Vue spot retinoscope
- lensometer
- membrane
- noncontact tonometer
- ophthalmodynamometer
- radius gauge
- refractor
- retinoscope
- slit lamp

Reichling's corneal scissors
Reiger's syndrome
reinervation
Reis-Bücklers corneal dystrophy
Reiter's
- disease
- syndrome

rejection line
Rekoss disk
relative
- r. accommodation
- r. afferent pupillary defect
- r. amblyopia
- r. convergence
- r. divergence
- r. hemianopia
- r. hyperopia
- r. scotoma
- r. size
- r. strabismus

relaxing incision
relucency
REM — rapid eye movements
removal of foreign body
Remy's separator
renal retinitis
rent
replacer
- Green's r.

replicating
reposited
repositor
- Nettleship iris r.

resection
residual cortex
resorbed
restrictive syndrome
retardation
rete mirabile
reticula
reticular
- r. cell sarcoma
- r. keratitis
- r. plate

reticulum

retina
- coarctate r.
- Coat's r.
- leopard r.
- nasal r.
- physiological r.
- shot silk r.
- temporal r.
- tented up r.
- tigroid r.
- upper r.
- watered silk r.

retinal
- r. abiotrophy
- r. adaptation
- r. angiomatosis
- r. aplasia
- r. apoplexy
- r. arterial occlusion
- r. asthenopia
- r. break
- r. capillary bed
- r. circinate
- r. circulation
- r. commotio
- r. cone
- r. correspondence
- r. degeneration
- r. detachment
- r. dystrophy
- r. elements
- r. embolism
- r. ganglion
- r. gliosis
- r. ice ball
- r. image
- r. imbrication
- r. isomerase
- r. lattice degeneration
- r. migraine
- r. neurons
- r. pigment epitheliopathy
- r. pigment epithelium

retinal *(continued)*
- r. rivalry
- r. rods
- r. scatter photocoagulation
- r. spike
- r. staphyloma
- r. stress lines
- r. tacks
- r. telangiectasia
- r. tufts
- r. vasculature
- r. vein occlusion
- r. vessels
- r. visual cells

retinal detachment
- r.d. hook
- r.d. pencil
- r.d. syringe

retinascope

retinectomy

retinene isomerase

retinitis
- actinic r.
- AIDS-related r.
- albuminuric r.
- apoplectic r.
- central angioplastic r.
- r. centralis serosa
- r. circinata
- circinate r.
- Coat's r.
- cytomegalovirus r.
- diabetic r.
- r. disciformans
- exudative r.
- foveomacular r.
- r. gravidarum
- gravidic r.
- r. haemorrhagica
- hypertensive r.
- Jacobson's r.
- Jensen's r.

retinitis *(continued)*
- leukemic r.
- metastatic r.
- r. nephritica
- Pick's r.
- r. pigmentosa
- r. proliferans
- proliferating r.
- proliferative r.
- r. punctata albescens
- punctate r.
- renal r.
- rubella r.
- serous r.
- solar r.
- splenic r.
- r. stellata
- striate r.
- suppurative r.
- syphilitic r.
- uremic r.
- Wagener's r.

retinoblastoma
- bilateral sporadic r.
- familial r.
- r. locus
- unilateral sporadic r.

retinochiasmatic
retinochoroid
retinochoroidal layer
retinochoroidectomy
retinochoroiditis
retinocortical
retinocytoma
retinodialysis
retinograph
retinography
retinoid
retinoillumination
retinomalacia
retinomigraine
retinopapillitis
retinopathy

retinopathy *(continued)*
- arteriosclerotic r.
- bull's eye r.
- carbon monoxide r.
- carotid occlusive disease r.
- cellophane r.
- central angioplastic r.
- central disk-shaped r.
- central serous r.
- circinate r.
- chloroquine r.
- diabetic r.
- drug abuse r.
- exudative r.
- foveomacular r.
- hemorrhagic r.
- hypertensive r.
- inflammatory r.
- Keith-Wagener r.
- leukemic r.
- pigmentary r.
- prematurity r.
- proliferative r.
- Purtscher's angiopathic r.
- radiation r.
- renal r.
- sickle cell r.
- solar r.
- stellate r.
- syphilitic r.
- vascular r.
- venous stasis r.
- X-linked juvenile r.

retinopexy
retinoschisis
- juvenile r.
- senile r.

retinoscope
- Keeler's r.
- Reichert's r.
- spot r.
- streak r.

retinoscopy
retinosis
retinotomies
retinotomy
retinotopic
retinotoxic
retraction syndrome
retractor
- Agrikola's lacrimal sac r.
- Alexander-Ballen r.
- Amenabar's iris r.
- Amoils' r.
- Arruga's r.
- Ballen-Alexander orbital r.
- Barraquer-Krumeich Swinger r.
- Berens' lid r.
- Blair's r.
- Brawley's r.
- Bronson-Turz r.
- Campbell's r.
- Castallo's r.
- Castroviejo's r.
- Coleman's r.
- Conway's lid r.
- Coston-Trent iris r.
- Desmarres' lid r.
- Drews-Rosenbaum iris r.
- Eliasoph's lid r.
- Elschnig's r.
- Ferris Smith r.
- Ferris-Smith-Sewall r.
- Fink's lacrimal r.
- Fisher's lid r.
- Forker's r.
- Givner's lid r.
- Goldstein's lacrimal sac r.
- Gradle's r.
- Graither's r.
- Groenholm's r.
- Gross' r.
- Harrison's r.

retractor *(continued)*
- Hartstein's r.
- Hill's r.
- Hillis' r.
- Jaeger's r.
- Jaffee-Givner lid r.
- Keeler Fison tissue r.
- Keeler-Rodger iris r.
- Keitzer-Lancaster lid r.
- Kelman's iris r.
- Kirby's r.
- Knapp's lacrimal sac r.
- Kronfeld's r.
- Kuglein's r.
- lacrimal sac r.
- MacKool's r.
- MacVicar's double-end strabismus r.
- McGannon's r.
- Mueller's lacrimal sac r.
- Oklahoma iris wire r.
- Paul's lacrimal sac r.
- Payne's r.
- Phoropter r.
- Rizzuti's iris r.
- Rollet's r.
- Rosenbaum-Drews r.
- Sanchez-Bulnes lacrimal sac r.
- Sato's lid r.
- Schepens' r.
- self-retaining r.
- Senn's r.
- Stevenson's lacrimal sac r.
- Thomas' r.
- Ticho's pliable iris r.
- Vaiser-Cibis muscle r.
- Wilmer's r.

retrieval device
retrobulbar
- r. hemorrhage
- r. injection

retrobulbar *(continued)*
r. needle
r. neuritis
r. optic neuritis
r. space
retrochiasmatic region
retrocorneal membrane
retrodisplacement
retroilluminate
retroillumination
retroiridian
retrolaminar
retrolental fibroplasia
retrolenticular
retromembranous
retro-ocular
retro-orbital
retropupillary
retrotarsal fold
Reuss
color chart
table
Reverdin's needle
reverse
r. Marcus Gunn pupil
r. shape implant
reverse-cutting needle
reversible amblyopia
rhabdomyoma
rhabdomyosarcoma
rhegmatogenous retinal detachment
Rhese's position
rheumatoid
r. arthritis
r. related ulceration
r. sclerouveitis
rhinitis
acute catarrhal r.
atrophic r.
r. caseosa
chronic catarrhal r.
croupous r.

rhinitis *(continued)*
dyscrinic r.
fibrinous r.
gangrenous r.
hypertrophic r.
membranous r.
pseudomembranous r.
purulent r.
scrofulous r.
r. sicca
syphilitic r.
tuberculous r.
rhinoscleroma
rhodogenesis
rhodophylactic
rhodophylaxis
rhodopsin
rhytidosis
ribbon
synaptic r.
ribbon-like keratitis
Richard's pillow
Richet's operation
Riddoch's
phenomenon
syndrome
ridge
supraorbital r.
synaptic r.
rigidity
mydriatic r.
Ridley's anterior chamber lens implant
Ridley Mark II lens implant
Riedel's needle
Rieger's
anomaly
syndrome
Reisman's sign
Rifkind's sign
right
r. deorsumvergence
r. gaze

right *(continued)*
r. gaze verticals
r. hypertropia
r. sursumvergence
right angle prism
right-beating nystagmus
right/left hand corneoscleral scissors
Riley-Day syndrome
Riley-Smith syndrome
rim to disk ratio
rima
r. cornealis
r. palpebrarum
ring
abscess r.
Bonaccolto's scleral r.
Bores' twist fixation r.
Burr's corneal r.
Caspar's r.
cataract mask r.
centering r.
choroidal r.
ciliary r.
Coats' r.
collagenous trabecular r.
common tendinous r.
conjunctival r.
corneal r.
corneal transplant centering r.
D chromosome r. syndrome
Dollinger's tendinous r.
Donder's r.
fixation r.
fixation-anchor r.
Fleischer's keratoconus r.
Fleischer-Strumpell r.
Flieringa's fixation r.
Flieringa-LeGrand fixation r.
Girard's scleral expander r.

ring *(continued)*
glaucomatous r.
glial r.
greater r.
r. of iris
Kayser-Fleischer r.
Klein-Tolentino r.
Landers' vitrectomy r.
Landolt's r.
lenticular r.
lesser r.
Lowe's r.
Martinez's corneal transplant centering r.
Maxwell's r.
McKinney's fixation r.
posterior limiting r.
rust r.
Schwalbe's anterior border r.
Schwalbe's r.
scleral expander r.
scotoma r.
Soemmering's r.
symblepharon r.
Tolentino's r.
r. ulcer
Vossius' lenticular r.
Wessely's r.
Zinn's r.
ring-shaped cataract
Ringer's lactate solution
Riolan's muscle
Ripault's sign
ripe cataract
Risley's rotary prism
Ritter's fiber
rivalry
binocular r.
retinal r.
river blindness
rivus lacrimalis
Rizzuti's
expressor

Rizzuti's *(continued)*
- fixation forceps
- graft carrier spoon
- rectus forceps
- iris retractor
- refractor
- retractor

Rizzuti-Bonaccolto
Rizzuti-Fleisher
Rizzuti-Furness cornea holding forceps
Rizzuti-Kayser-Fleischer
Rizzuti-Lowe
Rizzuti-Maxwell
Rizzuti-McGuire corneal section scissors
Rizzuti-Soemmering
Rizzuti-Spizziri cannula knife
RK — radial keratotomy
RLF — retrolental fibroplasia
Robertson's sign
Robin's chalazion clamp
Rochat's test
Rochon-Duvigneaud bouquet of cones
rod
- r. cells
- r. granule
- Maddox r.
- r. monochromatism
- retinal r.
- vision r.

Rodenstock System
Rodin's orbital implant
rods and cones
Rolf's
- dilator
- forceps
- lacrimal probe
- lance

roll
- scleral r.

rolled up epithelium with wavy border
roller forceps
Rollet's
- irrigating/aspirating unit
- lacrimal probe
- refractor
- retractor
- syndrome

Romana's sign
Rommel's cautery
Rommel-Hildreth cautery
rongeur
- Cittelli's r.
- Kerrison's r.
- lacrimal sac r.

Ronne's nasal step
roof of orbit
root
- long r. of ciliary ganglion
- motor r.
- oculomotor r.
- sensory r.
- short r. of ciliary ganglion

Roper's
- alpha-chymotrypsin cannula

Roper-Hall localizer
ropy mucus
Rosa-Berens orbital implant
rosacea keratitis
rose bengal red solution
Rosenbaum's pocket vision screener
Rosenbaum-Drews retractor
Rosenburg's operation
Rosengren's operation
Rosenmüller's
- body
- gland

rosette
Rosner's tonometer
rotary
- r. cutting tip

rotary *(continued)*
- r. nystagmus
- r. prism

rotation nystagmus
rotator
- Jaffe-Bechert nucleus r.

Roth's spots
Roth-Bielschowsky syndrome
Rothmund's syndrome
Rothmund-Thomson syndrome
rotoextractor
- Douvas' r.

Rouget's muscle
round hemorrhage
Roveda's
- lid everter
- operation

Rowbotham's operation
Rowinski's operation
Rowland's keratome
RP — retinitis pigmentosa
RP hypertrophy
RPE — retinal pigment epithelium
rubber dam
Rubbrecht's operation
rubella retinitis
rubeola
rubeosis
- r. iridis
- r. retinae

Rubin-Holth punch
Rubinstein's cryoprobe
ruby diamond knife
rudiment lens
rudimentary eye
Ruedemann's
- eye implant
- lacrimal dilator
- operation
- tonometer

Ruedemann-Todd tendon tucker
ruffed canal
Ruggeri's reflex
Ruiz plano fundus lens implant
rupture
Russian forceps
rust ring
Rutherford's syndrome
rutidosis
Ruysch's tunic
Rycroft's operation

S

S — spherical lens
Sabouraud's media
Sabreloc needle
saburral amaurosis fugax
sac
- conjunctival s.
- lacrimal s.
- tear s.

saccade palsy
saccades
saccadic
- s. eccentric targets
- s. movements
- s. velocities

saccular
sacculated
sacculus lacrimalis
saccus
- s. conjunctivae
- s. conjunctivalis
- s. lacrimalis

Sach's disease
Saemisch's
- operation
- ulcer

Saenger's sign
Safar's operation

sagittal
    s. axis of eye
    s. axis of Fick
    s. depth
sagittalization
St. Martin–Franceschetti cataract hook
Sakler's erysiphake
salmon patch hue
salt and pepper appearance
salt and pepper fundus
Salus'
    arch
    sign
Salzmann's
    corneal dystrophy
    degeneration
    dystrophy
    nodular corneal degeneration
Samoan conjunctivitis
Sanchez-Bulnes lacrimal sac retractor
Sanders'
    disease
    operation
Sandhoff's disease
Sanfilippo's
    disease
    disorder
    syndrome
sanguineous cataract
Sanson's images
Sanyal's conjunctivitis
saponification
Sappey's fibers
sarcoid
sarcoma
sarcomatosum
    s. senilis
    s. spasticum
    s. uveae
satellite lesion
Sato's
    cataract needle
    corneal knife
    keratoconus
    lid retractor
    needle
    procedure
Sattler's
    layer
    veil
saucer-shaped
saucering of rims
saucerization
Sauer's
    corneal debrider
    forceps
    speculum
Sauflon lens
Sauvineau's ophthalmoplegia
Savin's procedure
Sayoc's procedure
SBV — single binocular vision
sc — without correction
scaffold for new vessel growth
scalloped contours
scalloping
scalpel
    Guardian s. with myoguard depth resistor
    Guyton-Lundsgaard s.
    Oasis feather micro s.
scaly plaque
scan
    CT s.
    CAT s.
    MRI s.
scanning
    s. electron microscopy
    s. prism
scaphoid
scar plate
scarification

scarified
scarifier
Desmarres' s.
Scarpa's staphyloma
scatter
s. pattern
s. photocoagulation
scattergram
scatterplot
Schaaf's forceps
Schacher's ganglia
Schachne-Desmarres lid everter
Schaedel's cross-action towel clamp
Schaefer's sponge holder
Schäfer's syndrome
Scheie's
akinesia
anterior chamber cannula
blade
cataract aspirating needle
cautery
classification
electrocautery
goniopuncture knife
knife
operation
technique
thermal sclerostomy
trephine
Scheie-Westcott corneal section scissors
schematic eye
Schepens'
electrode
Gelfilm
operation
ophthalmoscope
refractor
retinal detachment unit
retractor
scleral depressor
spoon
Schepens-Pomerantzeff
binocular indirect ophthalmoscope
scheroma
Schilder's disease
Schillinger's suture support
Schimek's operation
Schiötz's
tonofilms
tonometer
Schirmer's tear quality test
schisis
Schlemm's canal
Schlichting's dystrophy
Schmalz's operation
Schmid-Fraccaro syndrome
Schmidt's keratitis
Schnabel's atrophy
Schnyder's crystalline corneal dystrophy
Schöbl's scleritis
Schocket's scleral depressor
Schöler's treatment
Schön's theory
school myopia
Schumann's giant type eye magnet
Schwalbe's
anterior border ring
line
ring
space
Schwann's cells
Schweigger's
forceps
perimeter
scieropia
scimitar scotoma
scintillating
s. granules
s. scotoma
scintillation
scirrhophthalmia

scissors
- Aebli's corneal s.
- alligator s.
- anterior chamber synechiae s.
- Atkinson's corneal s.
- bandage s.
- Barraquer's iris s.
- Barraquer's vitreous strand s.
- Barraquer-DeWecker s.
- Becker's corneal section spatulated s.
- Berens' corneal transplant s.
- Berkley Bioengineering mechanized s.
- Birks Mark II Micro trabeculectomy s.
- canalicular s.
- capsulotomy s.
- Castroviejo's corneal section s.
- Castroviejo's corneal transplant s.
- Castroviejo's iridocapsulotomy s.
- Castroviejo's keratoplasty s.
- Castroviejo's synechiae s.
- Cohan-Vannas iris s.
- Cohan-Westcott s.
- conjunctival s.
- corneal s.
- corneal spatulated s.
- corneoscleral s.
- corneoscleral right/left hand s.
- DeWecker's iris s.
- DeWecker-Pritikin s.
- dissecting s.
- enucleation s.
- Fine's suture s.
- Frost's s.

scissors *(continued)*
- Giardet's corneal transplant s.
- Gill's s.
- Gill-Hess s.
- Girard's corneoscleral s.
- Grieshaber's vertical cut s.
- Grieshaber's vitreous s.
- Guist's s.
- Haenig's irrigating s.
- Harrison's s.
- Hoskins-Castroviejo corneal s.
- Hoskins-Westcott tenotomy s.
- House-Bellucci alligator s.
- Huey's s.
- iridectomy s.
- iridocapsulotomy s.
- iridotomy s.
- iris s.
- Irvine's probe pointed s.
- Irvine's s.
- Karakashian-Barraquer s.
- Katzin's s.
- Keeler's intravitreal s.
- keratectomy s.
- keratoplasty s.
- Kirby's s.
- Knapp's iris s.
- Kreiger-Spitznas vibrating s.
- Lagrange's s.
- Lawton's corneal s.
- Lister's s.
- Littler's dissecting s.
- Manson-Aebli corneal section s.
- Mattis' s.
- Maunoir's iris s.
- Mayo's s.
- McClure's iris s.

scissors *(continued)*
- McGuire's corneal s.
- McLean's capsulotomy s.
- McPherson-Castroviejo corneal section s.
- McPherson-Vannas micro iris s.
- McReynolds' pterygium s.
- mechanized s.
- mini-keratoplasty stitch s.
- Moore-Troutman corneal s.
- MPC automated intravitreal s.
- Nadler's superior radial s.
- Noyes' iridectomy s.
- Noyes' iris s.
- Nugent-Gradle s.
- pterygium s.
- radial iridotomy s.
- Reeh's s.
- Reichling's corneal s.
- right/left hand corneoscleral s.
- Rizzuti-McGuire corneal section s.
- Scheie-Westcott corneal section s.
- Shield's iridotomy s.
- Spencer's s.
- Spring's iris s.
- Stevens' tenotomy s.
- Storz-Westcott conjunctival s.
- strabismus s.
- superior radial tenotomy s.
- Sutherland-Grieshaber s.
- Thorpe's s.
- Thorpe-Castroviejo s.
- Thorpe-Westcott s.
- Twisk micro s.

scissors *(continued)*
- Vannas' s.
- Verhoeff's s.
- vibrating s.
- vitreous strand s.
- Walker's s.
- Walker-Apple s.
- Walker-Atkinson s.
- Werb's s.
- Westcott's s.
- Wilmer's s.

sclera
- blue s.

sclerae

scleral
- s. blade
- s. buckle
- s. buckling procedure
- s. crescent
- s. depressor
- s. expander ring
- s. hook
- s. fistula
- s. furrow
- s. grip
- s. icterus
- s. implant
- s. lamina cribosa
- s. lip
- s. marker
- s. patch graft
- s. plexus
- s. reinforcement
- s. resection knife
- s. rigidity
- s. roll
- s. search coil technique
- s. shell
- s. shortening clips
- s. sponge rod
- s. spur
- s. staphyloma
- s. supporter

scleral *(continued)*
 s. sulcus
 s. trabeculae
 s. tunnel
 s. twist
scleralization
scleratitis
sclerectasia
sclerectasis
sclerectoiridectomy
sclerectoiridodialysis
sclerectome
sclerectomy
scleriasis
scleriritomy
scleritis
 annular s.
 anterior s.
 brawny s.
 s. necroticans
 necrotizing s.
 nodular s.
 posterior s.
 Schobl's s.
sclerocataracta
sclerochoroiditis
 anterior s.
 posterior s.
scleroconjunctival
scleroconjunctivitis
sclerocornea
sclerocorneal
 s. junction
 s. sulcus
sclerocytes
scleroderma
scleroiritis
sclerokeratitis
sclerokeratoiritis
sclerokeratosis
scleroma respiratorium
scleromalacia perforans
scleronyxis
sclero-optic
sclerophthalmia
scleroplasty
sclerosed
sclerosing keratitis
sclerosis
sclerostomy
sclerotic
 s. scatter
 s. stroma
sclerotica
scleroticectomy
scleroticochoroidal canal
scleroticochoroiditis
scleroticonyxis
scleroticopuncture
scleroticotomy
sclerotitis
sclerotome
 Alvis-Lancaster s.
 Atkinson's s.
 Curdy's s.
 Guyton-Lundsgaard s.
 Lundsgaard's s.
 Lundsgaard-Burch s.
sclerotomy
 anterior s.
 s. with drainage
 s. with exploration
 foreign body s.
 posterior s.
 s. punch
 s. removal of foreign body
sclerouveitis
Scobee's muscle hook
scoop
 Arlt's s.
 Daviel's s.
 Knapp's s.
 Lewis' s.
 Mules' s.
 Wilder's s.

scope
- Bjerrum's s.
- tangent s.

scopolamine patch
scotodinia
scotoma(s)
- absolute s.
- annular s.
- altitudinal s.
- arc s.
- arcuate s.
- aural s.
- bitemporal hemianopic s.
- Bjerrum's s.
- cecocentral s.
- central s.
- centrocecal s.
- color s.
- comet s.
- congruous homonymous hemianopic s.
- cuneate-shaped s.
- eclipse s.
- equatorial ring s.
- flittering s.
- focal s.
- homonymous hemianopic s.
- ipsilateral centrocecal s.
- junctional s. of Traquair
- motile s.
- negative s.
- s. of Traquair
- paracentral s.
- peripapillary s.
- peripheral s.
- physiologic s.
- positive s.
- relative s.
- ring s.
- scintillating s.
- Seidel's s.
- superior arcuate s.
- unilateral altitudinal s.

scotomagraph
scotomameter
scotomata
scotomatous
scotometer
- Bjerrum's s.

scotometry
scotomization
scotopia
scotopic
- s. adaptation
- s. vision

scotopsin
scotoscope
scotoscopy
Scott No. 2 curved ruler
screen
- Bjerrum's s.
- tangent s.

scrofular
- s. conjunctivitis
- s. keratitis
- s. ophthalmia

scurf
scutum region
sea
- s. fans
- s. fronds

seam
- pigment s.

Searcy's
- anchor/fixation
- chalazion trephine
- erysiphake

sebaceous
- s. cell carcinoma
- s. gland of conjunctiva

seborrheic blepharitis
sebum palpebrale
seclusion
second
- s. cranial nerve
- s. grade fusion
- s. sight

secondary
s. axis
s. cataract
s. deviation
s. exotropia
s. eye
s. dye test
s. focal point
s. glaucoma
s. keratitis
s. positions
s. vitreous
section
Saemisch's s.
sector
s. cuts
s. defect
s. iridectomy
s. pallor
s. retinitis pigmentosa
secoria
sedimentary cataract
sedimentation rate
see-saw nystagmus
Seeligmüller's sign
Seidel's
scotoma
sign
test
self-adhering lid retractor
self-retaining
s. irrigating cannula
s. retractor
self-sealing scleral puncture
sella
empty s.
J-shaped s.
s. turcica
sellae
sellar
Selinger's operation
semilunar fold
semishell implant
senescence
senescent
s. cataract
s. cortical degenerative cataract
s. disciform macular degeneration
s. ectropion
s. elastosis
s. enophthalmus
s. entropion
s. halo
s. keratosis
s. macular degeneration
s. macular exudative choroiditis
s. macular hole
s. miosis
s. nuclear degenerative cataract
s. pruritus
s. ptosis
s. retinoschisis
Senn's retractor
senopia
sensation
light s.
sense
color s.
form s.
light s.
stereognostic s.
sensory
s. esotropia
s. exotropia
s. fusion
s. nerve
s. receptors
s. retina
s. root of ciliary ganglion
s. visual pathway
separate image test
separation difficulty
septate
septic retinitis

septicemia
septo-optic dysplasia
septum
- s. cavum pellucidum
- orbital s.
- s. orbitale
- sequela

sequelae
sequestered spaces
serofibrinous
serologic test
serous
- s. chorioretinopathy
- s. detachment
- s. iritis
- s. retinitis
- s. macular detachment
- s. membrane
- s. pigment epithelium

serpiginous
- s. choroiditis
- s. keratitis

serrafine
- s. clamp
- Dieffenbach's s.
- Lemoine's s.

Serratia marcescens
sessile
setting
- s. sun phenomenon
- s. sun sign

seventh cranial nerve
SFP — simultaneous foveal perception
shadow
- s. graph
- Purkinje's s.
- s. test

Shafer's sign
Shaffer's operation
shaft vision
shagreen
shallowing of chamber
Sharplan argon laser
Sharpoint
- knife
- microsurgical knife
- slit knife
- V-lance blade

Shearing's lens
sheath
- arachnoid s.
- bulbar s.
- eyeball s.
- optic nerve s.
- pial s.
- s. syndrome

sheathing of vessels
sheet
- foil s.
- Silastic s.
- Supramid s.
- Teflon s.

Sheets' lens
Sheey-Urban sliding lens adaptor
Sheiner's principle
shelf-type implant
shell
- s. implant
- s. prosthesis
- scleral s.

shelving
Shepard's
- iris hook
- reversed iris hook

Shepard-Reinstein forceps
Sheridan-Gardiner Isolated Letter Matching Test
Sherrington's law
shield
- Barraquer's s.
- Buller's s.
- Cartella's s.
- cataract mask s.
- eye s.

shield *(continued)*
Expo Bubble s.
Fox's s.
Green's s.
Hessburg's corneal s.
Mueller's s.
Paton's s.
plastic s.
pressure s.
Universal s.
Weck's s.
Shields' iridotomy scissors
shield-shaped
shift
Purkinje s.
shingles
shiny cellophane reflection
shipyard
s. conjunctivitis
s. disease
s. eye
s. keratoconjunctivitis
Shoch's suture
short
s. ciliary nerves
s. posterior ciliary arteries
s. root of ciliary ganglion
s. sight
shortsightedness
short-scale contrast
shot-silk
s. reflex
s. retina
shredded iris
Shugrue's operation
shunt vessels
sicca syndrome
Sichel's
disease
knife
Sichi's orbital implant
sickle
s. retinopathy
sickle-cell disease
side port cannula
side-cutting spatula needle
siderophone
sideroscope
siderosis
s. bulbi
s. cataract
s. conjunctivae
s. lentis
Sidler-Huguenin endothelioma
Siegrist-Hutchinson syndrome
sight
day s.
far s.
long s.
near s.
night s.
old s.
second s.
short s.
sign
Abadie's s.
Argyll-Robertson pupil s.
Arroyo's s.
Ballet's s.
Bard's s.
Barany's s.
Barre's s.
Battle's s.
Bekhterev's s.
Berger's s.
Bianchi's s.
Bjerrum's s.
Brickner's s.
Cantelli's s.
Collier's s.
Dalrymple's s.
doll's eye s.
Elliot's s.
Enroth's s.

sign *(continued)*
- Gianelli's s.
- Gifford's s.
- Gower's s.
- Graefe's s.
- Hutchinson's s.
- Jendrassik's s.
- Kestenbaum's s.
- Knie's s.
- Kocher's s.
- Larcher's s.
- Magendie's s.
- Magendie-Hertwig s.
- Mann's s.
- Marcus Gunn pupillary s.
- May's s.
- Mobius' s.
- Mobius-von Graefe-Stellway s.
- Munson's s.
- Parrot's s.
- Piltz's s.
- Prevost's s.
- pseudo-Graefe's s.
- Reisman's s.
- Rifkind's s.
- Ripault's s.
- Robertson's s.
- Romaña's s.
- Saenger's s.
- Salus' s.
- Seeligmüller's s.
- Seidel's s.
- setting sun s.
- Shafer's s.
- Skeer's s.
- Stellwag's s.
- Stimson's s.
- Suker's s.
- swinging flashlight s.
- Tellais' s.
- Theimich's s.
- Tournay's s.

sign *(continued)*
- von Graefe's s.
- Weber's s.
- Weber-Rinne s.
- Wernicke's s.
- Widowitz's s.
- Wilder's s.
- Woods' s.

silafilcon A

silafocon A

Silastic
- implant
- plate
- sheet
- T-tube

silicone
- s. button
- s. conformer
- s. eye sphere
- s. hemisphere
- s. implant
- s. lens
- s. lubricant
- s. oil tamponade
- s. strip
- s. tire

siliculose cataract

siliquose cataract

Silva-Costa operation

silver-wire
- s. arterioles
- s. reflex

Simcoe II PC
- aspirating needle
- double cannula
- lens
- nucleus delivery loop

simple
- s. glaucoma
- s. hyperopic astigmatism
- s. myopic astigmatism

Simpson's lacrimal probe

simultaneous
- s. foveal perception
- s. macular perception
- s. perception
- s. prism and cover test

single binocular vision
sinistrality
sinistrocular
sinistrocularity
sinistrogyration
sinistrotorsion
Sinskey's
- lens hook

sinus
- anterior chamber s.
- Arlt's s.
- s. circularis iridis
- s. of Maier
- scleral venous s.
- s. venosus sclerae

SITE TXR
- 2200 Microsurgical Unit
- I/A system
- Phaco System

sixth
- s. cranial nerve
- s. cranial nerve palsy

Sjögren's
- disease
- syndrome

Skeele's
- curet

Skeer's sign
skein
- Holmgren's s.
- s. test

skew deviation
ski needle
skiametry
skiascope
skiascopy
skin
skin *(continued)*
- s. hook
- s. wheal
- s. whorl

Sklar-Schiötz tonometer
slant muscle operation
sleeve
- Charles' anterior segment s.
- Charles' infusion s.
- implant s.
- Stevens-Charles s.
- Watzke's s.

sliding flap
sling for implant
slit-lamp biomicroscopy
slit-like
sloping isopters
slough
sloughing
sludging of circulation
SMD — senile macular degeneration
small aperture Steri-Drape
Smart's
- forceps
- scissors

Smith's
- expressor hook
- eyelid operation
- intraocular capsular amputator
- knife
- modification
- operation
- orbital floor implant
- speculum
- trabeculectomy

Smith-Fisher
- iris replacer
- knife
- spatula

Smith-Green knife

Smith-Kuhnt-Szymanowski operation
SMP — simultaneous macular perception
snail tracks
snare
  Banner's enucleation s.
  Castroviejo's enucleation s.
  enucleation wire s.
  Foster's enucleation s.
Snell's law
Snellen's
  chart
  implant
  letter
  operation
  ptosis operation
  reform eye
  test
  vectis
snow-blind
snow-blindness
snowball opacities
snowbanks
snowflake cataract
snowglasses
snowstorm cataract
SO — superior oblique
sodium hyaluronate
Soemmering's
  foramen
  ring
  ring cataract
  spot
soft
  s. cataract
  s. contact lens
  s. exudates
  s. lens
  s. tissue swelling
SOF — superior orbital fissure
solar
  s. burn
  s. keratoma
  s. maculopathy
  s. retinitis
  s. retinopathy
  s. urticaria
solid color
Sondermann's canal
Sonometric Ocuscan
Soria's operation
Soriano's operation
Sorsby's pseudoinflammatory macular dystrophy
soul blindness
sound
  lacrimal s.
Sourdille's
  keratoplasty operation
  ptosis operation
Sovereign bifocal lens
space
  circumlental s.
  corneal s.'s
  episcleral s.
  Fontana's s.
  interfascial s.
  interlamellar s's
  intervaginal s. of optic nerve
  s. of Fontana
  s. of iridocorneal angle
  perichorioidal s.
  perichoroidal s.
  periscleral s.
  prezonular s.
  retrobulbar s.
  retro-ocular s.
  Tenon's s.
  zonular s's
Spaeth's
  cystic bleb operation
  ptosis operation

Spanish silk suture
Spanlang-Tappeiner syndrome
spasm
  s. of accommodation
  facial s.
  nictitating s.
  winking s.
spasmodic
  s. mydriasis
  s. strabismus
spasmus nutans
spastic
  s. ectropion
  s. entropion
  s. lagophthalmos
  s. mydriasis
  s. pseudosclerosis
spatia
  s. anguli iridis
  s. anguli iridocornealis
  s. zonularis
spatial localization
spatium
  s. episclerale
  s. interfasciale
  s. intervaginale
  s. perichorioideale
  s. perichoroideale
spatula
  angulated iris s.
  Bangerter's iris s.
  Barraquer's irrigator s.
  Berens' s.
  Birks Mark II Micro s.
  capsule fragment s.
  Castroviejo's cyclodialysis s.
  Castroviejo's double end s.
  Castroviejo's s.
  Cleasby's s.
  corneal fascia lata s.
  Culler's iris s.

spatula *(continued)*
  cyclodialysis s.
  double s.
  Drews-Sato suture pickup s.
  Elschnig's s.
  Fisher-Smith s.
  French hook s.
  French lacrimal s.
  French pattern s.
  Gill-Welch s.
  Green's s.
  Hertzog's lens s.
  Hirschman's s.
  hook s.
  iris s.
  Jaffe's intraocular s.
  Kimura's s.
  Kirby's angulated iris s.
  Kirby's iris s.
  Knapp's iris s.
  Knapp's s.
  Laird's s.
  Lindner's s.
  Manhattan E & E s.
  Maumenee's vitreous sweep s.
  McPherson's s.
  McReynold's s.
  needle s.
  Olk's vitreoretinal s.
  Paton's double s.
  Paton's single s.
  Paton's transplant s.
  platinum probe s.
  platinum s.
  probe s.
  side-biting s.
  Smith-Fisher s.
  spoon s.
  suture pickup s.
  synechia s.
  Tooke's s.

spatula *(continued)*
 vitreous sweep s.
 Wheeler's s.
spatulated needle
SPC — simultaneous prism and cover test
spear developmental cataract
Speas operation
specificity
speckled corneal dystrophy
spectacles
 compound s.
 decentered s.
 divided s.
 Franklin's s.
 Hallauer's s.
 industrial s.
 Masselon's s.
 mica s.
 pantoscopic s.
 periscopic s.
 prismatic s.
 protective s.
 pulpit s.
 safety s.
 stenopeic s.
 tinted s.
 wire frame s.
spectrocolorimeter
spectrum
 fortification s.
 ocular s.
 visible s.
specula
specular
 s. image
 s. microscope
 s. reflection
Specular Reflex Slit Lamp
speculum
 Alfonso s.
 Barraquer-Colibri s.
 Barraquer's s.

speculum *(continued)*
 basket style scleral support s.
 Becker-Park s.
 Bercovici's wire lid s.
 Berens' s.
 Bronson-Park s.
 Burch-Lester s.
 Castroviejo's s.
 Clark's eye s.
 Cook's s.
 Douvas-Barraquer s.
 eye s.
 Fanta's s.
 fine wire s.
 Fox's s.
 Guist-Bloch s.
 Guyton-Maumenee s.
 Guyton-Park lid s.
 Hirschman's s.
 Iliff-Park s.
 Keeler-Pierse s.
 Keizer-Lancaster s.
 Knapp's s.
 Lancaster's s.
 Lancaster-O'Connor s.
 Lange's s.
 Lester-Burch s.
 lid s.
 Maumenee-Park s.
 McKinney's lid s.
 McPherson's s.
 Mellinger's s.
 Metcher's s.
 Moria's one piece s.
 Mueller's s.
 Murdock-Wiener s.
 Park's s.
 Park-Guyton s.
 Park-Guyton-Callahan s.
 Park-Guyton-Maumenee s.
 Paton's single s.

speculum *(continued)*
- Paton's transplant s.
- pediatric s.
- Sauer's s.
- Smith's s.
- stop s.
- Sutherland-Grieshaber s.
- Weeks' s.
- Weiss' s.
- Wiener's s.
- Williams' s.

Spencer's scissors
Spencer-Watson
- operation
- Z-plasty

Spero's forceps
sph. — spherical lens
sphenoccipital fissure
sphenoid bone
sphenoidal fissure
sphenomaxillary fissure
spheno-occipital
spheno-orbital suture
sphenorbital
sphere
- Doherty's s.
- s. implant
- s. introducer
- Mules' vitreous s.
- Pyrex eye s.

spherical
- s. aberration
- s. equivalent
- s. implant
- s. lens

spherocylinder
spherocylindrical lens
spherocytosis
spherolith
spherophakia
spherule
- rod s.

sphincter
- s. iridis
- s. muscle
- s. oculi
- s. oris
- s. pupillae

sphincterectomy
sphincterolysis
sphingolipidoses
sphingomyelin lipidosis
spicule
spider
- s. angioma
- s. vasculature

Spielmeyer-Vogt disease
spin-cast lens
spina trochlearis
spinal mydriasis
spindle
- Axenfeld-Krukenberg s.
- cataract s.
- Krukenberg's s.

spindle-shaped
- s. area
- s. cells

spiral
- s. field
- s. of Tillaux

Spirilla
splenic retinitis
splenium of corpus callosum
splitting of lacrimal papilla
SPK — superficial punctate keratitis
spoke
spoke-like sutural cataracts
sponge
- Custodis s.
- s. implant
- Krukenberg's s.
- lens s.
- Lincoff's s.
- Microsponge Teardrop s.

sponge *(continued)*
- Pro-Ophtha s.
- Vaiser s.
- vitrectomy s.
- Weck-cel s.

sponge-like

spongioblast

spongy iritis

spontaneous
- s. congenital iris cyst
- s. ectopia lentis

spoon
- Bunge's evisceration s.
- Castroviejo's s.
- Culler's lens s.
- Cutler's lens s.
- Daviel's s.
- Elschnig's s.
- enucleation s.
- evisceration s.
- Fisher's s.
- graft carrier s.
- Hess' s.
- Kalt's s.
- Kirby's intracapsular lens s.
- Knapp's lens s.
- lens s.
- needle s.
- Rizzuti's graft carrier s.
- Schepens' s.
- spatula s.

spot
- acoustic s.
- ash leaf s.
- Bitot's s.
- blind s.
- Brushfield's s.
- cherry red s.
- cotton-wool s.
- cribriform s.
- Elschnig's s.

spot *(continued)*
- eye s.
- Forster-Fuchs black s.
- Fuchs' s.
- Gaule's s.
- Horner-Trantas s.
- Mariotte's s.
- Maxwell's s.
- s. retinoscope
- Roth's s.
- Soemmering's s.
- Tay's s.
- white s.
- Wies' s.
- yellow s.

spot retinoscope
- Ful-Vue s.r.
- Reichert's s.r.

spotty corneal opacities

Spratt mastoid curet

spring
- s. conjunctivitis
- s. ophthalmia
- s. pupil

Spring iris scissors

spud
- Alvis' s.
- Bahn's s.
- Corbett's s.
- Davis' s.
- Dix's s.
- Ellis' s.
- Fisher's s.
- foreign body s.
- Francis' s.
- golf club s.
- gouge s.
- Hosford's lacrimal s.
- LaForce's s.
- Levine's s.
- needle s.
- O'Brien's s.

spud *(continued)*
    Plange's s.
    Walter's s.
    Walton's s.
spur
    scleral s.
Spurway's syndrome
Sputnik Russian razor blade
squamous
    s. seborrheic blepharitis
    s. cell carcinoma
squashed tomato appearance
Squid instrument/apparatus
squint
    accommodative s.
    angle s.
    comitant s.
    convergent s.
    deviation s.
    divergent s.
    downward s.
    s. hook
    noncomitant s.
    upward s.
squirrel plague conjunctivitis
SR — superior rectus
SRNV — subretinal neovascularization
SSPE — subacute sclerosing panencephalitis
Stahli's
    caliper
    line
    pigment line
    nucleus expressor
stain
    acid mucopolysaccharide s.
    acid-Schiff s.
    alcian blue s.
    alkali Congo red s.
    diastase s.

stain *(continued)*
    eosin s.
    Gram s.
    hematoxylin s.
    lead citrate s.
    mucicarmine s.
staining
    corneal s.
stalk
    optic s.
Stallard's
    eyelid operation
    flap operation
Stallard-Liegard suture
staphylococcal
    s. blepharitis
    s. blepharoconjunctivitis
    s. conjunctivitis
Staphylococcus
    S. aureus
    S. epidermidis
staphyloma
    annular s.
    anterior s.
    ciliary s.
    s. corneae
    s. corneae racemosum
    corneal s.
    equatorial s.
    intercalary s.
    posterior s.
    s. posticum
    projecting s.
    retinal s.
    Scarpa's s.
    scleral s.
    uveal s.
staphylomatous
star(s)
    s. formation
    lens s.
    Winslow's s.

star-shaped field
stare
    hyperthyroid s.
starfold
Stargardt's
    disease
    syndrome
Starr's fixation forceps
stasis
    papillary s.
static
    s. perimeters
    s. refraction
stationary cataract
statometer
stave
steepest meridian
Steinhauser electro-mucotome
stella
    s. lentis hyaloidea
    s. lentis iridica
stellate cataract
Stellwag's
    brawny edema
    sign
    symptom
stenocoriasis
stenosis
    s. canaliculus
    punctum s.
stenopeic
    s. disk
    s. iridectomy
    s. spectacles
stenophotic
stenosal
stenosed
stenosis
stenotic
stent
step
    corneal graft s.
    Ronne's nasal s.
Step-Knife diamond blade knife
Stephenson's needle holder
stepwise fashion
stereo acuity
Stereo-Orthopter
stereocampimeter
stereogram
stereo-ophthalmoscope
stereophoroscope
stereopsis test
stereoscope
stereoscopic vision
Steri-Drape
sterile
    s. adhesive bubble chamber
    s. endophthalmitis
Steriseal disposable cannula
Stevens'
    forceps
    hook
    needle holder
    tenotomy hook
    tenotomy scissors
Stevens-Charles sleeve
Stevens-Johnson syndrome
Stevenson's
    lacrimal sac retractor
    refractor
Stickler's syndrome
Stifel's figure
stiff
    s. pupil
    s. retina
    s. retinal folds
stigmata
stigmatometer
stigmatoscope
stigmatoscopy
Stiles-Crawford effect
stiletto
    Berkley Bioengineering s.

stiletto
knife s.
Still's disease
stillicidium lacrimarum
Stilling's color test
Stilling-Turk-Duane syndrome
Stimson's sign
stimulus
stippling and staining
stitch
bow-tie s.
cuticular s.
s. removing knife
shoelace s.
triple throw square knot s.
s. with twists
zipper s.
Stock's operation
Stock-Spielmeyer-Vogt syndrome
Stocker's
line
needle
operation
Stocker-Holt-Schneider dystrophy
Stokes' lens
Stone's implant
stop speculum
Storz's
cataract knife
corneal bur
corneoscleral punch
keratome
Microvit magnet
Microvit vitrector
Storz-Atlas hand eye magnet
Storz-Bell erysiphake
Storz-Duredge steel cataract knife
Storz-Utrata forceps
Storz-Walker retinal detachment unit
Storz-Westcott conjunctiva scissors
strabismic
s. amblyopia
s. deviation
strabismometer
strabismus
A-pattern s.
absolute s.
accommodative s.
alternating s.
bilateral s.
binocular s.
Braid's s.
comitant s.
concomitant s.
convergent s.
constant s.
convergent s.
cyclic s.
s. deorsum vergens
divergent s.
dynamic s.
external s.
s. fixus
incomitant s.
intermittent s.
internal s.
kinetic s.
latent s.
manifest s.
mechanical s.
mixed s.
monocular s.
monolateral s.
muscular s.
noncomitant s.
nonconcomitant s.
nonparalytic s.
paralytic s.
periodic s.

strabismus *(continued)*
- relative s.
- spasmodic s.
- suppressed s.
- s. sursum vergens
- unilateral s.
- uniocular s.
- vertical s.

strabometer
strabometry
strabotome
strabotomy
Straith's eyelid operation
Strampelli's lens implant
Strampelli-Valvo operation
stratified
stratum
- cerebral s. of retina
- s. cerebrale retinae
- ganglionic s. of optic nerve
- ganglionic s. of retina

strawberry hemangiomas
streak(s)
- angioid s.
- Knapp's s.
- s. retinoscope
- s. retinoscopy

Streatfield's operation
Streatfield-Fox operation
Streatfield-Snellen operation
Streptococcus pneumoniae
streptotrichosis
stria
striae
- s. ciliaris
- Knapp's s.

striascope
striatal nigral degeneration
striate
- s. keratitis
- s. melanokeratosis
- s. opacities
- s. retinitis

striated
striation
striatum
string of pearls
stroboscopic disk
stroma
- s. of cornea
- s. of iris
- s. plexus
- vitreous s.
- s. vitreum

stromal
- s. bed
- s. blood vessel
- s. haze
- s. keratitis
- s. matrix
- s. melting
- s. mucopolysaccharide
- s. opacities
- s. splitting
- s. strands
- s. thickness
- s. vascularization

strumous ophthalmia
Stryker's frame
Sturge-Weber syndrome
Sturm's
- conoid
- interval

stuttering velocities
sty
- meibomian s.
- zeisian s.

stye
styes or sties (pl. of sty)
Suarez-Villafranca operation
subacute sclerosing panencephalitis
subarachnoid bleed
subcapsular
- s. cataract
- s. plaque

subchoroidal

Subco needle
subconjunctiva
subconjunctival
  s. emphysema
  s. hemorrhage
  s. injection
  s. needle
subconjunctivally
subcortical alexia
subcutaneous fat atrophy
subduct
subduction
subendothelial
subepithelial
  s. punctate corneal infiltrate
subfoveal
subhyaloid hemorrhage
subinternal
subjective refraction test
subjectoscope
sublatio retinae
subluxation of lens
subluxed lens
subnormal vision
suboptimal vision
suborbital
subpigment epithelial space
subretinal
  s. fluid
  s. neovascularization
  s. space
subscleral
subsclerotic
subsector
substance
  cortical s. of lens
  corneal s.
  s. exophthalmos
  s. of lens
  scleral s.
substantia
  s. corticalis lentis
  s. lentis

substantia *(continued)*
  s. propria
  s. propria corneae
substrate
succulent vessel
sugar-loaf cornea
Suker's sign
sulcus
  chiasmal s.
  infraorbital s. of maxilla
  s. infraorbitalis maxillae
  infrapalpebral s.
  s. infrapalpebralis
  intramarginal s.
  lacrimal s.
  optic s.
  orbital s.
  s. orbitales lobi frontalis
  s. sclerae
  scleral s.
  sclerocorneal s.
  supraorbital s.
Summerskill's operation
sunburst
  s. dial
  s. effect
sunburst-type lesions
sunflower cataract
sunglasses
sunrise syndrome
Super Pinky Ball
Superblade
  No. 75
  trapezoid
supercilia
superciliary arch
supercilium
superduct
superduction
superficial punctate keratitis
superimposition
superior
  s. arcade
  s. canaliculus

superior *(continued)*
- s. cervical ganglion
- s. fornix
- s. limbic keratoconjunctivitis
- s. myokymia
- s. nasal artery
- s. nasal vein
- s. oblique
- s. oblique palsy
- s. oblique tendon sheath syndrome
- s. ophthalmic vein
- s. orbital fissure
- s. orbital fissure syndrome
- s. palsy
- s. punctum
- s. quadrantanopia
- s. radial tenotomy scissors
- s. rectus
- s. sector iridectomy
- s. tarsus
- s. temporal artery
- s. temporal vein
- s. tendon of Lockwood
- s. tendon sheath syndrome
- s. vascular arcade

superioris
superonasal
superonasally
superoccipital
supertraction conus
superversion
suppressed strabismus
suppression amblyopia
suppuration
suppurative
- s. choroiditis
- s. keratitis
- s. retinitis

suprachoroid lamina
suprachoroidal
suprachoroidea
supraciliary canal
supraduction
Supramid
- Allen implant
- bridle collagen suture
- lens implant
- sheet
- suture

supranuclear pathways
supraocular
supraoptic
- s. canal
- s. commissure

supraorbital
- s. arch of frontal bone
- s. artery
- s. canal
- s. foramen
- s. margin of orbit
- s. nerve
- s. neuralgia
- s. notch
- s. point
- s. reflex
- s. ridge
- s. sulcus
- s. vein

suprascleral
suprasellar meningioma
supratrochlear nerve
supraversion
surface
- s. analgesia
- s. breakdown
- s. implant

Surg-E-Trol I/A/R System
Surgamid
surgical
- s. gut suture
- s. patch grafting

Surgidev
intraocular lens
suture
Surgikos drape
surplus field
sursumduction
sursumvergence
sursumversion
suspension
suspensory ligament
Sussman 4-mirror gonioscope
Sutherland Rotatable Microsurgery Instruments
Sutherland-Grieshaber
scissors
speculum
sutura
s. ethmoidolacrimalis
s. ethmoidomaxillaris
s. frontolacrimalis
s. infraorbitalis
s. lacrimoconchalis
s. lacrimomaxillaris
s. palato-ethmoidalis
s. palatomaxillaris
s. spheno-ethmoidalis
s. sphenofrontalis
s. spheno-orbitalis
sutural
s. cataract
s. developmental cataract
suture
absorbable s.
Alcon s.
Atroloc s.
black braided nylon s.
black braided silk s.
braided silk s.
braided Vicryl s.
chromic catgut s.
chromic collagen s.
coated Vicryl s.
Custodis s.

suture *(continued)*
Dacron s.
Davis-Geck s.
Deknatel silk s.
Dermalon s.
Dexon s.
double-armed s.
Ethicon Atroloc s.
Ethicon Micro-Point s.
Ethicon Sabreloc s.
Ethilon s.
Faden s.
Foster s.
frontolacrimal s.
frontosphenoid s.
Frost s.
Gaillard-Arlt s.
infraorbital s.
lacrimoconchal s.
lacrimo-ethmoidal s.
lacrimomaxillary s.
lacrimoturbinal s.
lancet s.
Look s.
Mannis s.
McLean s.
Mersilene s.
Micro-Point s.
monofilament nylon s.
nonabsorbable s.
Nurolon s.
nylon 66 s.
nylon s.
palatomaxillary s.
s. pickup spatula
plain catgut s.
plain collagen s.
polyester s.
polyglactin s.
Prolene s.
Quickert s.
Shoch s.
Spanish silk s.

suture *(continued)*
- sphenofrontal s.
- spheno-orbital s.
- Supramid bridle collagen s.
- Supramid s.
- Surgamid s.
- surgical gut s.
- Surgidev s.
- Swiss silk s.
- transverse s. of Krause
- twisted virgin silk s.
- Vicryl s.
- virgin silk s.
- white braided silk s.

suturing needle

Swan's
- discission knife
- incision
- knife
- lancet
- needle
- syndrome

Sweet's
- locator
- method
- original magnet

swelling
- Soemmering's crystalline s.

Swets goniotomy knife cannula

swimming pool conjunctivitis

swinging flashlight test

swinging light test

Swiss
- bladebreaker
- silk suture

sycosiform

sycosis tarsi

syllabic blindness

Sylva's
- anterior chamber irrigator

Sylva's *(continued)*
- irrigator and aspirator unit

Sylvian's aqueduct syndrome

symblepharon
- anterior s.
- posterior s.
- s. ring
- total s.

symblepharopterygium

symmetric surgery

sympathetic
- s. iridoplegia
- s. nervous system
- s. ophthalmia
- s. pathway
- s. uveitis

sympathizing eye

sympatholytic

symptom
- Anton's s.
- Berger's s.
- Haenel's s.
- halo s.
- Liebreich's s.
- Magendie's s.
- rainbow s.
- Stellweg's s.
- Wernicke's s.

symptomatic

synaphymenitis

synathroisis

syncanthus

synchesis
- s. corporis vitrei
- s. scintillans

syndectomy

syndesmitis

syndrome
- A and V s.
- accommodative effort s.
- adherence s.
- adhesive s.

syndrome *(continued)*
- Adie's s.
- Ahlström's s.
- Aicardi's s.
- Albright's s.
- Alezzandrini's s.
- Alport's s.
- Alström-Olsen s.
- Anderson's s.
- Andosky's s.
- Angelucci's s.
- anterior chamber cleavage s.
- Anton's s.
- Anton-Babinski s.
- aortic arch s.
- Apert's s.
- Ascher's s.
- ataxia-telangiectasia s.
- Axenfeld's s.
- BADS s.
- Balint's s.
- Bamatter's s.
- Bardet-Biedl s.
- Bassen-Kornzweig s.
- Batten-Mayou s.
- Beal's s.
- Behçet's s.
- Behr's s.
- Benedict's s.
- Bernard's s.
- Bernard-Horner s.
- Bielschowsky-Lutz-Cogan s.
- Bietti's s.
- blepharophimosis ptosis s.
- Bloch-Stauffer s.
- Block-Sulzberger s.
- Bonnet-Dechaume-Blanc s.
- Bonnier's s.
- brittle cornea s.

syndrome *(continued)*
- Brown's vertical retraction s.
- Brushfield-Wyatt s.
- capsular exfoliation s.
- cat's eye s.
- cavernous sinus s.
- Cestan's s.
- Cestan-Chenais s.
- Chandler's s.
- Charlin's s.
- Chédiak-Higashi s.
- Claude Bernard-Horner s.
- chiasma s.
- chiasmatic s.
- Cockayne's s.
- co-contraction s.
- Cogan's s.
- Collins' s.
- Conradi's s.
- craniofacial s.
- cri-du-chat s.
- Crouzon's s.
- Cushing's s.
- de Mosier's s.
- DeGrouchy's s.
- Dejean's s.
- dorsal midbrain s.
- Down's s.
- Doyne's s.
- dry eye s.
- Duane's s.
- D trisomy s.
- E s.
- Edwards' s.
- Ehlers-Danlos s.
- Elschnig's s.
- Fabry's s.
- fetal alcohol s.
- Fisher's s.
- Fitz-Hugh-Curtis s.
- Foix's s.

syndrome *(continued)*
- Forsius-Eriksson s.
- Forssman's carotid s.
- Foster-Kennedy s.
- Foville's s.
- Foville-Wilson s.
- Franceschetti's s.
- Franceschetti-Klein s.
- Francois' s.
- Friedenwald's s.
- Fuchs' s.
- Fuchs-Kraupa s.
- Gerstmann's s.
- Goldenhar's s.
- Goldmann-Favre s.
- Goltz-Gorlin s.
- Gradenigo's s.
- Graefe's s.
- Gregg's s.
- Greig's s.
- Gronblad-Strandberg s.
- Guillain-Barré s.
- Gunn's s.
- Hallermann-Streiff s.
- Hallermann-Streiff-Francois s.
- Harada's s.
- Heerfordt's s.
- Heidenhaim's s.
- hereditary benign intraepithelial s.
- heredodegenerative neurologic s.
- Hermansky-Pudlak s.
- Hertwig-Magendie s.
- Hippel-Lindau s.
- histoplasmosis s.
- Homén's s.
- Horner's s.
- Horner-Bernard s.
- Horton's s.
- Hunter's s.
- Hunter-Hurler s.

syndrome *(continued)*
- Hurler's s.
- Hurler-Scheie s.
- Hutchinson's s.
- hyperophthalmopathic s.
- Irvine-Gass s.
- Jansky-Bielschowsky s.
- jaw-winking s.
- Johnson's s.
- Kearns-Sayre s.
- Kennedy's s.
- Kiloh-Nevin s.
- Kimmelstiel-Wilson s.
- Klinefelter's s.
- Klippel-Feil s.
- Koeppe's s.
- Koerber-Salus-Elschnig s.
- Krause's s.
- Kufs' s.
- Kurz's s.
- lateral medullary s.
- Laurence-Moon-Biedl s.
- Lawford's s.
- Leber's s.
- Letterer-Siwe s.
- Lignac-Fanconi s.
- Louis-Bar s.
- Lowe's s.
- Lowe-Terry-Machlachan s.
- Lyle's s.
- Marchesani's s.
- Marcus Gunn s.
- Marcus Gunn jaw-winking s.
- Marfan's s.
- Marinesco-Sjögren s.
- Maroteaux-Lamy s.
- Melkersson's s.
- Melkersson-Rosenthal s.
- Menkes' s.
- Mikulicz's s.
- Millard-Gubler s.

syndrome *(continued)*
- Miller's s.
- Möbius' s.
- Monakow's s.
- monofixation s.
- monosomy G s.
- morning glory s.
- Morquio's s.
- Morquio-Brailsford s.
- nephrotic s.
- oculocerebrorenal s.
- oculoglandular s.
- Osler-Rendu-Weber s.
- Ota's nevus s.
- overwear s.
- Parinaud's s.
- Parinaud's oculoglandular s.
- Patau's s.
- Petzetakis-Takos s.
- Pierre-Robin s.
- Posner-Schlossman s.
- Potter's s.
- Prader-Willi s.
- Raeder's s.
- Raymond-Cestan s.
- Recklinghausen's s.
- Reese's s.
- Reiter's s.
- retraction s.
- Richner-Hanhart s.
- Riddoch's s.
- Rieger's s.
- Riley-Day s.
- Riley-Smith s.
- Ring D chromosome s.
- Rollet's s.
- Rot-Bielschowsky s.
- Roth's spot s.
- Rothmund's s.
- Rothmund-Thomson s.
- Rutherford's s.
- Sanfilippo's s.

syndrome *(continued)*
- Schafer's s.
- Scheie's s.
- Schmid-Fraccaro s.
- Shea's s.
- sheath s.
- sicca s.
- Siegrist-Hutchinson s.
- Sjögren's s.
- Spanlang-Tappeiner s.
- Spurway's s.
- Stargardt's s.
- Stevens-Johnson s.
- Stickler's s.
- Stilling-Turk-Duane s.
- Stock-Spielmeyer-Vogt s.
- Sturge-Weber s.
- Sturge-Weber-Dimitri s.
- sunrise s.
- Swan's s.
- Sylvian aquaduct s.
- tectal midbrain s.
- tegmental s.
- Terry's s.
- Terson's s.
- Thompson's s.
- Thomson's s.
- Tolosa-Hunt s.
- Touraine's s.
- Treacher-Collins s.
- Turner's s.
- Usher's s.
- uveitis-vitiligo-alopecia-poliosis s.
- Uyemura's s.
- van der Hoeve's s.
- vitreous wick s.
- Vogt's s.
- Vogt-Koyanagi s.
- Vogt-Koyanagi-Harada s.
- von Graefe's s.
- von Recklinghausen's s.
- Vs.

- syndrome *(continued)*
  - Waardenburg's s.
  - Waardenburg-Klein s.
  - Wallenberg's s.
  - Weber's s.
  - Weber-Dubler s.
  - Weill-Marchesani s.
  - Werner's s.
  - Wernicke's s.
  - white dot s.
  - Wilson's s.
  - wipe-out s.
  - Wiskott-Aldrich s.
  - Wolf's s.
  - Wyburn-Mason s.
  - Zellweger's s.
- synechia
  - annular s.
  - anterior s.
  - circular s.
  - iris s.
  - peripheral anterior s.
  - posterior s.
  - s. spatula
  - total anterior s.
  - total posterior s.
- synechiae
- synechialysis
- synechiotome
- synechiotomy
- synechotome
- synechotomy
- synephris
- syneresis
- synergist
- synizesis
- synkinesis
  - external pterygoid-levator s.
  - s. pupillae
- synkinetic
  - s. movements
  - s. near reflex
- synophrys
- synophthalmia
- synophthalmus
- synoptophore
- synoptoscope
- syphilis
- syphilitic
  - s. episcleritis
  - s. ocular disease
  - s. optic perineuritis
  - s. retinitis
  - s. scleritis
- syringe
  - Anel's s.
  - probe s.
- system
  - dioptric s.
- systemic
  - s. lupus erythematosus
  - s. sclerosis
- Szymanowski's operation
- Szymanowski-Kuhnt operation

t

- 3-M small aperture Steri-Drape
- T — tension
- T-tube
  - cul-de-sac irrigation T.
  - Houser cul-de-sac irrigator T.
  - lacrimal duct T.
  - polyethylene T.
  - Pyrex T.
  - Silastic T.
  - vinyl T.
- table
  - Reuss' t.
- taco test
- tactile

Taillefer's valve
Takahashi's forceps
Takayasu's disease
Takata laser
talantropia
Talbot's unit
tamponade
tamponage
tangency
tangent screen
tangential
Tangier's disease
Tansley's operation
tantalum
    t. clips
    t. mesh implant
TAP — tension applanation
taper-cut needle
taper-point needle
tapetal light reflex
tapetochoroidal dystrophy
tapetoretinal degeneration
tapetoretinopathy
tapetum
    t. choroideae
    t. lucidum
    t. nigrum
    t. oculi
tapioca iris melanoma
tarsadenitis
tarsal
    t. arteries
    t. canal
    t. gland
    t. muscle
    t. plate
tarsalis
tarsectomy
tarsi
tarsitis
tarsocheiloplasty
tarsomalacia
tarso-orbital
tarsoplasia
tarsoplasty
tarsorrhaphy
tarsotomy
tarsus
    inferior t. palpebrae
    t. osseus
    superior t. palpebrae
Tasia's operation
tattoo
tattooed
tattooing
    t. needle
    t. of cornea
tax double needle
Tay's
    choroiditis
    spot
Tay-Sachs disease
Teale-Knapp operation
tear
    giant t.
    horseshoe t.
    t. break-up time
    t. drainage system
    t. duct patency
    t. film
    t. film break-up time
    t. gas
    t. lake
    t. meniscus
    t. puncta
    t. sac
tear at 11 o'clock
tear-induced retinal detachment
teardrop pupil
tears
    crocodile t.
technique
    Atkinson's t.
    bare scleral t.
    Brockhurst's t.
    feeder-frond t.

technique *(continued)*
- letterbox t.
- McLean's t.
- Okamura's t.
- Schepens' t.
- Van Lint's t.

tectal midbrain syndrome
Teflon
- implant
- plates
- plug
- sheet

tegmental syndrome
teichopsia
tela
- t. cellulosa
- t. conjunctiva
- t. elastica

telangiectasia
- essential t.
- spider t.

telangiectatic
telea
telebinocular
telecanthus
teleopsia
Telfa dressing
Tellais' sign
TE-MOO mode beam laser
temple length
temporal
- t. arcade
- t. arteriole of retina
- t. arteritis
- t. artery biopsy
- t. artery pallor
- t. bulbar conjunctiva
- t. crescent
- t. hemianopia
- t. island of visual field
- t. lobe
- t. loop
- Myer's t. loop

temporal *(continued)*
- t. raphe
- t. retina
- t. venule of retina
- t. wedge

temporalis muscle
temporoparietal lobe
tenaculum
tenectomy
tendinous insertion
tendo
- t. oculi
- t. palpebrarum

tendon
- Brown's t.
- Lockwood's t.
- superior oblique t.
- Zinn's t.

tendon tucker
- Bishop's t.t.
- Bishop-Peter t.t.
- Burch's t.t.
- Burch-Greenwood t.t.
- Fink's t.t.
- Ruedemann-Todd t.t.

tendotome
tendotomy
Tennant's lens
Tenner's
- lacrimal cannula
- titanium suturing forceps

tenonectomy
tenonitis
- brawny t.

tenonometer
tenonotomy
Tenon's
- capsule
- fascia bulbi
- membrane
- space

tenosynovitis
tenotome

tenotomist
tenotomize
tenotomy
  curb t.
  free t.
  t. hook
  intrasheath t.
  t. of ocular tendon
tensile strength of vessels
Tensilon test
tension
  t. by applanation
  intraocular t.
  t. of eye
  tactile t.
  t. test
tensor insertion
tenting
tentorii ramus
Tenzel elevator
teratoma
terminus
Terrien's
  degeneration
  ulcer
Terry's
  keratometer
  silicone capsule polisher
  syndrome
Terson's operation
tertiary
  t. positions
  t. vitreous
tessellated fundus
Tessier's clefting
test
  cocaine t.
  DIVA t.
  Jaeger's t.
  letter t.
  pilocarpine t.
  Snellen's t.

test *(continued)*
  Tensilon t.
  Titmus stereoacuity t.
test card
  stigmometric t.c.
Tests and materials. *See instrument section.*
tetartanope
tetartanopia
tetartanopic
tetartanopsia
tetrachromic
tetrafilcon A
tetranopsia
tetrastichiasis
text blindness
thalamolenticular
thalamus
thaw-freeze
Theimich's lip sign
thelaziasis
Theobald's probe
Theodore's keratoconjunctivitis
theory
  Hering's t.
  Ladd-Franklin t.
  opponent colors t.
  Schon's t.
  Young-Helmholtz t.
therapeutic iridectomy
thermal
  t. adhesions
  t. burns
thermosclerostomy
thermosclerotomy
thermosector
third
  t. cranial nerve
  t. grade fusion
  t. nerve palsy
Thomas'
  brush
  cannula

Thomas' *(continued)*
 cryopter
 cryoretractor
 fixation forceps
 Kapsule Instruments
 operation
 retractor
Thompson's syndrome
Thomson's syndrome
Thorpe's
 caliper
 forceps
 scissors
Thorpe-Castroviejo
 caliper
 corneal forceps
 fixation forceps
 goniolens
 scissors
 vitreous foreign body forceps
Thorpe-Westcott scissors
Thrasher lens implant forceps
threat reflex
three-mirror lens
three-snip punctum
three-step test
three-way stopcock
threshold
 achromatic t.
 displacement t.
 t. of visual sensation
thrombi
thrombocytopenia
thrombosed artery
Thygeson's
 keratitis
 superficial punctate keratopathy
thymoma
thyroid
 t. lid retraction
 t. orbitopathy
 t. stare
thyrotoxic exophthalmos
thyrotropic exophthalmos
tic
 local t.
 motor t.
tic douloureux
Ticho's
 pliable iris retractor
 zonule sweeper
t.i.d. — three times a day
tie-over dressing
tigroid
 t. background
 t. fundus
 t. retina
Tilderquist's needle holder
Tillaux's spiral
Tillett's operation
Tillyer's bifocal lens
tilt of sella
tilted disk
tinea
 t. capitis
 t. facei
 t. tarsi
tinted lens
tire
 276 t.
 implant t.
 silicone t.
 Watzke's t.
tisiris. See phthiriasis
tissue
 episcleral t.
 sustentacular t.
titanium
 t. needle
 t. suturing forceps
Titmus
 stereoacuity test
 test
 vision test
titrated
titration

TN — tension
TNO stereo test
tobacco/alcohol amblyopia
TOD — tension of right eye
Todd's
 cautery
 gouge
 paralysis
Tolentino's vitreous cutter
Tolentinoo's ring
Tolosa-Hunt syndrome
Tomas'
 iris hook
 suture hook
tomography
tonic
 t. accommodation
 t. convergence
 t. lids
 t. pupil
tonofibrils
 t. tendinous xanthoma
 t. tuberous xanthoma
tonofilaments
tonogram
tonograph
tonography
tonometer
 air-puff contact t.
 Alcon t.
 Allen-Schiotz t.
 applanation t.
 Aus Jena-Schiotz t.
 Berens' t.
 Carl Zeiss t.
 Challenger's t.
 Coburn's t.
 Digilab t.
 electronic t.
 Goldmann's applanation t.
 Harrington's t.
 impression t.
 indentation t.
tonometer *(continued)*
 Intermedics intraocular t.
 Keeler's t.
 Lombert's t.
 MacKay-Marg electronic t.
 McLean's t.
 noncontract t.
 Perkins' applanation t.
 pneumotonometer
 Pulsair t.
 Reichert's t.
 Rosner's t.
 Ruedemann's t.
 Schiotz's t.
 Sklar-Schiotz t.
 Storz's t.
 Tono-Pen t.
tonometry
 applanation t.
 digital t.
 indentation t.
Tooke's
 knife
 spatula
Tooke-Johnson corneal knife
Topcon's
 aspheric lens
 camera
 chart projector
 digital lensmeter
 LM P5 digital lensmeter
 lensometer
 perimeter
 refractometer
 refractor
 slit lamp
 vision tester
tophi
topical anesthesia
topographic agnosia
toric lens
toricity
torpor retinae

torque
torsion
torsional diplopia
torticollis
    ocular t.
tortuosity
tortuous
TOS — tension of left eye
tosis. See ptosis
total
    t. astigmatism
    t. blindness
    t. cataract
    t. hyperopia
    t. hyphema
    t. posterior synechia
    t. symblepharon
Toti's operation
Toti-Mosher operation
Touraine's syndrome
Touton's giant cells
Townley-Paton operation
toxic
    t. amblyopia
    t. cataract
    t. conjunctivitis
Toxocara canis
toxocariasis
Toxoplasma gondii
toxoplasmic retinochoroiditis
toxoplasmosis
    ocular t.
TPI test — treponema pallidum immobilization test
trabecular
    t. membrane
    t. meshwork
    t. network
trabeculectomy
trabeculitis
trabeculodysgenesis
trabeculoplasty
    laser t.
trabeculopuncture
trabeculotome
    Allen-Burian t.
    Harms' t.
    McPherson's t.
trabeculotomy
trachoma
    Arlt's t.
    t. body
    brawny t.
    gland t.
    t. inclusion conjunctivitis
trachomata
trachomatous
    t. conjunctivitis
    t. keratitis
tracks
    bear t.
    snail t.
Tracor Northern
Tracoustic RV275
tract
    optic t.
    uveal t.
traction
    t. band
    t. detachment
    t. suture
tractional
    t. retinal degeneration
    t. retinal detachment
Trainor-Nida operation
trampoline
transcleral
transconjunctival
transducer
transferred ophthalmia
transfixion of iris
transient
    t. early exophthalmos
    t. obscuration of vision

transient *(continued)*
t. vertebrobasilar ischemia
t. visual obscuration
transillumination test
transilluminator
Finnoff t.
transition zone
translimbal
translucent
transocular
transorbital leukotomy
trans pars plana
transplant
corneal t.
ocular muscle t.
Transpore eye tape
transposition
transverse axis of Fick
transverse suture of Krause
transvitreal
transynaptic
Trantas'
dots
operation
trap door technique
trap incision
trapezoid
trapezoidal incision
Traquair
scotoma of T.
traumatic
t. amblyopia
t. cataract
t. corneal abrasion
t. corneal cyst
t. degenerative cataract
t. glaucoma
t. hyphema
t. ptosis
t. scleral cyst
Treacher-Collins syndrome
treatment

treatment *(continued)*
Imre's t.
Scholer's t.
trematode infection
tremulous
t. cataract
t. iris
trepanation
corneal t.
trephination
open-sky t.
trephine
Arruga's lacrimal t.
automatic t.
Bard-Parker t.
Barraquer's t.
Barron's epikeratophakia t.
Bonaccolto's t.
Boston's t.
Brown-Pusey corneal t.
Castroviejo's corneal transplant t.
chalazion t.
corneal t.
Davis' t.
Dimitry chalazion t.
Elliott's t.
Elschnig's t.
Gradle's corneal t.
Green's t.
Grieshaber's corneal t.
Guyton's corneal transplant t.
Hessburg-Barron vacuum t.
Iliff's lacrimal t.
Katena's t.
King's corneal t.
lacrimal t.
Lichtenberg's corneal t.
Martinez's disposable corneal t.

trephine *(continued)*
Mueller's electric corneal t.
Paton's corneal t.
Paufique's t.
Scheie's t.
Searcy's chalazion t.
Treponema pallidum
triad
Charcot's t.
Hutchinson's t.
t. of retinal cone
triangle
color t.
frontal t.
Wernicke's t.
triangular capsulotomy
trichiasis
trichinosis
trichoma
trichomatopsia
trichomatous
trichophytosis
trichosis carunculae
trichromasy
trichromat
trichromatic
trichromatism
trichromatopsia
trichromic
trifacial neuralgia
trifocal lens
trigeminal
t. nerve
t. neuralgia
t. neuropathic keratopathy
trigeminus reflex
trigone
Müller's t.
trilamellar
triopathy
Tripier's operation
triple
t. throw square knot
t. vision
triple-facet tip needle
triplokoria
triplopia
tripod
triptokoria
trisomy D
trisomy 13
trisomy 18
trisomy 21
tristichia
tritan
tritanomal
tritanomalous
tritanomaly
tritanope
tritanopia
tritanopic
tritanopsia
trochlea
t. musculi obliqui superioris bulbi
t. musculi obliqui superioris oculi
t. of superior oblique muscle
trochlear
t. fovea
t. muscle
t. nerve
troland
Troncoso's
gonioscope
gonioscopic lens implant
trophic retinal degeneration
tropia deviation
tropometer
troposcope
trough level
Troutman's
bladebreaker

Troutman's *(continued)*
- cannula
- conjunctiva scissors
- corneal knife
- implant
- lens loupe
- microsurgical scissors
- needle holder
- operation
- punch
- rectus forceps
- suture scissors
- tenotomy trephine
- trephine
- tying forceps

Troutman-Barraquer corneal fixation forceps
Troutman-Castroviejo corneal fixation forceps
Troutman-Katzin corneal transplant scissors
Troutman-Llobera fixation forceps
Truc's
- flap
- operation

true
- t. exfoliation
- t. hemianopia

Trump's solution
T-tube
tube
- Bowman's t.
- corneal t's
- fil d'Arion t.
- fusion t's
- Guibor's Silastic t.
- Houser's cul-de-sac irrigator t.
- Jones Pyrex t.
- L. T. Jones tear duct t.
- Moulton's lacrimal duct t.
- polyethylene t.

tube *(continued)*
- Quickert-Dryden t.
- silicone t.
- vinyl t.

tuber
- frontal t.

tubercle
- lacrimal t.
- lateral orbit t.
- lateral palpebral t.
- trochlear t.
- Whitnall's t.

tuberculosis
tuberous sclerosis
tubular visual fields
tuck procedure
tucker
- Burch-Greenwood t.
- Green's muscle t.
- Green's strabismus t.

Tudor-Thomas graft
tufts
tularemia
- t. conjunctivitis
- oculoglandular t.

Tulevech cannula
tumbling
- in t. fashion
- t. procedure
- t. technique

tumefaction
tumor
- cerebellar astrocytoma t.
- choristoma t.
- cystic hydrocystoma t.
- ependymona t.
- fibro-osseous t.
- medulloblastoma t.
- mucinous adenocarcinoma t.
- papilliform t.
- phakomatous choristoma t.

tumor *(continued)*
- pilomatrixoma t.
- retinal anlage t.
- springoma t.
- trichofolliculoma t.
- waxy t.

tunable dye laser
tunic
- fibrous t.
- Ruysch's t.

tunica
- t. adnata oculi
- t. albuginea oculi
- t. conjunctiva bulbi oculi
- t. conjunctiva palpebrae
- t. fibrosa bulbi
- t. fibrosa oculi
- t. interna bulbi
- t. nervea of Brücke's
- t. nervosa oculi
- t. ruyschiana
- t. sclerotica
- t. senoria bulbi
- t. uvea
- t. vascularis oculi
- t. vasculosa bulbi
- t. vasculosa lentis
- t. vasculosa oculi

tunicary
tunnel vision
tunneled implant
turbidity
Turk's line
Turkish saddle
Turner's syndrome
tutamina oculi
TVA — true visual acuity
twelfth nerve palsy
twilight
- t. blindness
- t. vision

twin cone
Twisk micro scissors
twist fixation hook
twisted virgin silk suture
two-angled polypropylene loops
two-way
- t. cataract aspirating cannula
- t. syringe
- t. towel clip

Tycos manometer
tylosis ciliaris
tylotic
Tyndall's effect
typhlology
typhlosis
typical coloboma
typoscope
Tyrell's
- iris hook
- tympanic membrane hook

U

ubiquitous
UGH syndrome — uveitis glaucoma hyphema syndrome
Ulanday's double cannula
ulcer
- catarrhal corneal u.
- central u.
- corneal u.
- dendriform u.
- dendritic u.
- hypopyon u.
- Jacob's u.
- marginal u.
- Mooren's u.
- pneumococcus u.

ulcer *(continued)*
ring u.
Saemisch's u.
serpiginous corneal u.
suppurative u.
ulcera
ulcerate
ulceration
ulcerative
ulcerogenic
ulcerogranuloma
ulceromembranous
ulcerous
ulcus serpens corneae
ulectomy
ulerythema ophryogenes
Ulloa's operation
Ultex lens implant
Ultra-Image
A scan
SCAN
Ultramatic
Project-O-Chart
Rx master phoroptor
ultrascan
Digital B System
ultrasonic
u. cataract removal lancet
u. Micrometer
ultrasonographic
ultrasonogram
A scan u.
B scan u.
Doppler u.
gray-scale u.
ultrasonography
ultrasound
UltraThin surgical blades
ultraviolet
u. radiation
u. ray ophthalmia
umbrella iris
uncinate process of lacrimal bone
uncrossed diplopia
undine
undulate
unguis
unharmonious ARC
unifocal optic nerve lesion
unilateral
u. altitudinal scotoma
u. arcus
u. hemianopia
u. microtremor
u. proptosis
u. strabismus
uniocular
u. hemianopia
u. strabismus
uniplanar
unit
Bovie u.
Mira u.
United Sonics J shock phaco fragmentor system
Universal
conformer
eyeshield
unrefined refraction
unstained wet mount
up-gaze
upbeat nystagmus
upper
u. canaliculus
u. hemianopia
u. punctum
u. retina
upside down
u.d. ptosis
u.d. reversal of vision
urate band keratopathy
uratic conjunctivitis
uremic
u. amaurosis

uremic *(continued)*
- u. amblyopia
- u. retinitis

Uribe's orbital implant
Usher's syndrome
UV Nova Curve lens
uvea
uveal
- u. effusion
- u. framework
- u. juvenile xanthogranuloma
- u. melanoma
- u. staphyloma
- u. tract

uveitic
uveitides
uveitis
- anterior u.
- aspergillosis u.
- Förster's u.
- granulomatous u.
- heterochromic u.
- lens-induced u.
- nongranulomatous u.
- phacolytic u.
- phacotoxic u.
- posterior u.
- sympathetic u.
- toxoplasmic u.
- tuberculous u.
- vitiligo u.

uveitis-vitiligo-alopecia-poliosis syndrome
uveolabyrinthitis
uveomeningitis
uveoneuroaxitis
uveoparotid
uveoparotitis
uveoplasty
uveoretinitis
uveoscleritis
Uyemura's syndrome

V

V slit lamp
V syndrome
V-lance
- blade/knife
- knife
- Sharpoint

V-pattern
- esotropia
- exotropia

VA — visual acuity
VA magnetic orbital implant
vaccinia
- blepharoconjunctivitis v.
- v. gangrenosa
- generalized v.
- v. infection
- progressive v.

vaccinial keratitis
Vactro perilimbal suction apparatus
vacuolar
vacuolation
vacuole
- cortical v.

vaginae
- v. bulbi
- v. externa nervi optici
- v. interna nervi optici
- v. nervi optici
- v. oculi

Vaiser sponge
Vaiser-Cibis muscle retractor
Valilab cautery
valve
- Beraud's v.
- Bianchi's v.
- Bochdalek's v.
- Foltz's v.
- Hasner's v.

valve *(continued)*
- Huschke's v.
- Krause's v.
- Rosenmüller's v.
- Taillefer's v.
- Van Herick's v.

van der Hoeve's
- disease
- syndrome

Van Herick's
- modification
- valve

Van Heuven's retinopathy

Van Lint's
- akinesia
- block
- flap
- injection
- modified technique
- technique

Van Lint–Atkinson lid akinetic block

Van Milligen eyelid repair technique

Vannas'
- capsulotomy
- scissors

Vari bladebreaker

variable strabismus

variation diurnal

Varicella
- v. iridocyclitis
- v. keratitis
- v. zoster ophthalmicus

varices

varicoblepharon

varicose ophthalmia

varicula

Varigray lens

Varilux lens implant

varix

vasa sanguinea retinae

Vasco-Posada orbital retractor

vascular
- v. arcade
- v. cataract
- v. circle of optic nerve
- v. fronds
- v. funnel
- v. keratitis
- v. loop
- v. tree
- v. trunks
- v. tunic

vascularization
- corneal v.

vascularized tortuosity

vasculitis retinae

vasculonebulous keratitis

vasoactive amines

vasodilatation

VECP — visual evoked cortical potential

vectograph

vectis
- Anis' irrigating v.
- aspirating/irrigating v.
- Pierce's irrigating v.

veil
- Sattler's v.
- vitreous v.

vein
- angular v.
- anterior ciliary v.
- anterior conjunctival v.
- aqueous v.
- Ascher's v.
- central retinal v.
- choroid v.
- ciliary v.
- cilioretinal v.
- conjunctival v.
- corticose v.
- episcleral v.
- facial v.
- frontal diploic v.

vein *(continued)*
- inferior ophthalmic v.
- inferior palpebral v.
- Kuhnt's postcentral v.
- lacrimal v.
- muscular v.
- nasofrontal v.
- ophthalmic v.
- ophthalmomeningeal v.
- palpebral v.
- posterior ciliary v.
- posterior conjunctival v.
- retinal v.
- superior ophthalmic v.
- superior palpebral v.
- supraorbital v.

velonoskiascopy

velum
- corneal v.

vena

venae
- v. angularis
- v. anteriores conjunctivales
- v. centralis retinae
- v. choroideae oculi
- v. ciliares anteriores
- v. ciliares posteriores
- v. conjunctivales
- v. diploica frontalis
- v. episclerales
- v. facialis
- v. lacrimalis
- v. musculares
- v. nasofrontalis
- v. ophthalmica inferior
- v. ophthalmica superior
- v. ophthalmomeningea
- v. palpebrales
- v. palpebrales inferiores
- v. palpebrales superiores
- v. posteriores conjunctivales
- v. vorticosae

venous
- v. engorgement
- v. hemangioma
- v. laminar
- v. sinuses
- v. stasis
- v. stasis retinopathy
- v. stenosis retinopathy

venter frontalis musculi occipitofrontalis

venula
- v. macularis inferior
- v. macularis superior
- v. medialis retinae
- v. nasalis retinae inferior
- v. nasalis retinae superior
- v. retinae medialis
- v. temporalis retinae inferior
- v. temporalis retinae superior

venulae
- medial v. of retina
- nasal v. of retina inferior
- nasal v. of retina superior
- temporal v. retina inferior
- temporal v. retina superior

VEP — visual evoked potential

VER — visual evoked response

vergence
- ability v.
- power v.
- reflux v.

Verhoeff's
- expressor
- forceps
- operation
- scissors
- stain

Verhoeff-Chandler capsulotomy

vermiform contractions
vernal
v. catarrh
v. conjunctivitis
v. keratoconjunctivitis
vernier
v. acuity
v. stimulus
v. visual acuity
verruca filiformis
verrucae
verrucous shape
version
deorsumversion
dextroversion
levoversion
sursumversion
versions and ductions
vertex
v. of cornea
v. of distance
v. of power
vertical
v. axis of eye
v. axis of Fick
v. comitant deviations
v. diplopia
v. divergence
v. ductions
v. gaze center
v. hemianopia
v. meridian
v. nystagamus
v. parallax
v. phoria
v. retraction syndrome
v. strabismus fixus
v. tropia
v. vergence
v. vertigo
verticillata cornea
vertigo
benign paroxysmal positional v.
vertigo *(continued)*
benign paroxysmal postural v.
ocular v.
special sense v.
vertical v.
Verwey's eyelid operation
vesicle
compound v.
kerionic v.
lens v.
lenticular v.
multiocular v.
ocular v.
ophthalmic v.
optic v.
vesicula ophthalmica
vesiculae
vesicular keratitis
vesiculation
eyelid v.
vesiculobullous
vesiculosis linear endothelial
vessel
ciliary v.
episcleral blood v.
ghost v.
vestibular
v. nystagmus
v. pupillary reaction
v. system
vestibulo-ocular
v. reflex
v. response
vestibulopathy
VG slit lamp
vibrating scissors
vibration
photoelectric v.
Vicker's needle holder
Vickerall round ringed forceps
Vicrosurgery
Vicryl suture
video specular microscope

Viers'
- cannula
- erysiphake
- needle
- operation
- rod
- trocar

Vieth-Mueller horopter

view
- Caldwell's v.
- Caldwell-Waters v.
- Waters' v.

Villasensor ultrasonic pachymeter

vinyl T-tube

violaceous

violet vision

viral
- v. conjunctivitis
- v. keratoconjunctivitis

virgin silk suture

virtual
- v. focus
- v. image

virus

VISC — vitreous infusion suction cutter

viscoelastic

VISCOFLOW cannula

viscous
- v. fluid
- v. ochre fluid
- v. xanthochromic fluid

visible spectrum

visile

visio oculus
- v.o. dextra
- v.o. sinister
- v.o. uterque

vision
- achromatic v.
- artificial v.
- best corrected v.

vision *(continued)*
- binocular v.
- blue v.
- central v.
- central keyhole v.
- chromatic v.
- color v.
- cone v.
- day v.
- decreasing v.
- dichromatic v.
- direct v.
- double v.
- eccentric v.
- facial v.
- false v.
- finger v.
- foveal v.
- green v.
- half v.
- halo v.
- haploscopic v.
- indirect v.
- iridescent v.
- keyhole v.
- linear v.
- low v.
- misty
- monocular v.
- multiple v.
- night v.
- nul v.
- obscure v.
- oscillating v.
- peripheral v.
- phantom v.
- photopic v.
- Pick's v.
- pseudoscopic v.
- rainbow v.
- red v.
- rod v.
- scoterythrous v.

vision *(continued)*
- scotoptic v.
- shaft v.
- solid v.
- stereoscopic v.
- subjective v.
- triple v.
- tubular v.
- tunnel v.
- twilight v.
- violet v.
- word v.
- yellow v.

Visitec
- 1624 irrigating/aspirating cannula
- angled lens hook
- aspiration unit
- capsule polisher curet
- corneal shield
- cortex extractor
- cystotome
- double cutting cystotome
- intraocular lens dialer
- irrigating/aspirating cannula
- iris retractor
- lens pusher
- micro double iris hook
- micro hook
- micro iris hook
- nucleus removal loop
- RK zone marker
- straight lens hook
- vico manipulator

visual
- v. acuities
- v. acuity
- v. agnosia
- v. angle
- v. association areas
- v. attentiveness
- v. axis

visual *(continued)*
- v. cone
- v. corkscrew defects
- v. cortex
- v. defects
- v. direction
- v. efficiency
- v. evoked cortical potential
- v. evoked potential
- v. evoked response
- v. field
- v. hallucinations
- v. image
- v. line
- v. organ
- v. preservation
- v. plane
- v. point
- v. purple
- v. receptor

Visual-Tech machine

visualization
- contrast v.
- double-contrast v.

visualize

Visulab System

Visulas
- argon C laser
- argon/YAG laser
- YAG C laser
- YAG E laser
- YAG S laser

visuoauditory

visuognosis

visuolexic

visuometer

visuopsychic

visuosensory

visuospatial

Visuscope
- motor test
- ophthalmoscope

Visuscope
    sensory test
Vitallium implant
vitelliform
    Best's v. macular dystrophy
    v. macular degeneration
vitiligo iridis
vitiligoidea
vitreal
    v. bleed
    v. cells
    v. veil
vitrectomy
    anterior v.
    core v.
    open-sky v.
    pars plana v.
    port v.
    posterior v.
    Weck-cel v.
vitrector
    Alcon v.
    Charles' v. with sleeve
    CILCO v.
    CooperVision v.
    Frigitonics v.
    Kaufman's v.
    Microvit v.
    Peyman's v.
    SITE Guillotine v.
    Storz Microvit v.
vitreitis
vitreocapsulitis
vitreolysis
vitreoretinal
    v. infusion cutter
    v. traction syndrome
vitreoretinopathy
vitreous
    v. abscess
    v. aspirating cannula
    v. aspirating needle

vitreous *(continued)*
    v. aspiration
    v. base
    v. block
    v. block glaucoma
    v. body
    v. bulge
    v. cavity
    v. chamber
    v. coloboma
    v. contraction
    v. cutter
    v. detachment
    v. face
    v. fibers
    v. floater
    v. fluff
    v. fluorophotometry
    v. forceps
    v. gel
    v. haze
    v. hemorrhage break-through
    v. herniation
    v. humor
    liquified v.
    v. membrane
    v. neovascularization
    v. nibbled away
    v. opacity
    v. pencil
    primary persistent hyperplastic v.
    v. prolapse
    v. retraction
    secondary v.
    v. seeding
    v. skirt
    v. strands
    v. strand scissors
    v. stroma
    v. sweep spatula
    v. tap

vitreous *(continued)*
    tertiary v.
    v. touch
    v. traction
    v. transplant needle
    v. veil
    v. wick syndrome
vitreous cutter
    Buettner-Parel v.c.
    Douvas' v.c.
    Kloti's v.c.
    Maguire-Harvey v.c.
    O'Malley-Heintz v.c.
    Parel-Crock v.c.
    Tolentino's v.c.
    VISC v.c.
vitreum corpus
vitreus humor
vitrina
    v. ocularis
    v. oculi
vitritis
Vitrophage-Peyman unit
vitrosi
VOD — visio oculus dexter
Vogt's
    cataract
    cornea
    degeneration
    disease
    operation
    syndrome
    white limbal girdle
Vogt-Barraquer corneal needle
Vogt-Koyanagi syndrome
Vogt-Koyanagi-Harada syndrome
Vogt-Spielmeyer disease
Volk's conoid lens implant
volumetric
voluntary
    v. convergence

voluntary *(continued)*
    v. eye movements
    v. nystagmus
Von Ammon's operation
von Blaskovics–Doyen operation
von Gierke's disease
von Graefe's
    cataract knife
    cautery
    cystotome
    fixation forceps
    iris forceps
    knife
    knife needle
    muscle hook
    operation
    sign
    strabismus hook
    syndrome
    tissue forceps
von Hippel's
    disease
    operation
    retinal angioma
von Hippel–Landau disease
von Monakow's fibers
von Mondak's forceps
von Noorden's incision
von Recklinghausen's disease
von Willebrandt's
    knee
    optic nerve fibers
VOR — vestibulo-ocular response
vortex
    corneal v. dystrophy
    v. dystrophy
    Fleischer's v.
    v. lentis
    v. system
    v. veins
vortex-like clumps

vortices
VOS — visio oculus sinister (vision left eye)
Vossius's lenticular ring
VOU — visio oculus uterque (vision both eyes)
VSR — venous stasis retinopathy
Vuero Meter
Vygantas-Wilder retinal drainage probe

W

W4D Test
Waardenburg's syndrome
Waardenburg-Klein syndrome
Wachendorf's membrane
Wadsworth's lid forceps
Wadsworth-Todd cautery
Wagener's retinitis
Wagner's disease
Wainstock's suturing forceps
waking ptosis
Waldeau's forceps
Waldenstrom's macroglobulinemia
Waldeyer's glands
Waldhauer's operation
Walker's
    coagulator
    electrode
    lid everter
    micro pin
    pin
    scissors
    trephine
Walker-Apple scissors
Walker-Atkinson scissors
Walker-Lee sclerotome
Wallach's cryosurgical pencil
Wallenberg's syndrome
walleye
walleyed
Walser's corneoscleral punch
Walter's spud
Walter Reed implant
Walton's
    punch
    spud
wart
    Hassall-Henle w's
water
    w. drinking test
    w. fissures
    w. provocative test
watered-silk
    w. reflex
    w. retina
Waters' view
Watt's stave bender
Watzke's
    band
    cuff
    forceps
    operation
    sleeve
    tire
wave edge knife
wax and wane
Weaver's
    chalazion forceps
    trocar introducer
Weber's
    knife
    sign
    syndrome
Weber-Elschnig lens loupe
Weber-Rinne sign
Weck's
    eyeshield
    microscope
Weck-cel
    sponge
    vitrectomy

Wedl cells
Weeker's operation
Weeks'
    bacillus
    needle
    operation
    speculum
Wegener's granulomatosis
Weigert's ligament
Weil's
    disease
    lacrimal cannula
Weill-Marchesani syndrome
Weisinger's operation
Weiss'
    chalazion forceps
    reflex
    speculum
Welch 4-drop device
Welch Allyn Pocket Scope
welder's conjunctivitis
Welland's test
Wells' enucleation spoon
Welsh's
    cannula
    cortex stripper cannula
    erysiphake
    flat olive tip double cannula
    iris retractor
    olive tipped cannula
    pupil spreader forceps
Werb's
    operation
    scissors
Wergeland's
    double cannula
    double needle
Werner's syndrome
Wernicke's
    encephalopathy
    sign
    symptom
Wernicke's *(continued)*
    syndrome
    triangle
Wesley Jessen lens
West's
    gouge
    lacrimal cannula
    lacrimal sac chisel
    operation
Westcott's
    tenotomy scissors
    test
Westergren sedimentation rate
Westphal-Piltz reflex
Westphal-Strumpell disease
wet
    bedewing to w.
    w. dressing
    w. field cautery
    w. mount
Wet-cote
Weve's
    electrode
    operation
Wharton-Jones operation
Whatman's filter
wheal
wheel rotation
Wheeler's
    cyclodialysis system
    cystotome
    discission knife
    implant
    knife
    operation
    spatula
Whipple's disease
white
    w. braided silk suture
    w. cells
    w. cord
    w. dot syndrome
    w. of the eye
    w. reflex

white *(continued)*
w. retinal necrosis
w. sclera
w. stromal infiltrate
w. tunica fibrosa oculi
visual w.
w. without pressure
White's glaucoma pump shunt
Whitnall's
ligament
sling operation
Whitney's superior rectus forceps
whorl lens
whorl-shaped
Wicherkiewicz's eyelid operation
wicking
w. glue patch
w. patch
wide-angle glaucoma
wide field eyepiece
Widmark's conjunctivitis
Widowitz's sign
Wieger's ligament
Wiener's
corneal hook
keratome
operation
speculum
Wies'
chalazion forceps
procedure
Wilbrand's prism test
Wild's operating microscope
Wilder's
band spreader
cystotome
dilator
lens loop
scleral depressor
scoop
sign
Wildgen-Reck localizer
Wilkerson's
forceps
intraocular lens insertion forceps
Willebrandt's knee
Williams'
probe
speculum
Willis' circle
Wills'
cautery
forceps
Wilmer's
conjunctiva scissors
operation
refractor
retractor
scissors
Wilmer-Bagley expressor
Wilson's
degeneration
disease
Wincor's enucleation scissors
window defect
wing cell
Wing test
winking
Winslow's stars
wipe-out syndrome
wire frame spectacles
wire mesh implant
Wirt's
4 dot test
stereo test
Wiskott-Aldrich syndrome
with
w. correction
w. motion
w. the rule astigmatism
without correction
Wolf's syndrome
Wolfe's
forceps

Wolfe's *(continued)*
graft
operation
Wolff's ptosis operation
Wolff-Eisner test
Wolfring's gland
Woods'
light examination
sign
Wooten's needle
word
w. blindness
w. vision
working distance
Worst's
corneal bur
medallion lens
needle
pigtail probe
Worth's
forceps
4-dot test
ptosis operation
stereopsis test
strabismus forceps
Wrattan's filter
Wright's
fascia needle
operation
wrinkle
Wucherer's conjunctivitis
Wullstein-House cup forceps
Wundt-Lamansky law

X

x — axis of Fick
X — exophoria
X chromosome
X-linked
X-linked *(continued)*
X. blue cone monochromatism
X. inheritance
X. recessive disorder
xanthelasma
xanthelasmatosis
x. bulbi
x. iridis
xanthism
xanthochromic fluid
xanthocyanopsia
xanthogranuloma, juvenile
xanthokyanopy
xanthoma
x. elasticum
x. palpebrarum
x. planum
xanthomata
xanthomatosis
x. bulbi
x. corneae
x. iridis
xanthophane
xanthophyll pigment
xanthopia
xanthopsia
xanthopsin
xenon
x. arc laser
x. photocoagulator
xenophthalmia
xeroderma
x. of Kaposi
x. pigmentosum
xerodermatic
xeroma
xeromycteria
xerophthalmia
xerophthalmus
xerosis
x. conjunctivae
conjunctival x.
x. corneae

xerosis *(continued)*
corneal x.
x. parenchymatosa
x. superficialis
xerotic keratitis
XT — exotropia
X(T) — intermittent exotropia
Xylocaine

Y

Y axis of Fick
Y sutures
YAG laser
Biophysic Medical Y.l.
Carl Zeiss Y.l.
CILCO Y.l.
Coherent Medical Y.l.
CooperVision Y.l.
neodymium (Nd) Y.l.
SITE Y.l.
Yale Luer-Lok
needle
syringe
Yazujian bur
yellow
y. light reflex
y. point
y. spot of retina
visual y.
yoke muscles
Young's operation
Young-Helmholtz theory
YS — yellow spots of retina

Z

Z axis of Fick
Z marginal tenotomy
Z myotomy
Z tenotomy
Z-plasty
Zeis glands
zeisian gland
zeisian sty
Zeiss'
cine adaptor
colposcope
Fiber Optic Illumination System
fundus camera
gonioscope
lens
loupe
microscope
operating field loupe
photocoagulator
slit lamp
Vertex refractionometer
Zeiss-Barraquer
cine microscope
surgical microscope
Zeiss-Gullstrand loupe
zero vergence
Ziegler's
cautery
cilia forceps
dilator
forceps
knife
knife needle
lacrimal dilator
operation
probe
puncture
speculum
zinc encrustations
Zinn's
circlet
corona
ligament
membrane

Zinn's *(continued)*
- tendon
- zonule

zipped angle
zipper stitch
Zollner's lines
zona
- blur z.
- ciliary z.
- z. ciliaris
- z. ophthalmica

zone
- extravisual z.
- inferior z. of retina
- interpalpebral z.
- nuclear z.
- z. of discontinuity
- pupillary z.
- retinal z.
- superior z. of retina
- temporal z. of retina
- transition z.
- visual z.
- z. of Zinn

zonula
- z. adherens
- z. ciliaris
- z. occludens

zonulae
zonular
- z. band
- z. cataract
- z. fibers
- z. keratitis
- z. pulverulent cataract
- z. stripper
- z. tension
- z. tetany

zonule
- ciliary z.
- lens z.
- Zinn's z.

zonulitis
zonulolysis
zonulotomy
zonulysis
zoster ophthalmicus
zygoma
zygomatic
- z. foramen of Arnold
- z. fracture
- z. nerve
- z. orbital foramen

zygomatico-orbital
- z. artery
- z. foramen
- z. process of the maxilla

Zylik's operation

SECTION FOUR

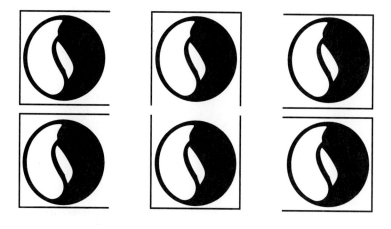

SURGICAL EQUIPMENT AND MATERIALS

a

- A & B scan ultrasonography
- A-scan
- abrader
  - Howard a.
- absorbable suture
- Accommodation Rule
- ACS needle
- Acuiometer
- acuity visual projector
- Acuscan Transducer 400
- adaptometer
  - color a.
- Adson's forceps
- Aebli's corneal scissors
- aftercataract bur
- Agnew's
  - canaliculus knife
  - keratome
  - tattooing needle
- Agrikola's
  - lacrimal sac retractor
  - refractor
  - tattooing needle
- air
  - a. injection cannula
  - a. puff tonometer
- Aker's lens pusher
- Alabama-Green needle holder
- Alcon's
  - aspirator
  - cautery
  - cryophake
  - Cryosurgical System
  - hand cautery
  - I-knife
  - irrigation/aspiration unit
  - Microsponge
  - phacoemulsification unit
  - suture
  - vitrectomy probe
- Alexander-Ballen retractor
- Alfonso's
  - guarded bur
  - speculum
- Allen's
  - cyclodialysis
  - orbital implant
- Allen-Barkan forceps
- Allen-Braley
  - forceps
  - implant
- Allen-Burian trabeculotome
- Allen-Schiøtz tonometer
- Allen-Thorpe
  - gonioscopic prism
  - lens
- Allergan
  - lensometer
  - Medical Optics photokeratoscope
- Allergan-Humphrey
  - laser
  - perimeter
  - refractor
- alligator scissors
- Allport cutting bur
- Aloe reading unit
- Alpar implant
- alpha-chymotrypsin cannula
- alternate cover/uncover test
- Alvis'
  - curet
  - spud
- Alvis-Lancaster sclerotome
- Amenabar's
  - capsule forceps
  - counterpressor
  - discission hook
  - iris retractor
  - lens loop
- American
  - Hydron Instruments
  - Medical Optics
  - Optical photocoagulator

Amoils'
- cryoextractor
- cryopencil
- cryophake
- cryoprobe
- cryosurgical unit
- refractor

Amsler's
- aqueous transplant needle
- chart
- grid test
- marker
- needle
- scleral marker

angled
- a. capsule forceps
- a. counterpressor
- a. discission hook
- a. iris hook and IOL dialer
- a. iris retractor
- a. iris spatula
- a. left/right cannula
- a. lens loop
- a. nucleus removal loop
- a. probe
- a. suction tube
- a. Vico manipulator

angulated iris spatula

Anis' irrigating vectis

anterior chamber
- a.c. cannula
- a.c. irrigating vectis
- a.c. irrigator
- a.c. synechia scissors

Anthony's orbital compressor

A-O Reichert Instruments
- applanation tonometer
- binocular indirect ophthalmoscope
- Ful-Vue diagnostic unit

A-O Reichert Instruments *(continued)*
- lensmeter
- Project-O-Chart

applicator
- Gifford's a.

aqueous transplant needle

AR 1000 refractor

arc perimeter

argon
- a. blue
- Britt a. pulsed laser
- CILCO/Lasertek a. laser
- Coherent 920 a. laser
- a. green
- LPK-80 II a. laser
- Ophthalas a. laser
- Sharplan a. laser

Argyll Robertson Instruments

Arlt's
- loop
- scoop

Arroyo's
- expressor
- forceps
- implant
- protector
- trephine

Arruga's
- expressor
- implant
- lacrimal trephine
- lens
- needle holder
- retractor
- trephine

Arruga-Moura-Brazil implant

Ascher's
- glass
- rod

Ascon Instruments

Aseptron II

aspheric viewing lens
aspirator
 Cavitron a.
 Cooper a.
 Kelman a.
 Nugent a.
 SITE a.
Assi's cannula
astigmagraph
astigmatometer
astigmatoscope
Athens' suture spreader
Atkinson's
 25-G short curved cystotome
 corneal scissors
 needle
 retrobulbar needle
 sclerotome
 single bevel blunt tip needle
 tip peribulbar needle
Atroloc suture
autofunduscope
autokeratometer
automated
 a. hemisphere perimeter
 a. refractor
 a. trephine
Autoswitch System
auto-ophthalmoscope
Auto-Plot
auto-refractor
Avit handpiece
awl
 lacrimal a.
 Mustarde a.
Axisonic II ultrasound
axometer
axonometer
Ayer's chalazion forceps
Ayerst Instruments

b

B-mode handpiece
B-scan
 ultrasonogram
 ultrasonography
B-VAT acuity test
Backhaus clamp
Bagley-Wilmer expressor
Bagolini's lens
Bahn's spud
Bailey's lacrimal cannula
Bailliart's
 goniometer
 ophthalmodynamometer
 ophthalmoscope
ball
 Pinky b.
 Super Pinky b.
Ballen-Alexander orbital retractor
bandage
 binocle b.
 binocular b.
 Borsch b.
 b. contact lens
 b. lens
 monocular b.
 b. scissors
Bangerter's iris spatula
Banner's enucleation snare
Bard-Parker
 keratome
 knife
 razor
 trephine
Barkan's
 goniolens
 gonioscopic lens
 goniotomy knife
 infant implant

Barkan's *(continued)*
- knife
- light

Baron-Bietti
Barraquer's
- cannula
- corneal dissector
- erysiphake
- eyeshield
- implant
- iris scissors
- irrigator spatula
- knife
- lens
- needle
- needle carrier
- needle holder
- razor bladebreaker
- scissors
- shield
- spatula
- speculum
- trephine
- vitreous strand scissors

Barraquer-Colibri speculum
Barraquer-DeWecker scissors
Barraquer-Krumeich test
Barraquer-Vogt needle
Barrier's
- drape
- Phaco Extracapsular Pack
- sheet

Barron's epikeratophakia trephine
base-down prism
base-in prism
base-out prism
base-up prism
basket-style scleral supporter speculum
BAT — Brightness Acuity Test
Bausch-Lomb-Thorpe slit lamp
BD — base-down prism
Beard's knife
Beaupre's forceps
Beaver's
- blade
- cryoextractor
- discission blade
- keratome
- knife
- Ocu-1 curved cystotome

Beaver-Lundsgaard blade
Beaver-Okamura blade
Beaver-Zeigler blade
Becker's
- corneal section spatulated scissors
- goniogram

Becker-Park speculum
Beckerscope Binocular Microscope
Becton Dickinson AcuteCare
Beebe's loupe
Beer's
- cataract knife
- knife

Bell's erysiphake
Bellows' cryoextractor
Bennett's forceps
bent blunt needle
Bercovici's wire lid speculum
Berens-Tolman ocular hypertension indicator
Berens'
- cataract knife
- corneal dissector
- corneal transplant scissors
- corneoscleral punch
- dilator
- electrode
- expressor
- forceps
- glaucoma knife

Berens' *(continued)*
- implant
- iridocapsulotomy scissors
- keratome
- keratoplasty knife
- lens loop
- lid everter
- marking caliper
- muscle clamp
- muscle forceps
- orbital compressor
- pinhole and dominance test
- prism bar
- ptosis knife
- punch
- refractor
- retractor
- scissors
- scleral hook
- spatula
- speculum
- suturing forceps
- test object
- Three Character Test
- tonometer

Berens-Rosa implant

Berke's
- clamp
- forceps
- lid everter

Berkley Bioengineering
- bipolar cautery
- brass scleral plug
- infusion terminal port
- mechanized scissors
- Ocutome

Berman's
- foreign body locator
- localizer

BI — base-in prism

bi-prism application tonometer

Bi-prong muscle marker

Bicap Biometer

biconcave lens

biconvex lens

Bielschowsky's test

Bielschowsky-Parks head-tilt three-step test

Binkhorst's
- collar stud lens implant
- four-loop iris fixated implant
- two-loop lens

binocle bandage

binocular
- b. bandage
- Reichert's Ful-Vue b. ophthalmoscope

binophthalmoscope

binoscope

biomicroscope

Bio-Pen biometric ruler

Biophysic laser

Bioptics
- camera
- specular microscope

Bio-Rad Laboratory

Birch-Hirschfeld lamp

Birch-Harmon irrigator

Birks Mark II
- micro cross-action holder
- micro push/pull
- micro spatula
- micro trabeculectomy scissors
- push/pull
- spatula

Bishop-Harmon
- anterior chamber irrigator
- bladebreaker
- cannula
- forceps
- irrigator

Bishop-Harmon *(continued)*
  knife
  Superblade
Bishop-Peter tendon tucker
Bjerrum's
  scotometer
  screen
BKS Refractive System
black braided
  nylon suture
  silk suture
blade
  Bard-Parker b.
  Beaver's discission b.
  Beaver-Lundsgaard b.
  Beaver-Okamura b.
  Beaver-Zeigler b.
  Beer's b.
  bent blunt b.
  Berens' b.
  broken razor b.
  Castroviejo's razor b.
  CooperVision Surgeon-Plus Ultra Thin b.
  Curdy-Hebra b.
  Curdy's b.
  diamond dusted knife b.
  GSA-9 b.
  Hebra's b.
  Hoskins' razor fragment b.
  Keeler's retractable b.
  Lange's b.
  Martinez's corneal trephine b.
  McPherson-Wheeler b.
  miniature b.
  MVR b.
  myringotomy b.
  razor b.
  replaceable b.
  Scheie's b.
blade *(continued)*
  Superblade No.75 b.
  trephine b.
bladebreaker
  Barraquer's razor b.
  knife b.
  Swiss b.
  Troutman b.
Blair's
  head drape
  retractor
  stiletto
Blaydes' forceps
bleb cup
Blenderm tape
blepharostat
  McNeill-Goldmann b.
blunt needle
BO — base-out prism
boat hook
  Katena's b.h.
Boberg-Ans lens implant
Bodkin thread holder
Bonaccolto's
  forceps
  monoplex orbital plant
  orbital implant
  scleral ring
  trephine
Bonaccolto-Flieringa scleral ring
bone-biting
  forceps
  punch
  trephine
Bonn's forceps
Bores' twist fixation ring
Borsch's bandage
Boston's trephine
Botvin-Bradford enucleator
bougie
Bovie
  cautery

Bovie *(continued)*
electrocautery unit
electrosurgical unit
retinal detachment unit
wet field cautery
Bowman's
cataract needle
needle
probe
stop needle
tube
Boyce's needle holder
Boyd's orbital implant
Boynton's needle holder
Bracken's
cannula
forceps
braided
silk suture
Vicryl suture
brass scleral plug
Brawley's
refractor
retractor
Brawner's orbital implant
Brightness Acuity Test
Britt's
argon laser
BL-12 laser
krypton laser
pulsed argon laser
Brombach's perimeter
Bronson-Magnion
eye magnet
forceps
Bronson-Park speculum
Bronson-Turner foreign body locator
Bronson-Turz
refractor
retractor
Brown's sterile adhesive
Brown-Dohlman Silastic corneal implant
Brown-Pusey corneal trephine
brush
Barraquer's sable b.
Haidinger's b.
Thomas' b.
BU — base-up prism
Buettner-Parel vitreous cutter
build-up implant
bulldog clamp
Buller's shield
Bunge's evisceration spoon
Bunker's implant
bur
after-cataract b.
Alfonso's guarded b.
Allport's cutting b.
Burwell's b.
corneal b.
corneal foreign body b.
cutting b.
diamond b.
foreign body b.
lacrimal sac b.
Storz's corneal b.
Yazujian's b.
Burch's
caliper
pick
tendon tucker
Burch-Greenwood tucker
Burch-Lister speculum
Burr's
butterfly needle
corneal ring
silicone button
Burwell's bur
button tip manipulator

C

C-loop posterior chamber lens
Calhoun's needle
Calhoun-Hagler lens needle
Calhoun-Merz needle
caliper
- Berens' marking c.
- Burch's c.
- Castroviejo's c.
- Green's c.
- Jameson's c.
- John Green c.
- Stahl's c.
- Thorpe's c.
- Thorpe-Castroviejo c.

Callahan's
- fixation forceps
- lens loop

Campbell's
- refractor
- retractor
- slit lamp

campimeter
canalicular scissors
cannula
- air injection c.
- alpha-chymotrypsin c.
- angled left/right c.
- anterior chamber c.
- Assi's c.
- Bailey's lacrimal c.
- Barraquer's c.
- Bishop-Harmon c.
- Bracken's c.
- Castroviejo's cyclodialysis c.
- cyclodialysis c.
- DeLavega's vitreous aspirating c.

cannula *(continued)*
- double irrigating/aspirating c.
- Drews' c.
- Fasanella's lacrimal c.
- Galt's aspirating c.
- Gans' c.
- Gass' cataract aspirat- ing c.
- Gills' double Luer-Lok c.
- Goldstein's c.
- goniotomy knife c.
- Gormley's double c.
- Heyner's double c.
- Hilton's self-retaining infusion c.
- iris hook c.
- irrigating/aspirating c.
- Johnson's double c.
- J-shaped irrigating/aspirating c.
- Karickhoff's double c.
- Keeler-Keislar lacrimal c.
- Kelman's cyclodialysis c.
- Klein's curved c.
- knife c.
- Kraff's cortex c.
- lacrimal c.
- liquid vitreous aspirating c.
- Maumenee's knife goniotomy c.
- Moncrieff's c.
- O'Gawa's cataract aspirating c.
- Oaks' double straight c.
- Pierce's coaxial irrigating/aspirating c.
- Peczon's irrigating/aspirating c.
- Randolph's cyclodialysis c.
- reed aspiration c.

cannula *(continued)*
- Roper's alpha-chymotrypsin c.
- Scheie's anterior chamber c.
- self-retaining irrigating c.
- side port c.
- Simcoe double c.
- Steriseal disposable c.
- Swets' goniotomy knife c.
- Tenner's lacrimal c.
- Thomas' c.
- two-way cataract aspirating c.
- Ulanday's double c.
- Veirs' c.
- VISCOFLOW c.
- Welsh's cortex stripper c.
- Welsh's flat olive tip double c.
- Wergeland's double c.

Canon CF-60U fundus camera

capsule fragment spatula

capsule polisher
- Kraff's c.p. curet
- Terry silicone c.p.

capsulotome
- Darling's c.

capsulotomy scissors

Cardona's
- corneal prosthesis forceps
- corneal prosthesis trephine
- fiberoptic diagnostic lens
- focalizing fundus lens implant
- gonio-focalizing lens implant
- threading forceps

Carl Zeiss Instruments

Cartella's eye shield

Carter's
- sphere
- sphere introducer

Castallo's
- refractor
- speculum

Castroviejo's
- acrylic implant
- aspirator
- blade
- bladebreaker
- caliper
- capsule forceps
- clip
- compressor
- corneal dissector
- corneal holding forceps
- corneal scissors with inside stop
- corneal section scissors
- corneal transplant marker
- corneal transplant scissors
- corneal transplant trephine
- corneoscleral punch
- cyclodialysis cannula
- cyclodialysis spatula
- discission knife
- double end spatula
- electro-keratotome
- enucleation snare
- erysiphake
- fixation forceps
- forceps
- implant
- iridocapsulotomy scissors
- keratome
- keratoplasty scissors
- knife
- lacrimal dilator
- lacrimal sac probe

Castroviejo's *(continued)*
- lens loupe
- lens spoon
- lid clamp
- lid retractor
- needle holder
- orbital aspirator
- punch
- razor blade
- refractor
- retractor
- scissors
- scleral shortening clip
- sclerotome
- snare
- spatula
- speculum
- spoon
- suture forceps
- synechia scissors
- trephine
- twin knife
- vitreous aspirating needle

Castroviejo-Arruga forceps
Castroviejo-Galezowski dilator
Castroviejo-Kalt needle holder
Castroviejo-Scheie cyclodiathermy
CAT scan — computed axial tomography scan
cataract
- c. aspirating needle
- c. mask ring
- c. pencil

catheter
- Lincoff's balloon c.

cautery
- Alcon's hand c.
- Berkley Bioengineering bipolar c.
- bipolar c.
- Bovie wet field c.
- Concept disposable c.
- Concept hand-held c.
- disposable c.
- Fine's micropoint c.
- Geiger's c.
- Gonin's c.
- Hildreth's c.
- Mentor's wet field c.
- Mira c.
- Mueller's c.
- NeoKnife c.
- Op-Temp c.
- Parker-Heath c.
- Prince's c.
- Rommel's c.
- Rommel-Hildreth c.
- Scheie's c.
- Todd's c.
- Valilab c.
- von Graefe's c.
- Wadsworth-Todd c.
- wet field c.
- Ziegler's c.

Cavitron irrigation/aspiration system
Cavitron-Kelman irrigation/aspiration system
CCT — computed corneal tomography
CD-5 needle
centering ring
chalazion
- c. clamp
- c. curet
- c. forceps
- c. trephine

Challenger Digital Applanation Tonometer
Chambers' sterile adhesive bubble
Chan's wrist rest
Chandler's forceps

Charles'
anterior segment sleeve
infusion sleeve
intraocular lens
needle
vacuuming needle
chart
astigmatic dial c.
Bailey-Lovie Log MAR c.
Donders c.
Ferris c.
Guibor c.
Illiterate c.
Kindergarten c.
Lancaster-Regan dial 1 c.
Lancaster-Regan dial 2 c.
Landolt broken ring c.
Landolt C c.
Lebensohn c.
Randot c.
reading c.
Reuss color c.
Snellen c.
sunburst dial c.
vectograph c.
cheiroscope
chisel
lacrimal sac c.
Choyce
Mark VIII implant
chromatoptometer
chromatoskiameter
chromic
c. catgut suture
c. collagen suture
Cibis'
electrode
needle
ski needle
CILCO
argon laser
Frigitronics
Hoffer Laseridge
CILCO *(continued)*
krypton laser
Lasertek A/K laser
Sonometric A-SCAN
Ultrasound Unit
Cine-Microscope
Citelli's rongeur
clamp
Berke's c.
bulldog c.
Castroviejo's lid c.
cross-action c.
Erhardt's c.
Gladstone-Putterman
entropion c.
muscle c.
Prince's muscle c.
Putterman's levator
resection c.
Putterman's ptosis c.
Putterman-Müller
blepharoptosis c.
Robin's chalazion c.
Schaedel's cross-action
towel c.
serrefine c.
Clark's eye speculum
Clayman's intraocular lens
Cleasby's spatulated needle
Clerf's needle holder
Clinitex Charles endophotocoagulator probe
clinometer
clinoscope
clip
c. applying forceps
double tantalum c.
holding c.
tantalum c.
clock dial
coagulating electrode
coated Vicryl suture
Coburn's

Coburn's *(continued)*
- camera
- irrigation/aspiration system
- lensometer
- refractor

Coburn-Meditec
Coburn-Rodenstock slit lamp
cocaine test
Codman/Micra
Cohan-Barraquer microscope
Cohan-Vannas iris scissors
Cohan-Westcott scissors
Cohen's
- corneal forceps
- needle holder

Coherent radiation
- argon/krypton laser
- Fluorotron

Coleman's retractor
Colibri's forceps
Collins 140 color adaptometer
Color Vision Test
colposcope
Comberg's localization
Combiline System
compressor
- Anthony's orbital c.
- Berens' orbital c.

Computon Microtonometer
Concept
- disposable cautery
- hand-held cautery

conformer
- Fox's c.
- McGuire's c.
- silicone c.
- Universal c.

Confrontation Visual Field Test
conical implant
conjunctiva
- c. scissors
- c. spreader

contact
- c. bandage lens
- hard c. lens
- c. lens
- long-wearing c. lens
- soft c. lens

Contact A and B scan
convergiometer
Conway's lid retractor
Cook's speculum
Cooper's
- implant
- irrigating/aspirating unit
- laser

CooperVision
- camera
- imaging perimeter
- irrigation/aspiration unit
- laser
- microscope
- refractive surgery photokeratoscope
- Surgeon-Plus Ultrathin blades
- ultrasound

Copeland's
- implant
- intraocular lens
- streak retinoscope

Coquille's plano lens
Corbett's spud
Corboy's
- hemostat
- needle holder

cordless monocular indirect ophthalmoscope
cornea
- c. abrader
- c. chisel
- c. holding forceps

corneal
- c. bur
- c. debrider

corneal *(continued)*
c. dissector
c. erysiphake
c. fascia lata spatula
c. fixation forceps
c. foreign body bur
c. implant
c. knife dissector
c. needle
c. prosthesis forceps
c. prosthesis trephine
c. scissors
c. section spatulated scissors
c. spatulated scissors
c. transplant marker
c. trephine
c. tube
corneoscleral
c. punch
c. right/left hand scissors
c. scissors
cosmetic contact shell implant
Costenbader's incision spreader
Coston-Trent iris retractor
counterpressor
Amenabar's c.
Gill's c.
cover/uncover test
Crawford's
forceps
lacrimal set
needle
stripper
Crile's needle holder
cross-action
c. capsule forceps
c. towel clamp
cryoextractor
Alcon's c.
Amoils' c.
Bellows' c.
Keeler's c.
cryoextractor *(continued)*
Kelman's c.
Rubinstein's c.
Thomas' c.
cryophake
Amoils' c.
Alcon's c.
Bellow's c.
Keeler's c.
Kelman's c.
Rubinstein's c.
cryoprobe
Amoils' c.
cryoptor c.
Rubinstein's c.
Thomas' c.
Cryostylet 2000
cryosurgical unit
Alcon's c.u.
Frigitronics c.u.
Keeler's c.u.
Kelman's c.u.
N_2O c.u.
Cryo-Barrages vitreous implant
CT scan — computed tomography scan
CUA needle
cuff
Watzke's c.
Cuignet's test
cul-de-sac
c. irrigating vectis
c. irrigation T-tube
Culler's
iris spatula
lens spoon
muscle hook
cup
Galin's bleb c.
Curdy's
blade
sclerotome
Curdy-Hebra blade

curet
- Alvis' c.
- chalazion c.
- Fink's c.
- Gifford's c.
- Gill-Welch c.
- Green's c.
- Heath's chalazion c.
- Hebra's c.
- Kraff's capsule polisher c.
- Meyhoeffer's chalazion c.
- Skeele's c.

Curran's knife needle
Cusick's goniotomy knife
Custodis
- sponge
- suture

Cutler's
- implant
- lens spoon

cutter
- Buettner-Parel c.
- Douvas' c.
- Kloti's c.
- Machemer's c.
- Maguire-Harvey c.
- O'Malley-Heintz c.
- Parel-Crock c.
- Tolentino's c.

cutting bur
cyanoacrylate tissue adhesive
cyanographic contrast material
cyanographin contrast material
cyclodialysis spatula
cyclodiathermy electrode
cyclogram
cyclophorometer
cylindrical lens
cystotome
- Graefe's c.
- Kelman's c.
- Lewicky's formed c.

cystotome *(continued)*
- Nevyas' double sharp c.
- von Graefe's c.
- Wheeler's c.
- Wilder's c.

Czermak's keratome

d

dacryocystorhinostomy
- Moria-France d. clamp

dacryolith
- Desmarres' d.

Dailey's cataract needle
Danberg's forceps
Dannheim's eye implant
Darin's lens
Darling's capsulotome
DaSilva's dermatome
Daviel's
- lens spoon
- scoop

Davis'
- knife needle
- spud
- trephine

Davis-Geck suture
Dean's
- iris knife
- knife holder
- needle

debrider
- Sauer's d.

deep blunt rake retractor
DeKnatel's silk suture
DeLavega's vitreous aspirating cannula
depressor
- Schepens' scleral d.

depressor
Schocket's scleral d.
Derf's needle holder
Dermalon suture
dermatome
DaSilva's d.
Descemet's membrane punch
Desmarres'
corneal dissector
fixation pick
forceps
knife
lid clamp
lid elevator
lid retractor
marker
refractor
scarifier
DeVilbiss' irrigating/aspirating unit
DeWecker's scissors
DeWecker-Pritikin scissors
diamond
d. blade knife
d. bur
d. dusted knife
diathermy
Mira d.
d. tip
Digilab tonometer
Digital B System
dilator
Berens' d.
Castroviejo's lacrimal d.
Castroviejo-Galezowski d.
French's lacrimal d.
Galezowski's lacrimal d.
Heath's d.
Hosford's lacrimal d.
House's lacrimal d.
Jones' d.
dilator *(continued)*
Muldoon's lacrimal d.
Nettleship-Wilder d.
punctum d.
pupil d.
Ruedemann's lacrimal d.
Wilder's d.
Dimitry's
chalazion trephine
erysiphake
Dimitry-Bell erysiphake
Dimitry-Thomas erysiphake
diopsimeter
diopter prism
Dioptimum System
dioptrometer
dioptroscope
direct ophthalmoscope
director
grooved d.
discission knife
disposable cautery
dissecting scissors
dissector
Barraquer's corneal d.
Berens' corneal d.
corneal knife d.
Desmarres' corneal d.
Green's corneal d.
knife d.
Martinez's d.
dissimilar
d. image test
d. target test
DIVA Test
Dix's spud
Dix-Hallpike test
Docustar fundus camera
Doherty's sphere implant
Dohlman's plug
Donaldson's eye patch
Donders' chart

double
- d. cutting sharp cystotome
- d. freeze/thaw cryopexy
- d. irrigating/aspirating cannula
- d. Maddox rod test
- d. spatula

double-arm suture

Doughtery's irrigating/aspirating unit

Douvas'
- rotoextractor
- vitreous cutter

Draeger's
- high vacuum erysiphake
- tonometer

drape
- 3-M Steri-Drape d.
- Alcon's disposable d.
- Barrier d.
- Blair's head d.
- Eye-Pak d.
- Hough's d.
- mini ophthamic d.
- Opraflex d.
- Steri-Drape d.
- Surgikos disposable d.
- VISIFLEX d.

dressing
- binocular d.
- Blenderm tape d.
- bolus d.
- Borsch's d.
- collodion d.
- compression d.
- crepe bandage d.
- Elastoplast d.
- Expo-Bubble d.
- eye pad d.
- fine moistened mesh gauze d.
- fluff d.

dressing *(continued)*
- fluffed gauze d.
- monocular d.
- pressure patch d.
- ribbon gauze d.
- sterile adhesive bubble d.
- Telfa plastic film d.
- tie-over Sellotape d.
- tulle gras d.
- wet d.
- saline saturated wool d.

Drew's
- irrigating/aspirating unit
- lens

Drew-Rosenbaum
- iris retractor
- irrigating/aspirating u.

dropper
- Undine d.

DS-9 needle

Dualoop

Duane's
- accommodation chart
- retractor

duction test

Duke-Elder lamp

Dulaney's lens

Dupuy-Dutemps dacryocystorhinostomy dye test

Dyonics syringe injector

e

echogram

echo-ophthalmogram

Echorule Ultrasonic Biometer

EchoScan by Nidek

Ehrmann's test

Elastoplast
- bandage
- dressing
- eye occlusor

Eldridge-Green lamp

electrocautery
- Prince's e.
- Fine's micropoint e.
- Geiger's e.
- Hildreth's e.
- Mentor's wet-field e.
- Mira e.
- Mueller's e.
- Op-Temp disposable e.
- ophthalmic e.
- Parker-Heath e.
- Rommel's e.
- Rommel-Hildreth e.
- Scheie's e.
- Todd's e.
- Valilab e.
- von Graefe's e.
- Wadsworth-Todd e.
- wet field e.
- Ziegler's e.

electrode
- diathermy e.
- Gradle's e.
- Kronfeld's e.
- Pischel's e.
- Weve's e.

electro-keratome

electro-mucotome

electron
- e. microscopy
- e. volt — eV

electronystagmograph

electroretinography

electroretinogram — ERG

elevator
- Desmarres' lid e.
- Joseph's e.

Eliasoph's lid retractor

ELISA test

Elliot's corneal trephine

Ellis'
- foreign body spud
- needle holder
- needle probe

Elschnig's
- capsule forceps
- cataract knife
- corneal knife
- cyclodialysis spatula
- fixation forceps
- forceps
- knife
- pterygium knife
- refractor
- retractor
- spatula
- spoon

Elschnig-O'Brien forceps

Empac-Cavitron irrigation/
aspiration unit

Endo-Set by Haag-Streit

enucleation
- e. scissors
- e. scoop
- e. spoon
- e. wire snare

enucleator
- Banner's snare e.
- Botvin-Bradford e.
- Bradford's snare e.
- Castroviejo's snare e.
- Foerster's snare e.
- Foster's snare e.
- snare e.

epilator

Epstein's collar stud acrylic lens

erbium laser

Erhardt's lid forceps

erysiphake
- Barraquer's e.
- Bell's e.

erysiphake *(continued)*
- Castroviejo's e.
- Dimitry's e.
- Dimitry-Bell e.
- Dimitry-Thomas e.
- Draeger high vacuum e.
- Esposito's e.
- Floyd-Grant e.
- Harrington's e.
- Johnson's e.
- Johnson-Bell e.
- Kara's e.
- L'Esperance's e.
- Maumenee's e.
- New York e.
- Nugent-Green-Dimitry e.
- oval cup e.
- Post-Harrington e.
- Sakler's e.
- Searcy's e.
- Storz-Bell e.
- Veirs' e.
- Welch's rubber bulb e.
- Welsh's Silastic e.

Eschenback Optik

Esposito's erysiphake

Esterman's scale

ether guard

Ethicon
- Atroloc suture
- Micro-Point suture
- Sabreloc suture
- suture

Ethilon suture

ethyl cyanoacrylate

euthyscope

eV — electron volt

Evergreen Lasertek
- laser
- coagulator

everter
- Berens' e.
- lid e.
- Roveda's e.

everter *(continued)*
- Schachne-Desmarres e.
- Struble's e.
- Walker's e.

evisceration spoon

Excimer laser

exophthalmometer
- Hertel's e.
- Luedde's e.

Expo Bubble
- eye cover
- eye shield

expressor
- Arruga's e.
- Berens' e.
- Heath's e.
- hook e.
- Hosford's e.
- Kirby's hook e.
- lens e.
- McDonald's e.
- meibomian gland e.
- ring lens e.
- Rizzuti's e.
- Smith's e.
- Stahl's nucleus e.
- Verhoeff's e.

extended round needle

extractor
- Krwawicz's cataract e.
- roto e.

eye
- patch
- oval

Eye Con 5

eyelid

Eye Pak II
- cover
- drape

eyepiece
- comparison e.
- compensating e.
- demonstration e.
- huygenian e.

- eyepiece *(continued)*
  - negative e.
  - positive e.
  - Ramsden's e.
  - wide field e.
- eyeshield
  - Barraquer's e.
  - Buller's e.
  - Cartella's e.
  - Expo-Bubble e.
  - Fox's e.
  - Green's e.
  - Hessburg's e.
  - Mueller's e.
  - Paton's e.
  - plastic e.
  - ring cataract mask e.
  - Universal e.
  - Weck e.
- eye speculum
- eye wash

f

- Falco
- Farnsworth-Munsell 100 Hue Color Test
- fascia lata stripper
- Fechner's intraocular lens
- Federov's
  - 4-loop iris clip
  - type I implant
  - type II implant
- Feldman's
  - adaptometer
  - RK optical center marker
- Fenzle's
  - angled manipulating hook
  - manipulating hook
- Ferree-Rand perimeter
- Ferris Smith
  - refractor
  - retractor
- Ferris-Smith-Sewall retractor
- Fiberlite microscope
- fiberoptic pick
- fiberscope
- Fibra Sonics phaco aspirator
- filamentary keratome
- filter
  - interference f.
  - Millex f.
  - Millipore f.
  - neutral density f.
  - red free f.
  - UV blocking f.
  - Whatman f.
  - Wrattan f.
- Fine's
  - corneal carrying case
  - dissecting forceps
  - magnetic implant
  - micropoint cautery
  - toothed forceps
  - tying forceps
- Fine-Castroviejo forceps
- fine-toothed forceps
- Fink's
  - cataract aspirator
  - cul-de-sac irrigator
  - curet
  - hook
  - irrigator
  - lacrimal retractor
  - muscle hook
  - muscle marker
  - oblique muscle hook
  - retractor
  - tendon tucker
- Fink-Jameson muscle forceps
- Fink-Weinstein two-way syringe
- Finnoff's transilluminator
- Fisher's
  - lid retractor

Fisher's *(continued)*
- needle
- spoon
- spud

Fisher-Arlt iris forceps
Fison indirect binocular ophthalmoscope
fixation
- binocular f. forceps
- f. forceps
- f. hook
- f. pick
- f. ring

Flieringa's
- fixation ring
- scleral ring

Flieringa-Kayser fixation ring
Flieringa-LeGrand fixation ring
Floyd-Grant erysiphake
fluorescein
- f. angiogram test
- f. dye disappearance test

fluorophotometry
- vitreous f.

Föerster's
- enucleation snare
- forceps

foil sheet
forced duction test
forceps
- Adson's f.
- Alabama University utility f.
- Allen-Barkan f.
- Allen-Braley f.
- Allis' f.
- Alvis' fixation f.
- Ambrose's suture f.
- Amenabar's capsule f.
- Arruga's capsule f.
- Arruga-MacKool f.
- Asch's septal f.
- Ayer's chalazion f.

forceps *(continued)*
- B.B. shot f.
- Bailey's chalazion f.
- Baird's chalazion f
- Ballen-Alexander f.
- Bangerter's muscle f.
- Banner's f.
- Bard-Parker f.
- Barkan's iris f.
- Barraquer's cilia f.
- Barraquer's conjunctival f.
- Barraquer's corneal f.
- Barraquer's hemostatic mosquito f.
- Barraquer–von Mondak capsule f.
- bayonet f.
- beaked f.
- Beaupre's cilia f.
- Bennett's cilia f.
- Berens' corneal transplant f.
- Berens' muscle f.
- Berens' ptosis f.
- Berens' suturing f.
- Berke's ptosis f.
- Berkley Bioengineering ptosis f.
- Bettman-Noyes fixation f.
- bipolar f.
- Birks-Mathelone micro f.
- Birks Mark II Colibri f.
- Birks Mark II f.
- Birks Mark II grooved f.
- Birks Mark II micro needle holder f.
- Birks Mark II straight f.
- Birks Mark II suture tying f.
- Birks Mark II toothed f.
- Bishop-Harmon f.
- Blaydes' corneal f.

forceps *(continued)*
blepharochalasis f.
Bonaccolto's fragment f.
Bonaccolto's jeweler f.
Bonaccolto's magnet tip f.
Bonaccolto's utility f.
bone-biting f.
Bonn's f.
Boruchoff's f.
Botvin's iris f.
Bracken's fixation f.
Bracken's iris f.
Bronson-Magnion f.
Callahan's lens loop fixation f.
capsule f.
capsule fragment f.
Castroviejo's capsule f.
Castroviejo's clip applying f.
Castroviejo's fixation f.
Castroviejo's lid f.
Castroviejo's scleral fold f.
Castroviejo's suturing f.
Castroviejo's wide grip handle f.
Castroviejo-Arruga f.
chalazion f.
Chandler's iris f.
cilia f.
Clark's capsule fragment f.
Clark-Verhoeff capsule f.
Clayman's lens implant f.
clip applying f.
Cohen's corneal f.
Coleman-Taylor IOL f.
Colibri's f.
corneal fixation f.
corneal holding f.
corneal prosthesis f.

forceps *(continued)*
corneal splinter f.
corneoscleral f.
Crawford's f.
cross-action capsule f.
Culler's fixation f.
Dallas lens inserting f.
Dan's chalazion f.
Dan-Gradle cilia f.
Danberg's iris f.
Davis' f.
Desmarres' chalazion f.
Dixon-Thorpe vitreous foreign body f.
Douglas' cilia f.
dressing f.
Drews' cilia f.
Drews-Sato tying f.
Eber's needle holder f.
Ehrhardt's lid f.
Elschnig's capsule f.
Elschnig's fixation f.
Elschnig-O'Brien f.
Elschnig-O'Connor f.
entropion f.
Erhardt's lid f.
Ewing's capsular f.
Fine's dissecting f.
Fine's tying f.
Fine-Castroviejo suturing f.
fine-toothed f.
Fink-Jameson muscle f.
Fisher-Arlt iris f.
fixation/anchor f.
fixation binocular f.
fixed f.
Foerster's iris f.
fold f.
foreign body f.
Frances' spud chala- zion f.
Francis' f.

forceps *(continued)*
- Fuchs' capsule f.
- Fuchs' iris f.
- Furniss' cornea holding f.
- Gelfilm f.
- Gifford's fixation f.
- Gill-Arruga capsular f.
- Gill-Hess iris f.
- Girard's corneoscleral f.
- Gradle's cilia f.
- Graefe's fixation f.
- Graefe's iris f.
- Graefe's tissue f.
- Grayton's corneal f.
- Green's fixation f.
- Grieshaber's diamond coated f.
- Grieshaber's iris f.
- Guist's fixation f.
- Gunderson's muscle f.
- Guyton-Clark fragment f.
- Guyton-Noyes fixation f.
- Halberg's contact lens f.
- Halsted's mosquito hemostatic f.
- Harmon's fixation f.
- Harms' corneal f.
- Harms' tying f.
- Harms-Tubingen tying f.
- Hartmann's mosquito hemostatic f.
- Heath's chalazion f.
- hemostatic f.
- Hertel's stone f.
- Hess' f.
- Hess-Barraquer f.
- Hess-Horwitz f.
- Hirschman's lens f.
- Holth's f.
- Hoskins' beaked Colibri f.
- Hoskins' fine straight f.

forceps *(continued)*
- Hoskins' fixation f.
- Hoskins' micro straight f.
- Hoskins' miniaturized micro straight f.
- Hoskins' straight micro iris f.
- Hoskins' suture f.
- Hoskins Dallas intraocular lens inserting f.
- Hoskins-Luntz f.
- Hoskins-Skeleton fine f.
- Hoskins-Skeleton micro grooved broad-tipped f.
- host tissue f.
- Houses' miniature f.
- Hubbard's corneoscleral f.
- Hunt's chalazion f.
- Hyde's double curved f.
- Ilg's capsule f.
- Ilg's curved micro tying f.
- Ilg's insertion f.
- intraocular f.
- Iowa State fixation f.
- iris f.
- Jacobs' capsule fragment f.
- Jameson's muscle f.
- Jansen-Middleton septotomy f.
- Jensen's intraocular lens f.
- Jervey's capsule fragment f.
- Jervey's iris f.
- jeweler f.
- Jones' f.
- Judd's f.
- Kalt's f.

forceps *(continued)*
- Katena's f.
- Katzin-Barraquer f.
- Keeler's extended round tip f.
- Keeler's intraocular foreign body grasping f.
- Kerrison's f.
- Kevorkian-Young f.
- King-Prince muscle f.
- Kirby's capsule f.
- Kirby's corneoscleral f.
- Kirby's iris f.
- Kirby's tissue f.
- Knapp's f.
- Koby's cataract f.
- Kraff-Utrata capsulorrhexis f.
- Kraft's f.
- Kronfeld's f.
- Krukenberg's pigment spindle f.
- Kuhnt's fixation f.
- Kulvin-Kalt f.
- Lambert's chalazion f.
- large-angled f.
- Leakey's chalazion f.
- Leigh's capsule f.
- lens threading f.
- Lester's fixation f.
- lid f.
- Linn-Graefe iris f.
- Lister's f.
- Littauer's cilia f.
- Llobera's fixation f.
- Lordan's chalazion f.
- Lucae's dressing f.
- Manhattan E & E suturing f.
- marginal chalazion f.
- Maumenee's capsule f.
- Maumenee's corneal f.

forceps *(continued)*
- Maumenee's Suregrip f.
- Max Fine f.
- McCullough's suturing f.
- McGregor's conjunctiva f.
- McGuire's marginal chalazion f.
- McLean's capsule f.
- McLean's muscle recession f.
- McPherson's bent f.
- McPherson's corneal f.
- McPherson's micro iris f.
- McPherson's micro suture f.
- McPherson's tying iris f.
- Mentor-Maumenee Suregrip f.
- micro Colibri f.
- miniature f.
- Moehle's corneal f.
- mosquito hemostatic f.
- Neubauer's f.
- New Orleans E & E fixation f.
- Noble's f.
- Noyes' f.
- Nugent's rectus f.
- O'Brien's fixation f.
- O'Connor's sponge f.
- O'Connor-Elschnig fixation f.
- Ochsner's tissue/cartilage f.
- Ogura's tissue/cartilage f.
- Osher's foreign body f.
- Paton's anterior chamber lens implant f.
- Paton's capsule f.
- Paton's corneal transplant f.
- Paton's suturing f.

forceps *(continued)*
Paton's tying/stitch removal f.
Paufique's suturing f.
Pavlo-Colibri corneal f.
Penn-Anderson scleral fixation f.
Perritt's f.
Peyman-Green vitreous f.
Phillips' fixation f.
Pierse's corneal f.
Pierse's fixation f.
Pley's extracapsular f.
Pollock's f.
Primbs' suturing f.
Prince's muscle f.
ptosis f.
Puntenny's f.
pupil spreader/retractor f.
Quevedo's fixation f.
Quevedo's suturing f.
Quire's mechanical finger f.
Reese's muscle f.
Reisinger's lens extracting f.
ring f.
Rizzuti's fixation f.
Rizzuti's rectus f.
Rizzuti-Furniss cornea holding f.
Rolf's f.
Russian f.
Rycroft's tying f.
Sachs' tissue f.
Sanders-Castroviejo suturing f.
Sandt's f.
Sauer's suture f.
Schaaf's foreign body f.
Schaefer's fixation f.
Scheie-Graefe fixation f.

forceps *(continued)*
Schepens' f.
Schweigger's capsule f.
scleral twist grip f.
Scott's lens insertion f.
Shields' f.
silicone rod and sleeve f.
silicone sponge f.
Skeleton's fine f.
sleeve spreading f.
Smart's f.
Smith-Leiske cross-action intraocular lens f.
Snellen's entropion f.
Snyder's corneal spring f.
Spender's chalazion f.
Spero's f.
Starr's fixation f.
Stern-Castroviejo f.
Stevens' f.
Storz's capsule f.
Storz's cilia f.
Storz's corneal f.
Storz-Bonn suturing f.
Storz-Utrata f.
Strow's corneal f.
superior rectus f.
suturing f.
Takahashi's iris retractor f.
Tennant's titanium suturing f.
Terson's capsule f.
Terson's extracapsular f.
Thomas' fixation f.
Thorpe's f.
Thorpe-Castroviejo corneal f.
Thorpe-Castroviejo fixation f.
Thorpe-Castroviejo vitreous foreign body f.

forceps *(continued)*
- Thrasher's lens implant f.
- three toothed f.
- Troutman's f.
- tying and stitch removal f.
- Verhoeff's f.
- Vickers' f.
- vitreous foreign body f.
- von Graefe's f.
- von Mondak's f.
- Wadsworth's lid f.
- Wainstock's suturing f.
- Waldeau's f.
- Wies' chalazion f.
- Worth's strabismus f.
- Wullstein-House cup f.
- Ziegler's f.

foreign body
- f.b. bur
- Ellis' f.b. spud
- f.b. forceps
- Shoch's f.b. pickup
- f.b. spud

Foerster's enucleation snare

Forker's retractor

Foster's enucleation snare

Four Dot Test

four-loop iris fixated implant

Fox's
- aluminum shield
- conformer
- implant
- irrigating/aspirating unit
- shield
- sphere implant

fragmatome
- Gill-Hess f.
- Girard's f.

fragmentation/aspiration handpiece

fragmentor
- Lieberman's f.

Fragmatome flute syringe

Francis'
- forceps
- spud

Franklin's
- glasses
- spectacles

Freeman's solution

Freer's
- chisel
- elevator

freeze-thaw cryotherapy

French's
- needle holder
- hook spatula
- lacrimal dilator
- lacrimal probe
- lacrimal spatula
- pattern spatula

Fresnel
- lens
- prism

Frey's
- implant
- tunneled implant

Friedenwald's
- funduscope
- ophthalmoscope

Friedman's
- hand-held Hruby lens
- tantalum clip

Frigitronics
- cryosurgery apparatus
- freeze-thaw cryopexy probe

Fritz's vitreous transplant needle

Frog cortex remover

Frost's
- scissors
- suture

Fuchs'
- capsule forceps
- iris forceps

Fuchs' *(continued)*
lancet type keratome
retinal detachment syringe
two-way syringe
Ful-Vue
ophthalmoscope
spot retinoscope
streak retinoscope
funduscope
Furniss' cornea holding forceps
Fyodorov's lens

g

Galezowski's lacrimal dilator
Galin's
bleb cup
intraocular implant lens
gallium citrate contrast
Galt's aspirating cannula
Gamboscope
Gans' cannula
Ganzfeld's electroretinograph
Garcia-Ibanez camera
Garcia-Novito eye implant
Gass'
cannula
dye applicator
irrigating/aspirating unit
retinal detachment hook
scleral marker
scleral punch
vitreous aspirating cannula
Geiger's cautery
Gelfilm
cap
forceps
retinal implant
Geuder's keratoplasty needle
Giardet's corneal transplant scissors
Gibralter's headrest
Gibson's irrigating/aspirating unit
Gifford's
applicator
corneal curet
fixation forceps
iris forceps
needle holder
Gill's
blade
corneal knife
counterpressor
double Luer-Lok cannula
intraocular implant lens
iris forceps
knife
scissors
Gill-Fine corneal knife
Gill-Hess
blade
fragmatome
iris forceps
knife
scissors
Gill-Welch
curet
guillotine port
knife
scissors
Gilmore's intraocular implant lens
Girard's
anterior chamber needle
cataract aspirating needle
corneoscleral forceps
fragmatome
phakofragmatome
scleral expander ring
Gish's micro YAG laser

Givner's lid retractor
Gladstone-Putterman transmarginal rotation entropion
clamp
glass sphere implant
glasses
- bifocal g.
- contact g.
- crutch g.
- executive bifocal g.
- executive trifocal g.
- Franklin's g.
- Hallauer's g.
- Masselon's g.
- safety g.
- sun g.
- trifocal f.

glaucoma pencil
glue
- butyl cyanoacrylate g.
- ethyl cyanoacrylate g.
- histacryl g.
- methyl cyanoacrylate g.
- g. patch
- wicking g. patch

glued-on hard contact lens
Gold's sphere implant
Goldmann's
- 3-mirror lens
- applanation tonometer
- Coherent radiation
- contact lens prism
- goniolens
- multi-mirrored lens
- perimeter
- serrated knife

Goldmann-Weekers Dark
Adaptometer
Goldstein's
- anterior chamber syringe
- cannula
- golf club spud
- lacrimal sac retractor

Goldstein's *(continued)*
- lacrimal syringe
- refractor
- retractor
- syringe

golf club spud
Gonin's cautery
goniofocalizing lens
goniogram
- Becker's g.

goniolens
- 4-mirror g.
- Allen-Thorpe g.
- Goldmann's g.
- Koeppe's g.
- single-mirror g.
- Thorpe-Castroviejo g.

goniophotography
gonioprism
goniopuncture knife
gonioscope
- Lovac's g.
- Sussman's 4-mirror g.
- Zeiss' g.

gonioscopic
- g. lens
- g. prism

goniotomy
- g. knife
- g. needle holder

Gonnin's marker
Gonnin-Amsler marker
Good's retractor
Gormley's double cannula
gouge
- lacrimal sac g.
- spud g.
- Todd's g.

Gould's intraocular implant lens
Gradle's
- cilia forceps
- corneal trephine
- electrode

Gradle's *(continued)*
- forceps
- refractor
- retractor

Graefe's
- cataract knife
- cystotome
- forceps
- iris forceps
- knife
- strabismus hook

graft
- g. carrier spoon
- g. preservation solution

Graither's
- collar button
- refractor
- retractor

Grayson's corneal forceps

Green's
- caliper
- capsule forceps
- cataract knife
- chalazion forceps
- corneal dissector
- corneal knife
- curet
- dissector
- double spatula
- eye shield
- fixation forceps
- forceps
- hook
- iris replacer
- knife
- muscle hook
- muscle tucker
- needle holder
- refractor
- replacer spatula
- spatula
- strabismus hook
- strabismus tucker
- trephine

grid
- Amsler's g.

Gridley's intraocular lens

Grieshaber's
- corneal trephine
- keratome
- knife
- micro-bipolar coagulator
- needle
- needle holder
- power injector system
- ruby knife
- trephine
- vertical cutting scissors
- vitreous scissors

Groenholm's
- refractor
- retractor

groove
- g. silicone implant
- g. suture

Gross' retractor

Gruning's magnet

GS-9 needle

guard
- cataract knife g.
- eye knife g.
- forceps g.
- keratome g.
- scalpel g.

Guibor's
- chart
- duct tube
- shield

guillotine
- g. cutting tip
- g. vitrectomy instrument

Guist's
- enucleation hemostat
- enucleation scissors
- fixation forceps
- hemostat
- implant
- scissors

Guist's *(continued)*
- speculum
- sphere implant

Guist-Bloch speculum
Gullstrand's
- loupe
- ophthalmoscope
- slit lamp

Gunderson's muscle forceps
Guyton's
- corneal transplant trephine
- electrode

Guyton-Clark fragment forceps
Guyton-Friedenwald suture
Guyton-Lundsgaard
- cataract knife
- keratome
- scalpel
- sclerotome

Guyton-Maumenee speculum
Guyton-Minkowski Potential Acuity Meter
Guyton-Park speculum

h

Haab's
- knife needle
- magnet
- scleral resection knife

Haag-Streit slit lamp
Haenig's irrigating scissors
Hague's cataract lamp
Haidinger's brush
Haik's implant
Halberg's trial clip occluder
Hallauer's
- glasses
- spectacles

Hallpike's maneuver
halogen ophthalmoscope
halogram
Halsey's needle holder
Halsted's curved mosquito forceps
hand-held
- h. eye magnet
- h. fundus camera
- h. Hruby lens
- h. rotary prism

hand-motion visual acuity test
handle
- Beaver's h.

Hansel's stain
Hansen's
- keratome
- keratome guard

hapten
hard contact lens
Hardesty's tenotomy hook
Hardy's punch
Hardy-Rand-Littler plates
Harmon's forceps
Harms'
- corneal forceps
- trabeculotome

Harms-Tubingen tying forceps
Harrington's
- erysiphake
- retractor
- tonometer

Harrison's
- retractor
- scissors

Hartmann's
- forceps
- hemostatic forceps

Hartstein's
- irrigator
- refractor
- retractor

Hasner's lid forceps
head-tilt test

Heath's
    chalazion curet
    curet
    dilator
    expressor
    forceps
Hebra's
    blade
    curet
    hook
helium
    h. aiming ion laser
    h. neon aiming laser
hemisphere implant
hemostat
Hemovac
Hering-Bielschowsky after-image test
Hertel's exophthalmometer
Hertzog's
    lens spatula
    pliable probe
Hess'
    diplopia screen
    forceps
    screen test
    spoon
Hess-Barraquer forceps
Hess-Horwitz forceps
Hess-Lee screen
Hessburg's
    corneal shield
    intraocular lens glide
    subpalpebral lavage system
Hessburg-Barron vacuum trephine
heteroscope
Heyer-Schulte microscope
Heyner's
    curet
    cannula
    dilator
Heyner's *(continued)*
    double cannula
    expressor
    forceps
HGH laser
Hildreth's cautery
Hill's retractor
Hillis' retractor
Hilton's
    self-retaining infusion cannula
    sutureless infusion cannula
Hirschberg's
    magnet
    test
Hirschman's
    spatula
    speculum
hollow sphere implant
Holmgren's
    color test
    wool skein test
Holofax
Holth's
    forceps
    scleral punch
Honan's
    cuff
    manometer
hook
    Amenabar's discission h.
    anchor h.
    Berens' h.
    Birks Mark II h.
    boat h.
    corneal h.
    Culler's muscle h.
    discission h.
    Drews-Sato suture pickup h.
    expressor h.
    Fenzle's manipulating h.

hook *(continued)*
- Fink's muscle h.
- fixation h.
- flat h.
- Gass's retinal detachment h.
- Graefe's strabismus h.
- Green's muscle h.
- Green's strabismus h.
- Hardesty's tenotomy h.
- Hebra's h.
- Hunkeler's ballpoint h.
- iris h.
- Jameson's muscle h.
- Kirby's h.
- Knapp's iris h.
- Kuglein's h.
- Maumenee's iris h.
- McReynolds' lid retracting h.
- muscle h.
- Nugent's h.
- oblique muscle h.
- O'Conner's flat h.
- O'Conner's sharp h.
- Ochsner's h.
- Osher's h.
- Praeger's iris h.
- retinal detachment h.
- scleral h.
- sharp h.
- Shepard's iris h.
- Shepard's reversed iris h.
- Sinskey's lens h.
- Smith's expressor h.
- spatula h.
- squint h.
- St. Martin–Franceshetti cataract h.
- Stevens' tenotomy h.
- strabismus h.
- suture pickup h.
- tenotomy h.

hook *(continued)*
- Tomas' iris h.
- Tomas' suture h.
- twist fixation h.
- Tyrell's iris h.
- von Graefe's h.
- Wiener's h.

Hoopes' corneal marker
Hopkins' Rod Lens Telescope
horopter
- Vieth-Muller h.

Hosford's
- expressor
- lacrimal dilator
- spud

Hoskins' razor blade fragments
Hoskins-Castroviejo corneal scissors
Hoskins-Westcott tenotomy scissors
host tissue forceps
Hough's drape
House's
- knife
- lacrimal dilator
- miniature forceps
- myringotomy knife

House-Bellucci alligator scissors
House-Dieter nipper
House-Urban-Pentax camera
Houser's cul-de-sac irrigator T tube
Howard's abrader
Hruby's contact lens
Hubbard's forceps
Huey's scissors
Hughes' implant
Humphrey's
- automatic refractor
- perimeter

Hunkeler's ballpoint hook
Hunt's chalazion scissors
huygenian eyepiece

Hyde's
- forceps
- irrigator/aspirator unit

hydrodiascope
hyfrecator
hyperbolic glasses

I

Ialo's photocoagulator
IDI corneoscope
Ilg's
- lens loop
- micro needle holder
- needle
- probe
- push/pull

Iliff's
- lacrimal probe
- lacrimal trephine

Iliff-Park speculum
Iliff-Wright fascia needle
Illiterate Eye Chart
illuminated suction needle
implant
- 4-loop iris clip i.
- 4-loop iris fixated i.
- 45-degree bent reform i.
- acorn-shaped i.
- acrylic i.
- Allen's orbital i.
- Allen-Braley i.
- Alpar's i.
- Arruga's i.
- Arruga-Moura-Brazil i.
- Berens' conical i.
- Berens' pyramidal i.
- Berens-Rosa scleral i.
- Binkhorst's i.
- Boberg-Ans i.

implant *(continued)*
- Bonaccolto's orbital i.
- Boyd's orbital i.
- Brawner's i.
- Brown-Dohlman Silastic corneal i.
- build-up i.
- Bunker's i.
- Cardona's focalizing fundus i.
- Cardona's goniofocalizing i.
- Castroviejo's acrylic i.
- Choyce's i.
- Choyce Mark VIII i.
- Cogan-Boberg-Ans i.
- conical i.
- conventional shell i.
- Copeland's i.
- corneal i.
- cosmetic contact shell i.
- Cryo-Barrages vitreous i.
- Cutler's i.
- Dannheim's i.
- Dermostat's i.
- Doherty's i.
- Epstein's collar stud acrylic i.
- Federov's type I and II i.
- Ferguson's i.
- Fox's sphere i.
- Frey's i.
- Frey's tunneled i.
- front build-up i.
- full-dimpled Lucite i.
- Garcia-Novito i.
- Gelfilm i.
- glass sphere i.
- Gold's sphere i.
- Gold-Mules i.
- Goldmann's i.
- gonioscopic i.
- grooved silicone i.

implant *(continued)*
- Guist's i.
- Haik's i.
- hemisphere i.
- hollow sphere i.
- hook type i.
- Hruby's i.
- Hughes' i.
- Iowa i.
- Ivalon's sponge i.
- Jordon's i.
- King's i.
- Koeppe's i.
- Kryptok's i.
- Landegger's i.
- Lemoine's i.
- Levitt's i.
- Lincoff's scleral sponge i.
- Lovac 6-mirror i.
- Lucite sphere i.
- Lyda-Ivalon-Lucite i.
- magnetic i.
- McGhan's i.
- Melauskas' acrylic i.
- meridional i.
- methyl methacrylate i.
- motility i.
- Mulberger's i.
- Mules' i.
- Müller's i.
- Nocito's i.
- O'Malley's i.
- optic i.
- orbital floor i.
- peanut's i.
- plastic sphere i.
- Plexiglas i.
- polyethylene i.
- Radin-Rosenthal i.
- Rayner-Choyce i.
- reverse-shape i.
- Ridley's i.
- Ridley Mark II i.

implant *(continued)*
- Rodin's i.
- Rosa-Berens i.
- Ruedemann's i.
- Ruiz plano fundus i.
- Schepens' hollow hemisphere i.
- scleral i.
- semishell i.
- Severin's i.
- shelf-type i.
- shell i.
- Sichi's i.
- Silastic scleral buckler i.
- silicone i.
- sleeve i.
- Smith's orbital floor i.
- Snellen's conventional reform i.
- solid silicone with Supramid mesh i.
- sphere i.
- spherical i.
- sponge i.
- Stampelli's i.
- Stone's i.
- subperiosteal i.
- Supramid i.
- Supramid-Allen i.
- surface i.
- tantalum mesh i.
- Teflon i.
- Tennant's i.
- Tensilon i.
- tire i.
- Troncoso's gonioscopic i.
- Troutman's i.
- tunneled i.
- Ultex i.
- Uribe's i.
- VA magnetic i.
- Varigray i.
- Varilux i.

implant *(continued)*
- Vitallium i.
- Volk's conoid i.
- Walter Reed i.
- Wheeler's eye sphere i.
- wire mesh i.

impression tonometer
indirect ophthalmoscope
injector
- automatic twin syringe i.

InnoMed
INNOVA System 920
insulin pump CPI90-100
Intermedics Phaco I/A Unit
intraocular lens dialer
IntraOptics lensometer
introducer
- Carter sphere i.
- silicone i.
- sphere i.

IOCARE titanium needle
IOL — intraocular lens
IOLAB irrigating/aspirating photocoagulator
IOLAB Titanium Instruments
ion laser
IOPTEX
iridectomy scissors
iridodilator
iridotomy scissors
iris
- i. hook cannula
- i. scissors
- i. spatula

irrigating
- anterior chamber i. vectis
- i. cannula
- i. cul-de-sac i. vectis
- i. cystotome
- plastic disposable i. vectis

IRRIGATING/ASPIRATING UNITS

- Alcon's
- Bishop-Harmon
- Bracken's
- Cavitron
- Cavitron-Kelman
- Charles'
- Cooper's
- CooperVision
- DeVilbiss'
- Doughtery's
- Drews'
- Drews-Rosenbaum
- Fink's
- Fox's
- Gass'
- Gibson's
- Hartstein's
- Hyde's
- IOLAB
- Irvine's
- Kelman's
- Kelman-Cavitron
- McIntyre's
- Phaco Cavitron
- Rollet's
- SITE TXR System
- Surg-E-Trol System
- Sylva's
- Visitec

Irvine's
- irrigating/aspirating unit
- probe-pointed scissors
- scissors

Ishihara's
- Color Test
- I-Temp cautery
- IV slit lamp
- Pseudoisochromatic Plates

Ivalon's sponge implant

j

J-shaped irrigating/aspirating cannula
Jacob-Swann gonioscope
Jaeger's
- hook
- keratome
- lid plate
- retractor
- Visual Test

Jaffee's intraocular spatula
Jaffee-Bechert nucleus rotator
Jaffee-Givner lid retractor
Jameson's
- caliper
- forceps
- hook
- muscle hook

Javal's ophthalmometer
Jedmed A-Scan
Jenning's test
Jensen's
- capsule scratcher
- intraocular lens forceps

jeweler's tweezer
John Green's caliper
Johnson's
- double cannula
- evisceration knife

Johnson-Bell erysiphake
Johnson-Tooke corneal knife
Jones'
- dilator
- keratome
- Pyrex tube
- tear duct tube
- test

Jordon's implant
Joseph's elevator
Judd's forceps
Judson Smith manipulator

k

Kalt's
- corneal needle
- forceps
- needle holder
- spoon

Kamerling Capsular 90
Kara's
- cataract needle
- erysiphake

Karakashian-Barraquer scissors
Karickhoff's
- double cannula
- laser lens

Karl Ilg Instruments
Katena Products
Katzin's scissors
Katzin-Barraquer forceps
Kaufman's
- medium
- vitrector

Kayser-Fleischer ring
Kearney's side-notch IOL
Keeler's
- Catford needle holder with micro jaws
- cryophake
- cryosurgical unit
- extended round tip
- Fison tissue retractor
- intravitreal scissors
- lancet tip
- loupe
- micro round tip
- micro spear tip
- micro tip
- panoramic loupe

Keeler's *(continued)*
prism
Pulsair tonometer
puncture tip
razor tip
retractable blade
ruby knife
Specular Microscope
triple facet tip
ultrasonic cataract removal lancet
Keeler-Amoils
curved cataract probe
glaucoma probe
long shank retinal probe
Machemer retinal probe
micro curved cataract probe
Ophthalmic Cryosystem
retinal probe
straight cataract probe
vitreous probe
Keeler-Keislar lacrimal cannula
Keeler-Meyer diamond knife
Keeler-Pierse eye speculum
Keeler-Rodger iris retractor
Keitzer-Lancaster
eye speculum
lid retractor
Kelly Descemet's membrane punch
Kelman's
cannula
cryoextractor
cyclodialysis cannula
cystotome
iris retractor
irrigating/aspirating unit
irrigating handpiece
knife
lens
phacoemulsification unit
Kelman-Cavitron I/A unit
KeraCorneaScope
Kerascan
keratectomy scissors
keratoiridoscope
Kerato-Kontours Instruments
Keratolux fixation device
keratome
Agnew's k.
Bard-Parker k.
Beaver's k.
Berens' partial k.
Castroviejo's k.
Czermak's k.
Fuchs' lancet type k.
Grieshaber's k.
Guyton-Lundsgaard k.
Hansen's k.
Jaeger's k.
Jones' k.
Kirby's k.
Lancaster's k.
Martinez's k.
McReynolds' k.
Rowland's k.
Storz's k.
keratometer
keratoplasty scissors
keratoscope
Kerrison's
forceps
rongeur
Keystone Test
kibisitome
Kimura's platinum spatula
Kimwipes
Kindergarten Eye Chart
kinescope
King's
corneal trephine
orbital implant
King-Prince knife
Kirby's
angulated iris spatula

Kirby's *(continued)*
- cataract knife
- dislocator
- forceps
- hook
- intracapsular lens spoon
- intraocular lens loop
- iris forceps
- iris spatula
- keratome
- knife
- lens dislocator
- lens loop
- refractor
- retractor
- scissors
- spoon

Kirby-Bauer disk sensitivity test

Klein's
- curved cannula
- keratoscope

Kloti's vitreous cutter

Knapp's
- cataract knife
- eye speculum
- iris hook
- iris probe
- iris repositor
- iris scissors
- iris spatula
- knife
- knife needle
- lacrimal sac retractor
- lens spoon
- refractor
- retractor
- scissors
- spatula
- spoon

knife
- Agnew's canaliculus k.
- Alcon's surgical k.
- Bard-Parker k.

knife *(continued)*
- Barkan's goniotomy k.
- Barraquer's k.
- Beaver's k.
- Beer's cataract k.
- Berens' cataract k.
- Berens' glaucoma k.
- Berens' keratoplasty k.
- Berens' ptosis k.
- bladebreaker k.
- cannula k.
- Castroviejo's k.
- Castroviejo's twin k.
- corneal k.
- Cusick's goniotomy k.
- Desmarres' k.
- Deutschman's cataract k.
- diamond dusted k.
- discission k.
- dissector k.
- Duredge's k.
- Elschnig's k.
- Gill's k.
- Gill-Fine corneal k.
- Gill-Hess k.
- Gill-Welch k.
- Goldmann's serrated k.
- goniopuncture k.
- goniotomy k.
- Graefe's cataract k.
- Green's k.
- Grieshaber's ruby k.
- Guyton-Lundsgaard cataract k.
- Haab's scleral resection k.
- House's myringotomy k.
- I-Knife microsurgical k.
- Johnson's evisceration k.
- Johnson-Tooke corneal k.
- Keeler's ruby k.
- Keeler-Meyer diamond k.

knife *(continued)*
- Kelman's k.
- King-Prince k.
- Kirby's cataract k.
- Knapp's cataract k.
- KOI k.
- Lancaster's k.
- Lowell's glaucoma k.
- Lundsgaard's k.
- Martinez's k.
- McPherson-Wheeler k.
- McPherson-Ziegler k.
- McReynolds' pterygium k.
- Meyer Swiss Diamond lancet k.
- Meyer Swiss Diamond mini-angled k.
- Meyer Swiss Diamond wedge k.
- Microknife k.
- Myocure k.
- Parker's k.
- Paton's corneal k.
- Paufique's k.
- ptosis k.
- razor blade k.
- Reese's ptosis k.
- Rizzuti-Spizziri cannula k.
- ruby diamond k.
- ruby k.
- Sato's corneal k.
- Scheie's goniopuncture k.
- scleral resection k.
- Sharpoint k.
- Sichel's k.
- Smith-Green cataract k.
- Spizziri's cannula k.
- Step-Knife diamond blade k.
- stiletto k.

knife *(continued)*
- stitch removing k.
- Storz-Duredge steel cataract k.
- Storz's cataract k.
- Swan's discission k.
- Tooke's k.
- V-lance k.
- von Graefe's k.
- wave edge k.
- Weber's k.
- Wheeler's k.
- Ziegler's k.

Knolle's capsule polisher
Koeppe's lens
KOI diamond knife
Kollmorgen elements
koroscope
koroscopy
KOWA
- camera
- Fluorescein System
- Optimed slit lamp

Kraff's
- capsule polisher curet
- cortex cannula
- polisher

Kraff-Utrata capsulorrhexis forceps
Krasnov's lens
kratometer
Kratz
- diamond-dusted needle
- lens
- needle
- polisher/scratcher

Kratz-Johnson lens
Kreiger-Spitznas vibrating scissors
Krimsky Test
Krimsky-Prince Accommodation Rule
Kronfeld's

Kronfeld's *(continued)*
- electrode
- forceps
- refractor
- retractor

Krukenberg's sponge
Krwawicz's cataract extractor
Kryospray II
krypton laser
Kuglein's
- hook
- iris hook
- irrigating lens manipulator
- lens manipulator
- push/pull
- refractor

Kuhnt's forceps
Kulvin-Kalt forceps
Kwitko's conjunctival spreader

L

L. T. Jones tear duct tube
L'Esperance erysiphake
lacrimal
- awl
- cannula
- duct T-tube
- intubation probe
- probe
- sac bur
- sac chisel
- sac gouge
- sac retractor
- sac rongeur
- syringe
- trephine

lacrimotome
Lactoplate
LaForce's spud
Lagleyze's needle
Lagrange's scissors
Laird's spatula
Lambert's forceps
lamp
- Birch's l.
- Birch-Hirschfeld l.
- Duke-Elder l.
- Gullstrand's slit l.
- Haag-Streit slit l.
- Hague's cataract l.
- Rodenstock's l.
- slit l.
- Zeiss l.

Lancaster's
- eye magnet
- eye speculum
- keratome
- knife
- lid speculum
- magnet
- red-green test
- speculum

Lancaster-O'Connor speculum
Lancaster-Regan test
lance
- Rolf's l.

lancet
- suture l.
- Swan's l.

Landegger's implant
Landers' vitrectomy ring
Landolt's broken ring chart
Lane's needle
Lange's speculum
lantern test
LASAG microruptor
laser
- Allergan Humphrey l.
- AMO YAG 100 l.
- argon blue l.
- argon green l.

laser *(continued)*
- Biophysic Medical l.
- Britt argon/krypton l.
- Britt BL-l2 l.
- Britt pulsed argon l.
- Candela l.
- Cardona l.
- Carl Zeiss l.
- CILCO argon l.
- CILCO Frigitronics l.
- CILCO Hoffer Laseridge l.
- CILCO krypton l.
- CILCO Lasertek A-K l.
- CO_2 l.
- CO_2 Sharplan l.
- Coherent 7910 l.
- Coherent 920 argon/dye l.
- Coherent Radiation argon/krypton l.
- Cooper 2000 l.
- Cooper 2500 l.
- Cooper Laser Sonics l.
- CooperVision l.
- erbium l.
- Evergreen Lasertek l.
- Excimer l.
- Gish Micro YAG l.
- helium aiming ion l.
- helium neon aiming l.
- HGM l.
- ion l.
- krypton l.
- Lasertek l.
- liquid organic dye l.
- LPK-80 II argon l.
- Meditech l.
- Merrimac l.
- Microruptor II l.
- mode locked Nd:YAG l.
- molectron l.
- Nanolas Nd:YAG l.

laser *(continued)*
- Nd:YAG l.
- NdiYAG l.
- neodymium YAG l.
- Nidek Laser System l.
- oculocutaneous l.
- Ophthalas argon/krypton l.
- photodisrupting l.
- photovaporizing l.
- Q-switched neodymium YAG l.
- Q-switched ruby l.
- ruby l.
- Sharplan argon l.
- SITE l.
- Takata l.
- TE MOO mode beam l.
- tunable dye l.
- Visulas argon l.
- Visulas argon/YAG l.
- Visulas YAG C l.
- Visulas YAG E l.
- Visulas YAG S l.

LASER TERMS

- argon green laser
- argon laser
- axial length
- blanching
- continuous wave argon laser
- desired end-point
- double contiguous row
- duration
- dye laser
- end-point
- fluorescein angiogram
- gray white burn
- J — Joule's equivalent
- krypton laser

LASER TERMS *(continued)*
- krypton red laser
- luminosity
- meshwork
- microaneurysm
- microaneurysmal leakage
- micron/microns
- micron spot size
- mJ — millijoules
- mode-locked train
- msec — millisecond
- mv — millivolt
- mw — milliwatt
- Nd — neodymium
- nsec — nanosecond
- panretinal
- periphery
- photocoagulation
- psec — pulses per second
- pulse mode
- pulsers
- quadrants
- rarefied pigment
- retinal hole
- ruby laser
- spot placement
- spot size
- spots
- trabecular meshwork
- tunable dye laser
- w — watt
- xenon arc
- YAG laser

Lasertek laser
Lawton corneal scissors
lead-filled mallet
Lebensohn's Visual Acuity Chart
Leitz microscope
Leland refractor
Lemoine
- implant
- serrefine

Lemoine-Searcy fixation anchor loop
Lempert-Storz loupe
lens
- 3-mirror contact l.
- 4-mirror goniolens l.
- Abraham peripheral button iridotomy l.
- Accugel l.
- achromatic l.
- acrylic l.
- adherent l.
- Amenabar l.
- American Medical Optics Baron l.
- amnifocal l.
- Amsoft l.
- Anis staple l.
- aplanatic l.
- apochromatic l.
- Appolionio l.
- Aquaflex l.
- Aquasight l.
- Arruga l.
- aspheric cataract l.
- aspherical ophthalmoscopic l.
- auxillary l.
- Azar l.
- Bagolini l.
- bandage l.
- Barkan gonioscopic l.
- Baron l.
- Barraquer l.
- Bausch & Lomb Optima l.
- Bechert 7 mm l.
- Beebe l.
- biconcave contact l.
- biconvex l.
- bicylindrical l.
- Bietti l.
- bifocal l.

lens *(continued)*
- Binkhorst l.
- Binkhorst-Fyodorov l.
- bispherical l.
- Bi-Soft l.
- Boberg-Ans l.
- Boys-Smith laser l.
- Brucke l.
- Carl Zeiss l.
- cataract l.
- Centra-Flex l.
- Charles contact l.
- Choyce Mark VIII l.
- Cibasoft l.
- Cibathin l.
- CILCO-Simcoe II l.
- CILCO-Sonometrics l.
- Clayman l.
- clip l.
- Coburn l.
- concave l.
- concavoconcave l.
- concavoconvex l.
- condensing l.
- contact low-vacuum l.
- CooperVision PMMA-ACL Flex l.
- Copeland radial pan-chamber UV l.
- Coquille plano l.
- Crookes l.
- crystalline l.
- decentered l.
- diagnostic fiberoptic l.
- direct gonioscopic l.
- dispersing l.
- Doubra l.
- Dura-T l.
- Emery l.
- ERG-Jet disposable contact l.
- Eschenback Optik l.
- Feister Dualens l.

lens *(continued)*
- fiber optic diagnostic l.
- Flexlens l.
- FormFlex l.
- Frelex l.
- Frenzel l.
- Friedman hand-held Hruby l.
- fundus contact l.
- fundus focalizing l.
- fused bifocal l.
- Galin l.
- Genesis l.
- Gilmore l.
- Goldmann 3 mirror l.
- Goldmann macular contact l.
- goniofocalizing l.
- goniolens l.
- gonioscopic l.
- Gullstrand's l.
- hand-held Hruby l.
- Hessburg l.
- Hoffer LaserRidge intraocular l.
- Hruby l.
- Hunkeler l.
- Hydracon l.
- Hydrocurve l.
- Hydron l.
- Hydrosight l.
- immersion l.
- infant Karickhoff laser l.
- infant 3-mirror laser l.
- Intermedics l.
- Interspace YAG laser l.
- intraocular l.
- IOLAB 108B l.
- IOPTEX TabOptic l.
- iridocapsular l.
- iseikonic l.
- J loop PC l.
- Jaffe CILCO l.

lens *(continued)*
- Kamerling Capsular 90 l.
- Karickhoff laser l.
- Kearney side-notch l.
- Keeler panoramic l.
- Kelman flexible tripod l.
- Kelman Multiflex II l.
- Kelman Omnifit l.
- Kelman PC 27LB CapSul l.
- Koeppe l.
- Krasnov l.
- Kratz elliptical style l.
- Kratz/Johnson l.
- Krieger fundus l.
- Landers biconcave l.
- Landers contact l.
- Landers-Foulks temporary keratoprosthesis l.
- laser l.
- Laseridge Optics l.
- Layden infant l.
- Leiske l.
- Lempert-Storz l.
- Lems l.
- Lieb-Guerry l.
- Lindstrom Centrex l.
- Liteflex l.
- localizer
- loop l.
- loupe l.
- Lovac gonioscopic l.
- Machemer flat l.
- Machemer infusion contact l.
- Machemer magnifying l.
- macular contact l.
- Mainster retinal laser l.
- March laser l.
- Mark IX l.
- Mark II magni-Fouser l.
- McGhan l.
- McLean l.

lens *(continued)*
- medallion l.
- Meditec bandage contact l.
- meniscus concave l.
- meter l.
- minus l.
- Multi-Optics l.
- Neolens l.
- New Orleans l.
- Nova Aid l.
- Nova Soft II l.
- NOVACurve l.
- O'Malley-Pearce-Luma l.
- O'Shea l.
- Oculaid l.
- Ocular Gamboscope l.
- Ophtec Co. l.
- Optical Radiation l.
- Optiflex l.
- Opti-Vu l.
- Opt-Visor l.
- Osher l.
- P. F. Lee pediatric goniolens l.
- panchamber UV l.
- Pannu Type II l.
- PanoView Optics l.
- PBII blue loop l.
- pediatric Karickhoff laser l.
- pediatric 3-mirror laser l.
- Permalens l.
- Perspex CQ-Shearing-Simcoe-Sinskey l.
- Petrus single mirror laser l.
- Peyman l.
- Peyman-Tennant-Green l.
- Peyman wide field l.
- Pharmacia Visco J loop l.

lens *(continued)*
- Plano-Convex nonridge l.
- Platina clip l.
- Posner diagnostic l.
- Precision Cosmet l.
- prismatic contact l.
- prismatic gonioscopic l.
- prismatic goniotomy l.
- prosthetic l.
- punktal l.
- Rayner l.
- Red Reflex Lens Systems l.
- retroscopic l.
- Ridley l.
- Ritch trabeculoplasty laser l.
- Rodenstock panfundus l.
- Ruiz fundus l.
- Sauflon PW l.
- Schachar l.
- Scharf l.
- Severin l.
- Shearing l.
- Sheets l.
- short C loop l.
- Signet Optical l.
- silicone elastomer l.
- Silsoft contact l.
- Simcoe II PC l.
- Sinskey l.
- Soflens l.
- Stokes l.
- Strampelli l.
- Style S2 clear loop l.
- Surefit AC 85J l.
- Surgidev l.
- Sutherland l.
- T l.
- Tennant Anchorflex AC l.
- Tillyer l.
- Tolentino prism l.

lens *(continued)*
- Topcon l.
- Toric-Optima series l.
- trifocal l.
- Trokel l.
- Trokel-Peyman laser l.
- Uniplanar style PC II l.
- Urrets-Zavalia retinal surgical l.
- UVEX l.
- Varilux l.
- Viscolens l.
- Vision Tech l.
- Weber-Elsching l.
- Wild l.
- Wise iridotomy laser l.
- Wise iridotomy-sphincterotomy laser l.
- Woods Concept l.
- Yannuzzi fundus laser l.
- Yannuzzi l.
- Youens l.
- Zeiss l.
- Zeiss-Gullstrand l.

lensometer
- Allergan-Humphrey l.
- A-O Reichert l.
- Carl Zeiss l.
- Coburn l.
- IntraOptics l.
- Marco l.
- Reichert l.
- Topcon l.

Lens-Eze inserter

L'Esperance erysiphake

leukoscope

Levine's spud

Levitt's implant

Lewicky's
- formed cystotome
- self-retaining chamber maintainer

Lewis'

Lewis' *(continued)*
 lens loupe
 scoop
Lichtenberg's corneal trephine
lid everter
 Berens' l.e.
 Roveda's l.e.
 Schachne-Desmarres l.e.
 Struble's l.e.
 Walker's l.e.
lid speculum
Lieberman's
 fragmentor
 phaco crusher
Life-Tech Inc.
Lincoff's
 balloon catheter
 implant
 sponge
Linde's cryogenic probe
Lindner's spatula
linear visual acuity test
liquid
 l. organic dye laser
 l. vitreous aspirating cannula
Lister's
 forceps
 lens manipulator
 scissors
Lister-Burch speculum
Littauer's dissecting scissors
Littler's scissors
locator
 Berman's l.
 foreign body l.
 Roper-Hall l.
 Wildgren-Reck l.
Lombert's
 radiuscope
 tonometer
Londermann's corneal trephine
Look

Look *(continued)*
 capsule polisher
 cortex extractor
 cystotome
 I/A coaxial cannula
 irrigating lens loop
 irrigating vectis
 retrobulbar needle
 suture
loop
 angled nucleus removal l.
 Arlt's l.
 Berens' lens l.
 Elschnig-Weber l.
 Formflex lens l.
 Ilg's lens l.
 Kirby's intraocular lens l.
 Lemoine-Searcy fixation anchor l.
 nucleus delivery l.
 nucleus removal l.
 Pierse-Knoll irrigating lens l.
 Simcoe nucleus delivery l.
 two-angled polypropylene l.
Lordan's chalazion forceps
Loring's ophthalmoscope
Lotman Visometer
Lo-Trau side-cutting needle
loupe
 Amenabar's l.
 Beebe's l.
 Gullstrand's l.
 Keeler's panoramic l.
 Lempert-Storz l.
 Lewis l.
 Mark II Magni-Foscuser l.
 New Orleans l.
 Ocular Gamboscope l.
 Opt-Visor l.

- loupe *(continued)*
  - Weber-Elschnig l.
  - Zeiss l.
  - Zeiss-Gullstrand l.
- Lovac's
  - 6-mirror gonioscopic lens implant
  - fundus contact lens implant
- Lowell's glaucoma knife
- Lowry assay
- LPK-80 II argon laser
- L. T. Jones tear duct tube
- Lucite implant
- Luedde's
  - exophthalmometer
  - transplant rule
- Luer's
  - cannula lock
  - connections
  - tube
- Lumiwand light
- Lundsgaard's
  - knife
  - rasp
  - sclerotome
- Lundsgaard-Burch
  - corneal rasp
  - sclerotome
- Luxo Surgical Illuminator

m

- 3-M small aperture Steri-Drape
- M-TEC 2000 Surgical System
- Machemer's
  - caliper
  - cutter
  - vitreous cutter
- MacKay-Marg tonometer
- MacKool's capsule retractor
- MacVicar's double-end strabismus retractor
- Maddox's
  - prism
  - rod test
  - wing test
- magnet
  - Bronson-Magnion m.
  - Gruning's m.
  - Haab's m.
  - hand-held m.
  - Hirschberg's m.
  - implant m.
  - Lancaster's m.
  - original Sweet eye m.
  - rare earth m.
  - Schumann's giant type m.
  - Storz-Atlas hand m.
- magnifying loupe
- Maguire-Harvey vitreous cutter
- Mainster's retinal laser lens
- Malis Bipolar Coagulating/Cutting System
- Manhattan forceps
- manipulator
  - Judson-Smith m.
- manometer
  - Honan's m.
  - Tycos' m.
- manoptoscope
- March's laser sclerostomy needle
- Marco
  - chart projector
  - lensometer
  - perimeter
  - radius gauge
  - refractor
  - slit lamp
  - SurgiScope
- marker
  - Amsler's m.

marker *(continued)*
bi-prong muscle m.
Castroviejo's corneal transplant m.
corneal transplant m.
Desmarres' m.
Feldman RK optical center m.
Fink's bi-prong m.
Fink's muscle m.
Gass' scleral m.
Gonnin-Amsler m.
O'Brien's m.
radial keratotomy m.
Marlex mesh
Marlow's test
Martin Surefit lens pusher
Martinez
corneal transplant centering ring
corneal trephine blade
disposable corneal trephine
dissector
keratome
knife
Massachusetts Vision Kit
Masselon's
glasses
spectacles
Master's two-step test
Mattis' scissors
Maumenee's
erysiphake
iris hook
knife goniotomy cannula
vitreous aspirating needle
vitreous sweep spatula
Maumenee-Park speculum
Maunoir's iris scissors
Mauthner's test
Max Fine scissors
Mayo's scissors
McCannell's ocular pressure reducer
McCarey-Kaufman transport medium
McClure's iris scissors
McCullough's forceps
McDonald's expressor
McGannon's
refractor
retractor
McGhan's
3-M lens
implant
McGuire's
conformer
corneal scissors
forceps
I/A system
scissors
McIntyre's Irrigation/Aspiration System
McKinney's fixation ring
McLean's
forceps
scissors
suture
tonometer
McNeill-Goldmann blepharostat
McPherson's
forceps
needle holder
scissors
spatula
speculum
McPherson-Castroviejo scissors
McPherson-Vannas scissors
McPherson-Wheeler
blade
knife
McPherson-Ziegler knife
McReynolds'
hook

McReynolds' *(continued)*
keratome
knife
scissors
mechanized scissors
medallion lens
media
chondroitin sulfate m.
contrast m.
K-Sol m.
McCarey-Kaufman m.
Sabouraud's m.
mediaometer
Meditech laser
Melauska's orbital implant
Meller's
refractor
retractor
Mellinger's speculum
Mendez cystotome
Mentor
B-VAT II Video Acuity
Exeter ophthalmoscope
precut drain
wet field cautery
wet field eraser
Mentor-Maumenee Suregrip forceps
meridional implant
Merocel Surgical Spears
Mersilene suture
Mesco
mesh
Marlex m.
tantalum m.
Metcher's speculum
metric ophthalmoscope
metronoscope
Meyer's
Swiss diamond knife lancet
Swiss diamond mini-angled knife

Meyer's *(continued)*
Swiss diamond wedge knife
temporal loupe
Meyer-Schwickerath coagulator
Meyhoeffer's
chalazion curet
curet
mica spectacles
Michelson's counter pressure
Michel's pick
micro round-tip needle
microgonioscope
Microknife
Micro-Lite
micrometer
microphthalmoscope
Micropigmentation System
micro-point
m. needle
m. suture
Microruptor II laser
microscope
corneal m.
slit lamp m.
Wild M 690 m.
Zeiss m.
microspectroscope
Microsponge
Microvit
Probe System
vitrector
Miller-Nadler glare tester
Millex filter
Millipore filter
mini keratoplasty stitch scissors
mini ophthalmic drape
Mira
AGL-400
diathermy
endovitreal cryopencil
photocoagulator
Miracon

Miraflow
Mirasept
mirror haploscope
MK IV ophthalmoscope
mode-locked Nd:YAG laser
Moehle's
  cannula
  forceps
Moller's microscope
Moncrieff's cannula
monocular patch
monofilament nylon suture
Moore-Troutman corneal scissors
Moria's
  obturator
  one-piece speculum
  trephine
Moria-France dacryocystorhinostomy clamp
Mot-R-Pak vitrectomy system
motility
  ocular m. test
Moulton's lacrimal duct tube
MP Video endoscopic lens attachment
MPC automated intravitreal scissors
MRI scan
MTL trial frame
mucotome
Mueller's
  cautery
  electric corneal trephine
  lacrimal sac retractor
  refractor
  retractor
  shield
  speculum
  trephine
Muldoon's lacrimal dilator
Mules'
  implant

Mules' *(continued)*
  scoop
  vitreous sphere
Multilux
Murdock's speculum
Murdock-Wiener speculum
Mustarde
  awl
  graft
MVK — Massachusetts Vision Kit
MVR blade
MVS — Massachusetts XII Vitrectomy System
Myocure
  blade scalpel
  phacoblade
myoscope
myringotomy blade

n

N_2O Cryosurgical System
Nadler's superior radial scissors
Nagel's
  anomaloscope
  test
Nanolas Nd:YAG laser
nanometer
Nd:YAG laser
needle
  ACS n.
  Agnew's tattooing n.
  Alcon Surgical irrigating n.
  Alcon Surgical reverse cutting n.
  Alcon Surgical spatula n.
  Alcon Surgical taper cut n.

needle *(continued)*
- Alcon Surgical taper point n.
- Amsler's aqueous transplant n.
- aqueous transplant n.
- Atkinson's retrobulbar n.
- Barraquer's n.
- Barraquer-Vogt n.
- bent blunt n.
- blunt n.
- Bowman's cataract n.
- Bowman's n. stop
- Burr's butterfly n.
- butterly n.
- Calhoun's n.
- Calhoun-Hagler lens n.
- Calhoun-Merz n.
- cataract aspirating n.
- CD-5 n.
- Charles' n.
- Cibis' ski n.
- Cleasby's spatulated n.
- CooperVision irrigating n.
- CooperVision spatulated n.
- corneal n.
- CUA n.
- Curran's knife n.
- Dailey's cataract n.
- Davis' knife n.
- Dean's knife n.
- Drews' cataract n.
- DS-9 n.
- Ellis' foreign body n.
- Elschnig's extrusion n.
- extended round n.
- Fischer's n.
- flute n.
- Fritz's vitreous transplant
- Geuder's keratoplasty n.

needle *(continued)*
- Girard's cataract aspirating n.
- Girard's phacofragmatome n.
- Grieshaber's n.
- Haab's knife n.
- Heyner's double n.
- Ilg's n.
- Iliff-Wright fascia n.
- illuminated suction n.
- IOLAB irrigating n.
- IOLAB taper-cut n.
- IOLAB taper-point n.
- IOLAB titanium n.
- Kalt's corneal n.
- Kara's cataract n.
- Knapp's knife n.
- Lagleyze's n.
- Lane's n.
- Look's retrobulbar n.
- Lo-Trau side-cutting n.
- March's laser sclerostomy n.
- Maumenee's vitreous aspirating n.
- micro-point n.
- micro-round tip n.
- Oaks' double n.
- peribulbar n.
- probe n.
- puncture-tip n.
- razor-tip n.
- retrobulbar n.
- Reverdin's suture n.
- reverse-cutting n.
- Riedel's n.
- Sabreloc n.
- Sato's cataract n.
- Scheie's cataract aspirating n.
- sclerostomy n.
- side-cutting spatula n.

needle *(continued)*
- Simcoe aspirating n.
- SITE irrigating n.
- SITE taper-point n.
- SITE titanium n.
- spatulated n.
- spoon n.
- spud n.
- Stocker's n.
- Subco n.
- subconjunctival n.
- suturing n.
- Swan's n.
- taper-cut n.
- taper-point n.
- tattooing n.
- tax double n.
- titanium n.
- triple facet-tip n.
- Ultrasonic cataract removal lancet n.
- Viers' n.
- vitreous aspirating n.
- vitreous transplant n.
- Vogt-Barraquer corneal n.
- von Graefe's knife n.
- Weeks' n.
- Wergeland's double n.
- Worst's n.
- Wright's fascia n.
- Yale Luer-Lok n.
- Ziegler's knife n.

needle holder
- Alabama-Green n.h.
- Arruga's n.h.
- Barraquer's n.h.
- Birks Mark II Micro lock type n.h.
- Boyce's n.h.
- Boynton's n.h.
- Castroviejo's n.h.
- Castroviejo-Kalt n.h.

needle holder *(continued)*
- Clerf's n.h.
- Cohen's n.h.
- Crile's n.h.
- Derf's n.h.
- Gifford's n.h.
- Green's n.h.
- Grieshaber's n.h.
- Halsey's n.h.
- Ilg's micro n.h.
- Kalt's n.h.
- Keeler Catford micro jaws n.h.
- McPherson's n.h.
- Paton's n.h.
- Stephenson's n.h.
- Stevens' n.h.
- Tilderquist's n.h.
- Vickers n.h.

neodymium (Nd) YAG laser

Neolens

Nettleship's iris repositor

Nettleship-Wilder dilator

Neubauer's forceps

Nevyas' double sharp cystotome

New Orleans lens loupe

Nidek's laser system

nipper

Noble's forceps

Nocito's implant

Nokrome bifocal lens

nonabsorbable suture

noncontact tonometer
- Reichert's n.t.

Noyes'
- forceps
- iridectomy scissors
- iris scissors

nucleus
- n. delivery loop
- n. removal loop

Nugent's
- forceps
- hook
- soft cataract aspirator

Nugent-Gradle scissors
Nugent-Green-Dimitry erysiphake
Nurolon suture
nylon suture

O

O'Brien's
- forceps
- marker
- spud

O'Connor's
- depressor
- flat hook
- marker
- sharp hook

O'Donohue's angled DCR probe
O'Malley self-adhering lens implant
O'Malley-Heintz
- infusion cannula
- vitreous cutter

Oaks'
- double needle
- straight cannula

Oasis feather micro scalpel
oblique
- o. muscle hook
- o. prism device

Ochsner's forceps
Octopus
- 500 EZ
- 201 perimeter
- test

Oculab Tono-Pen
Ocular Gamboscope loupe
ocular
- o. motility test
- o. pressure reducer

oculocutaneous laser
oculoplasty corneal protector
Ocuscan 400 Transducer
Ocusoft scrub
Ocutome
- II Fragmentation System
- probe

O'Gawa's cataract aspirating cannula
Oklahoma iris wire retractor
Olivella-Garrigosa photocoagulator
Olk's
- vitreoretinal pick
- vitreoretinal spatula

OM
- 4 ophthalmometer
- 2000 operation microscope

OMNI Plus
OMS
- Empac Irrigation/Aspiration Unit
- Machemer/Parel VISC

Ophthalas
- argon laser
- krypton laser

Ophthascan
OpMi microscope
Opraflex drape
Optacon
Op-Temp cautery
Op-Temp disposable cautery
Opti-Pure System
Opt-Visor loupe
orbital compressor
original Sweet eye magnet
Ortho-Lite
OSCAR
Osher's hook

P

pachometer
- Packo pars plana cannula

Packysonic II

PAM — Potential Acuity Meter

Parel-Crock vitreous cutter

Parker's discission knife

Parker-Heath
- anterior chamber syringe
- cautery
- piggyback probe

Park's speculum

Park-Guyton-Callahan speculum

Park-Guyton-Maumenee speculum

Parks-Bielschowsky three-step head-tilt test

patch
- Donaldson eye p.
- Hutchinson's p.
- scopolamine p.
- Snugfit eye p.

Paton's
- corneal knife
- corneal trephine
- double spatula
- eye shield
- knife
- needle holder
- single spatula
- transplant spatula

Paufique's
- knife
- trephine

Paul's lacrimal sac retractor

Payne's retractor

Pierce's I/A
- cannula
- irrigating vectis
- tripod implant
- unit

Peczon I/A
- cannula
- unit
- vectis

pediatric speculum

pencil
- cataract p.
- glaucoma p.
- retinal detachment p.
- vitreous p.

peribulbar
- needle p.

perilimbal suction
- Vactro p.s.

perimeter
- Allergan-Humphrey p.
- Canon p.
- CILCO p.
- CooperVision p.
- Digilab p.
- Ferree-Rand p.
- Humphrey p.
- Marco p.
- Octopus 201 p.
- Schweigger's p.
- Topcon p.
- Tubingen p.

Perkins'
- applanation tonometer
- Brailler

Perritt's forceps

Petri dish

Peyman's vitrector

Phaco Emulsifier Cavitron Unit

phacoblade

Pharmacia Intermedics

phoropter retractor

photodisrupting laser

photokeratoscope
Allergan-Humphrey p.
CooperVision p.
photoptometer
Forster p.
Phototome System 2700
pick
Burch's p.
fixation/anchor p.
Michel's p.
Pickford-Nicholson anal-moscope
Pierse-Knoll irrigating lens loop
piggyback
p. contact lens
p. probe
pigtail probe
Pinhole and Dominance Test
Pinky Ball
Pischel's
electrode
micropins
pin
scleral rule
plain catgut suture
plastic
p. disposable irrigating vectis
p. prism
p. shield
p. sphere implant
plates
Ishihara's p.
isochromatic p.
pseudoisochromatic p.
Platina
clip lens
lens
platinum
p. probe spatula
p. spatula
pleoptics
Plexiglas implant
Pley's forceps
plug
Berkley Bioengineering brass scleral p.
Dohlman's p.
Eagle Vision-Freeman punctum p.
pneumotonometer
polarizing ophthalmoscope
polisher
Kraff's p.
Kratz's p.
Polle pod attachment for ophthalmoscope
polyester suture
polyethylene
p. implant
p. tube
p. T-tube
polyglactin suture
Post-Harrington erysiphake
Potential Acuity Meter — PAM
Potter-Bucky diaphragm
Powell's wand
Pram Occluder
Prince's
cautery
clamp
forceps
muscle clamp
rule
prism
A-O rotary p.
Allen-Thorpe goni-oscopic p.
apex p.
bar p.
base-down p.
base-in p.
base-out p.
base-up p.
Becker's gonioscopic p.
Berens' p.

prism *(continued)*
- p. diopter
- Fresnel's p.
- hand-held rotary p.
- Jacob-Swann gonioscopic p.
- Keeler's p.
- Maddox's p.
- oblique p.
- press-on p.
- right angle p.
- Risley's rotary p.
- scanning p.
- square p.
- Wolff-Eisner p.

prismatic gonioscopy lens

Pritikin's punch

probe
- Alcon's vitrectomy p.
- Anel's p.
- Bowman's p.
- Castroviejo's lacrimal sac p.
- Ellis' foreign body spud needle p.
- French's lacrimal p.
- Hertzog's pliable p.
- Iliff's p.
- Keeler-Amoils ophthalmic curved cataract p.
- Keeler-Amoils ophthalmic long shank p.
- Keeler-Amoils ophthalmic Machemer retinal p.
- Keeler-Amoils ophthalmic micro curved cataract p.
- Keeler-Amoils ophthalmic retinal p.
- Keeler-Amoils ophthalmic straight cataract p.
- Keeler-Amoils ophthalmic vitreous p.
- Knapp's iris p.
- lacrimal intubation p.
- Linde's cryogenic p.
- Manhattan E & E p.
- Mannis p.
- Microvit p.
- needle p.
- Ocutome p.
- Parker-Heath piggyback p.
- pigtail p.
- Quickert's lacrimal p.
- Quickert-Dryden p.
- Rolf's lacrimal p.
- Rollet's lacrimal p.
- Simpson's lacrimal p.
- spatula p.
- Theobald's p.
- Vygantas-Wilder retinal drainage p.
- Williams' p.
- Worst's p.
- Ziegler's p.

Pro-Koester wide field SCM microscope

Prolene suture

Pro-Ophtha
- drape
- dressing
- eye pad
- sponge
- sticks

pseudoisochromatic plates

pterygium scissors

ptosis
- knife
- scissors

punch
- Berens' corneoscleral p.
- Castroviejo's p.
- corneoscleral p.

punch *(continued)*
    Descemet's membrane p.
    Gass' sclerotomy p.
    Holth's p.
    Kelly Descemet's membrane p.
    Klein's p.
    Pritikin's p.
    Rubin-Holth p.
    sclerectomy p.
    Storz's corneoscleral p.
    Walton's p.
punctal dilator
puncture tip needle
pupillograph
pupillometer
pupilloscope
pupillostatometer
Purkinje's image tracker
push/pull
    Birks Mark II Micro Instruments p.
    Ilg's p.
    Kuglein's p.
pusher
    Martin-Surefit lens p.
Putterman's ptosis clamp
Putterman-Chaflin ocular asymmetry device
Putterman-Müller blepharoptosis clamp
Pyrex T-tube

q

Q-switched
    neodymium YAG laser
    ruby laser
Quad cutting tip
Quevedo's
    fixation forceps
    suturing forceps
Quickert's
    lacrimal probe
    suture
Quickert-Dryden
    probe
    tube

r

radial
    r. iridotomy scissors
    r. keratotomy marker
radiotherapy
Randolph's
    cyclodialysis cannula
    irrigator
Randot Dot E Stereotest
rasp
    Lundsgaard-Burch corneal r.
Rayner-Choyce implant
razor
    r. bladebreaker
    r. bladeknife
    r. tip needle
Reeh's scissors
reed aspiration cannula
Reese's
    forceps
    ptosis knife
reflectometer
refractometer
refractor
    Agrikola's r.
    Allergan-Humphrey r.
    Amoils' r.

refractor *(continued)*
- Berens' r.
- Brawley's r.
- Bronson-Turz r.
- Campbell's r.
- Canon's r.
- Castallo's r.
- Castroviejo's r.
- Coburn's r.
- CooperVision Diagnostic Imaging r.
- Desmarres' r.
- Elschnig's r.
- Ferris-Smith-Sewall r.
- Fink's r.
- Goldstein's r.
- Gradle's r.
- Graither's r.
- Green's r.
- Groenholm's r.
- Hartstein's r.
- Hillis' r.
- Kirby's r.
- Knapp's r.
- Kronfeld's r.
- Kuglein's r.
- McGannon's r.
- Marco's r.
- Meller's r.
- Mueller's r.
- Reichert's r.
- Rizzuti's r.
- Rollet's r.
- Schepens' r.
- Stevenson's r.
- Topcon's r.

regurgitation test

Reichert's
- binocular indirect ophthalmoscope
- camera
- Ful-Vue ophthalmoscope
- Ful-Vue spot retinoscope
- lensometer
- noncontact tonometer
- ophthalmodynamometer
- radius gauge
- refractor
- retinoscope
- slit lamp

Reichling's corneal scissors

Remy's separator

replacer
- Green's r.

repositor
- Nettleship iris r.

retinal detachment
- r.d. hook
- r.d. pencil
- r.d. syringe

retinoscope
- Keeler's r.
- Reichert's r.
- spot r.
- streak r.

retractor
- Agrikola's lacrimal sac r.
- Alexander-Ballen r.
- Amenabar's iris r.
- Amoils' r.
- Arruga's r.
- Ballen-Alexander orbital r.
- Barraquer-Krumeich-Swinger r.
- Berens' lid r.
- Blair's r.
- Brawley's r.
- Bronson-Turz r.
- Campbell's r.
- Castallo's r.
- Castroviejo's r.
- Coleman's r.

retractor *(continued)*
- Conway's lid r.
- Coston-Trent iris r.
- Desmarres' lid r.
- Drews-Rosenbaum iris r.
- Eliasoph's lid r.
- Elschnig's r.
- Ferris-Smith r.
- Ferris-Smith-Sewall r.
- Fink's lacrimal r.
- Fisher's lid r.
- Forker's r.
- Givner's lid r.
- Goldstein's lacrimal sac r.
- Gradle's r.
- Graither's r.
- Groenholm's r.
- Gross' r.
- Harrison's r.
- Hartstein's r.
- Hill's r.
- Hillis' r.
- Jaeger's r.
- Jaffee-Givner lid r.
- Keeler Fison tissue r.
- Keeler Rodger iris r.
- Keizer-Lancaster lid r.
- Kelman's iris r.
- Kirby's r.
- Knapp's lacrimal sac r.
- Kronfeld's r.
- Kuglein's r.
- lacrimal sac r.
- MacKool's r.
- MacVicar's double-end strabismus r.
- McGannon's r.
- Meller's lacrimal sac r.
- Mueller's lacrimal sac r.
- Oklahoma iris wire r.
- Paul's lacrimal sac r.
- Payne's r.
- Phoropter r.

retractor *(continued)*
- Rizzuti's iris r.
- Rollet's r.
- Rosenbaum-Drews r.
- Sanchez-Bulnes lacrimal sac r.
- Sato's lid r.
- Schepens' r.
- self-retaining r.
- Senn's r.
- Stevenson's lacrimal sac r.
- Thomas' r.
- Ticho's pliable iris r.
- Vaiser-Cibis muscle r.
- Wilmer's r.

retrieval device

retrobulbar needle

Reuss'
- color chart
- table

Reverdin's needle

reverse-cutting needle

reverse-shape implant

Richard's pillow

Ridley anterior chamber lens implant

Ridley Mark II lens implant

Riedel's needle

right angle prism

right/left hand corneoscleral scissors

ring
- Bonaccolto's scleral r.
- Bores' twist fixation r.
- Burr's corneal r.
- cataract mask r.
- centering r.
- corneal transplant centering r.
- fixation r.
- fixation-anchor r.
- Flieringa's fixation r.

ring *(continued)*
- Flieringa-LeGrand fixation r.
- Girard's scleral expander r.
- Landers' irrigating vitrectomy r.
- Martinez corneal transplant centering r.
- McKinney's fixation r.
- scleral expander r.

Ringer's solution
Risley's rotary prism
Rizzuti's
- expressor
- fixation forceps
- graft carrier spoon
- iris retractor
- rectus forceps
- refractor
- retractor

Rizzuti-Bonaccolto instruments
Rizzuti-Fleischer instruments
Rizzuti-Furniss cornea holding forceps
Rizzuti-Kayser-Fleischer instruments
Rizzuti-Lowe instruments
Rizzuti-Maxwell instruments
Rizzuti-McGuire corneal section scissors
Rizzuti-Soemmering instruments
Rizzuti-Spizziri cannula knife
Robin's chalazion clamp
Rochat test
Rodenstock System
Rodin's orbital implant
Rolf's
- dilator
- forceps
- lacrimal probe

Rolf's
- lance

roller forceps
Rollet's
- irrigating/aspirating unit
- lacrimal probe
- refractor
- retractor

Rommel's cautery
Rommel-Hildreth cautery
rongeur
- Citelli's r.
- Kerrison's r.
- lacrimal sac r.

Roper's
- alpha-chymotrypsin cannula

Roper-Hall localizer
Rosa-Berens orbital implant
Rosenbaum's pocket vision screener
Rosenbaum-Drews retractor
Rosner's tonometer
rotator
- Jaffe-Bechert nucleus r.

rotoextractor
- Douvas' r.

Roveda's lid everter
Rowland's keratome
Rubin-Holth punch
Rubinstein's cryoprobe
ruby diamond knife
Ruedemann's
- implant
- lacrimal dilator
- tonometer

Ruedemann-Todd tendon tucker
Ruiz
- plano fundus lens implant

Russian forceps

S

Sabouraud media
Sabreloc needle
St. Martin–Franceshetti cataract hook
Sakler's erysiphake
Sanchez-Bulnes lacrimal sac retractor
Sato's
- cataract needle
- corneal knife
- lid retractor
- needle

Sauer's
- corneal debrider
- forceps
- speculum

Sauflon lens
scalpel
- Guardian s. with depth resistor
- Guyton-Lundsgaard s.
- Oasis feather micro s.

scan
- CAT s.
- CT s.
- MRI s.

scanning prism
scarifier
- Desmarres' s.

scattergram
Schaaf's forceps
Schachne-Desmarres lid everter
Schaedel's cross-action towel clamp
Schaefer's sponge holder
Scheie's
- anterior chamber cannula
- blade

Scheie's *(continued)*
- cataract aspirating needle
- cautery
- electrocautery
- goniopuncture knife
- knife
- trephine

Scheie-Westcott corneal section scissors
schematic eye
Schepens'
- electrode
- ophthalmoscope
- refractor
- retinal detachment unit
- retractor
- scleral depressor
- spoon

Schepens-Pomerantzell binocular indirect ophthalmoscope
Schillinger's suture support
Schiøtz's
- tonofilms
- tonometer

Schirmer tear quality test
Schocket's scleral depressor
Schumann's giant type eye magnet
Schweigger's
- forceps
- perimeter

scissors
- Aebli's corneal s.
- alligator s.
- anterior chamber synechiae s.
- Atkinson's corneal s.
- bandage s.
- Barraquer's iris s.
- Barraquer's vitreous strand s.
- Barraquer-DeWecker s.

scissors *(continued)*
- Becker's corneal section spatulated s.
- Berens' corneal transplant s.
- Berkley Bioengineering mechanized s.
- Birks Mark II Micro trabeculectomy s.
- canalicular s.
- capsulotomy s.
- Castroviejo's corneal section s.
- Castroviejo's corneal transplant s.
- Castroviejo's iridocapsulotomy s.
- Castroviejo's keratoplasty s.
- Castroviejo's synechiae s.
- Cohan-Vannas iris s.
- Cohan-Westcott s.
- conjunctival s.
- corneal s.
- corneal spatulated s.
- corneoscleral s.
- corneoscleral right/left hand s.
- DeWecker's iris s.
- DeWecker-Pritikin s.
- dissecting s.
- enucleation s.
- Fine's suture s.
- Frost's s.
- Giardet's corneal transplant s.
- Gill's s.
- Gill-Hess s.
- Girard's corneoscleral s.
- Grieshaber's vertical cut s.
- Grieshaber's vitreous s.
- Guist's s.

scissors *(continued)*
- Haenig's irrigating s.
- Harrison's s.
- Hoskins-Castroviejo corneal s.
- Hoskins-Westcott tenotomy s.
- House-Bellucci alligator s.
- Huey's s.
- iridectomy s.
- iridocapsulotomy s.
- iridotomy s.
- iris s.
- Irvine's s.
- Irvine's probe pointed s.
- Karakashian-Barraquer s.
- Katzin's s.
- Keeler's intravitreal s.
- keratectomy s.
- keratoplasty s.
- Kirby's s.
- Knapp's iris s.
- Kreiger-Spitznas vibrating s.
- Lagrange's s.
- Lawton's corneal s.
- Lister's s.
- Littler's dissecting s.
- Manson-Aebli corneal section s.
- Mattis' s.
- Maunoir's iris s.
- Mayo's s.
- McClure's iris s.
- McGuire's corneal s.
- McLean's capsulotomy s.
- McPherson-Castroviejo corneal section s.
- McPherson-Vannas micro iris s.
- McReynolds' pterygium s.

scissors *(continued)*
- mechanized s.
- mini-keratoplasty stitch s.
- Moore-Troutman corneal s.
- MPC automated intravitreal s.
- Nadler's superior radial s.
- Noyes' iridectomy s.
- Noyes' iris s.
- Nugent-Gradle s.
- pterygium s.
- radial iridotomy s.
- Reeh's s.
- Reichling's corneal s.
- right/left hand corneoscleral s.
- Rizzuti-McGuire corneal section s.
- Scheie-Westcott corneal section s.
- Shield's iridotomy s.
- Spencer's s.
- Spring's iris s.
- Stevens' tenotomy s.
- Størz-Westcott conjunctival s.
- strabismus s.
- superior radial tenotomy s.
- Sutherland-Grieshaber s.
- Thorpe's s.
- Thorpe-Castroviejo s.
- Thorpe-Westcott s.
- Twisk micro s.
- Vannas' s.
- Verhoeff's s.
- vibrating s.
- vitreous strand s.
- Walker's s.
- Walker-Apple s.
- Walker-Atkinson s.
- Werb's s.

scissors *(continued)*
- Westcott's s.
- Wilmer's s.

scleral
- s. blade
- s. depressor
- s. expander ring
- s. hook
- s. implant
- s. marker
- s. resection knife
- s. shortening clips
- s. sponge rod

sclerotome
- Alvis-Lancaster s.
- Atkinson's s.
- Curdy's s.
- Guyton-Lundsgaard s.
- Lundsgaard's s.
- Lundsgaard-Burch s.

sclerotomy punch

Scobee's muscle hook

scoop
- Arlt's s.
- Daviel's s.
- Knapp's s.
- Lewis' s.
- Mules s.
- Wilder's s.

scotometer
- Bjerrum's s.

scotomagraph

scotometer
- Bjerrum's s.

scotoscope

Scott's No. 2 curved ruler

screen
- Bjerrum's s.
- tangent s.

Searcy's
- anchor/fixation
- chalazion trephine
- erysiphake

Seidel's test
self-adhering lid retractor
self-retaining
    s. irrigating cannula
    s. retractor
semishell implant
Senn's retractor
separate image test
serrefine
    s. clamp
    Dieffenbach's s.
    Lemoine's s.
Sharplan argon laser
sheet
    foil s.
    Silastic s.
    Supramid s.
    Teflon s.
Sheets' lens
Sheehy-Urban sliding lens adaptor
shelf-type implant
shell implant
Shepard's
    iris hook
    reversed iris hook
Shepard-Reinstein forceps
Sheridan-Gardiner Isolated Letter Matching Test
shield
    Barraquer's s.
    Buller's s.
    Cartella's s.
    eye s.
    Expo Bubble s.
    Fox's s.
    Green's s.
    Hessburg's corneal s.
    Mueller's s.
    Paton's s.
    plastic s.
    pressure s.
    ring cataract mask s.

shield *(continued)*
    Universal s.
    Visitec corneal s.
    Weck's s.
Shields' iridotomy scissors
Shoch's suture
side-cutting spatula needle
side port cannula
sideroscope
Silastic
    implant
    plate
    sheet
    T-tube
silicone
    s. button
    s. conformer
    s. eye sphere
    s. hemisphere
    s. implant
    s. lubricant
    s. strip
    s. tire
Simcoe II PC
    aspirating needle
    double cannula
    lens
    nucleus delivery loop
Simpson's lacrimal probe
Sinskey's lens hook
SITE TXR
    I & A System
    2200 Microsurgical Unit
    Phaco System
Skeele's curet
ski needle
skiameter
skiascope
Sklar-Schiotz tonometer
sleeve
    Charles' anterior segment s.
    Charles' infusion s.

sleeve *(continued)*
implant s.
Stevens-Charles s.
Watzke's s.
slit lamp
s.l. biomicroscopy
small aperture Steri-Drape
Smart's
forceps
scissors
Smith's
expressor hook
intraocular capsular amputator
knife
orbital floor implant
speculum
Smith-Fisher
iris replacer
knife
spatula
Smith-Green
cataract knife
snare
Banner's enucleation s.
Castroviejo's enucleation s.
enucleation wire s.
Foerster's enucleation s.
Foster's enucleation s.
Snellen's
chart
implant
letter
reform eye
soft contact lens
test
vectis
Sonometric Ocuscan
Sovereign bifocal lens
Spanish silk suture
spatula
angulated iris s.

spatula *(continued)*
Bangerter's iris s.
Barraquer's irrigator s.
Berens' s.
Birks Mark II Micro Instruments s.
capsule fragment s.
Castroviejo's cyclodialysis s.
Castroviejo's double end s.
Cleasby's s.
corneal fascia lata s.
Culler's iris s.
cyclodialysis s.
double s.
Drews-Sato suture pickup s.
Elschnig's s.
Fisher-Smith s.
French's hook s.
French's lacrimal s.
French's pattern s.
Gill-Welch s.
Green's s.
Hertzog's lens s.
Hirschman's s.
hook s.
iris s.
Jaffe's intraocular s.
Kimura's s.
Kirby's angulated iris s.
Kirby's iris s.
Knapp's
Knapp's iris s.
Laird's s.
Lindner's s.
Manhattan E & E s.
Maumenee's vitreous sweep s.
McPherson's s.
McReynolds' s.

speculum *(continued)*
- pediatric s.
- Sauer's s.
- Smith's s.
- stop s.
- Sutherland-Grieshaber s.
- Weeks' s.
- Weiss' s.
- Wiener's s.
- Williams' s.

Spencer's scissors
Spero's forceps
sphere
- Doherty's s.
- implant
- introducer
- Mules' vitreous s.
- Pyrex eye s.

spherical
- implant
- lens

spherocyclindrical lens
sponge
- Custodis s.
- implant
- Krukenberg's s.
- Lincoff's lens s.
- Microsponge Teardrop s.
- Pro-Ophtha s.
- Vaiser's s.
- vitrectomy s.
- Weck-cel s.

spoon
- Bunge's evisceration s.
- Castroviejo's s.
- Culler's lens s.
- Cutler's lens s.
- Daviel's s.
- Elschnig's s.
- enucleation s.
- evisceration s.
- Fisher's s.
- graft carrier s.

spoon *(continued)*
- Hess' s.
- Kalt's s.
- Kirby's intracapsular lens s.
- Knapp's lens s.
- lens s.
- needle s.
- Rizzuti's graft carrier s.
- Schepens' s.
- spatula s.

spot retinoscope
- Ful-Vue s.r.
- Reichert's s.r.

Spratt's mastoid curet
Spring's iris scissors
spud
- Alvis' s.
- Bahn's s.
- Corbett's s.
- Davis' s.
- Dix's s.
- Ellis' s.
- Fisher's s.
- foreign body s.
- Francis' s.
- golf club s.
- gouge s.
- Hosford's s.
- LaForce's s.
- Levine's s.
- needle s.
- O'Brien's s.
- Plange's s.
- Walter's s.
- Walton's s.

Sputnik Russian razor blade
squint hook
Stahli's
- caliper
- nucleus expressor

Starr's fixation forceps
Steinhauser's electro-mucotome

Stephenson's needle holder
Step-Knife diamond blade knife
stereopsis test
Steri-Drape
Steriseal disposable cannula
Stevens'
- forceps
- hook
- needle holder
- tenotomy hook
- tenotomy scissors

Stevens-Charles sleeve
Stevenson's
- lacrimal sac retractor
- refractor

stiletto
- Berkley Bioengineering s.
- knife

Stilling's color test
stitch removing knife
Stocker's needle
Stoke's lens
Stone's implant
stop speculum
Storz
- cataract knife
- corneal bur
- corneoscleral punch
- keratome
- microscope
- Microvit vitrector

Storz-Atlas hand eye magnet
Storz-Bell erysiphake
Storz-Duredge steel cataract knife
Storz-Utrata forceps
Storz-Walker retinal detachment unit
Storz-Westcott conjunctiva scissors
strabometer
streak retinoscope
striascope
Stryker's frame
Subco needle
subconjunctival needle
subjective refraction test
Super Pinky Ball
Superblade
- No. 75
- trapezoid

superior radial tenotomy scissors
Supramid
- Allen implant
- bridle collagen suture
- lens implant suture
- sheet

surface implant
SurgiMed
Surg-E-Trol I/A/R System
surgical gut suture
Surgidev
- lens
- suture

Surgikos drape
Sussman 4-mirror gonioscope
Sutherland Rotatable Microsurgery Instruments
Sutherland-Grieshaber
- scissors
- speculum

suture
- absorbable s.
- Alcon s.
- Atroloc s.
- black braided nylon s.
- black braided silk s.
- braided silk s.
- braided Vicryl s.
- chromic catgut s.
- chromic collagen s.
- coated Vicryl s.
- Custodis s.
- Dacron s.

suture *(continued)*
- Davis-Geck s.
- Deknatel silk s.
- Dermalon s.
- Dexon s.
- double-armed s.
- Ethicon Atroloc s.
- Ethicon Micro-Point s.
- Ethicon Sabreloc s.
- Ethilon s.
- Faden s.
- Foster s.
- Frost s.
- Gaillard-Arlt s.
- lancet s.
- Look s.
- Mannis s.
- McLean s.
- Mersilene s.
- Micro-Point s.
- monofilament nylon s.
- nonabsorbable s.
- Nurolon s.
- nylon s.
- nylon 66 s.
- pickup spatula s.
- plain catgut s.
- plain collagen s.
- polyester s.
- polyglactin s.
- Prolene s.
- Quickert s.
- Shoch s.
- Spanish silk s.
- Supramid bridle collagen s.
- SurgiMed s.
- surgical gut s.
- Surgidev s.
- Swiss silk s.
- twisted virgin silk s.
- Vicryl s.
- virgin silk s.
- white braided silk s.

suturing needle

Swan's
- discission knife
- knife
- lancet
- needle

Sweet's
- locator
- original magnet

Swets goniotomy knife cannula

swinging flashlight test

Swiss
- bladebreaker
- silk suture

Sylva
- anterior chamber irrigator
- irrigating/aspirating unit

symblepharon ring

synechia spatula

synechotome

synoptoscope

syringe
- Anel's s.
- probe s.

t

table
- Reuss' t.

taco test

Takata laser

tantalum
- t. clip
- t. mesh implant

taper-cut needle

taper-point needle

tattooing needle

tax double needle

TE-MOO mode beam laser
Teflon
- implant
- plates
- sheet
- plug

Telfa dressing
tendon tucker
- Bishop's t.t.
- Bishop-Peter t.t.
- Burch's t.t.
- Burch-Greenwood t.t.
- Fink's t.t.
- Ruedemann-Todd t.t.

Tennant's titanium suturing forceps
Tenner's lacrimal cannula
tenotomy hook
Tensilon test
Tenzel elevator
Terry's
- keratometer
- silicone capsule polisher

TESTS, EXAMINATIONS, MATERIALS

- acetylcholine receptor antibody level
- achromatic perimetry
- after-image t.
- air puff noncontact
- alternate cover and uncover t.
- Amsler chart
- Amsler grid t.
- anaglyph
- angiography
- applanation tonometry t.
- astigmatic dial chart
- automated visual field
- Bailey-Lovie Log Mar chart

TESTS, EXAMINATIONS, MATERIALS *(continued)*
- Barraquer-Krumeich Swinger refractive
- basic tear secretion t.
- BAT — Brightness Acuity Test
- Berens Pinhole and Dominance Test
- Berens three-character t.
- Berman locator t.
- Bielschowsky head-tilt t.
- Bielschowsky three-step head-tilt t.
- binocular indirect ophthalmoscope t.
- Birkhauser chart
- Bjerrum target screen visual field t.
- blindness t.
- Bruchner t.
- B-VAT acuity t.
- caloric t.
- cardinal position of gaze
- Challenger Digital Applanation
- cheiroscope t.
- cocaine t.
- color perimetry
- color vision t.
- confrontation visual field t.
- corneal reflex t.
- corneal staining t.
- cover t.
- cover/uncover t.
- Cuignet t.
- cyclodamia
- cycloplegic refraction
- dacryocystogram
- dark adaptation t.
- darkroom provocative t.
- direct light response
- dissimilar image t.

TESTS, EXAMINATIONS, MATERIALS *(continued)*

- dissimilar target t.
- Dix-Hallpike t.
- DIVA t.
- Donder chart
- double Maddox rod t.
- Duane accommodation chart
- duction t.
- duochrome
- Dupuy-Dutemps dye t.
- Dvorine t.
- dye t.
- E t.
- echogram
- echo-ophthalmography t.
- Ehrmann t.
- electroperimetry
- echoretinography t.
- ELISA t. — E t.
- edrophonium chloride t.
- EOG — electro-oculogram
- ERG — electroretinogram
- exophthalmometry t.
- FFF — flicker fusion frequency fields
- Farnsworth D100
- Farnsworth D15
- Farnsworth-Munsell 100 hue color vision t.
- Ferris chart
- fields of gaze
- finger-counting
- fluorescein angiogram
- fluorescein angiography t.
- fluorescein dye and stain solution
- fluorescein dye disappearance

TESTS, EXAMINATIONS, MATERIALS *(continued)*

- fluorophotometry
- fogging
- forced duction t.
- forced generation
- Four Dot t.
- Giemsa stain
- glare t.
- glarometer
- gonioscopy t.
- Graefe t.
- Gram stain
- Guibor chart
- hand-motion visual acuity t.
- hand-movement visual acuity t.
- Hardy-Rand-Littler plates
- Harrington-Flocks multiple pattern
- head-tilt t.
- Hering t.
- Hering-Bielschowsky after-image t.
- Hess screen t.
- Hirschberg t.
- Holmgren color t.
- Holmgren wool skein t.
- Illiterate Eye Chart
- indentation tonometry
- Ishihara color t.
- Ishihara pseudoisochromatic plates
- Jaeger t.
- Jenning t.
- Jones t.
- K-readings
- keratoscope
- Keystone t.
- Kindergarten Eye Chart
- kinetic perimetry

TESTS, EXAMINATIONS, MATERIALS *(continued)*

Kirby-Bauer disk sensitivity t.
Klein keratoscope t.
Krimsky t.
lacrimal irrigation t.
Lactoplate
Lancaster red-green t.
Lancaster-Regan dial 1 chart
Lancaster-Regan dial 2 chart
Landolt broken ring chart
lantern t.
Lebensohn chart
light and color perception t.
light perception t.
light projection t.
limulus lysate t.
linear visual acuity t.
macular function t.
macular photostress
Maddox rod t.
Maddox wing t.
manifest refraction
Marlow t.
Master two-step t.
materials primary dye
Mauthner's t.
Maxwell spot
monocular confrontation visual field t.
mydriatic provocative t.
Nagel t.
near point of conversion
neutral density filter t.
objective t.
occlusion t.
Octopus t.
ocular motility t.

TESTS, EXAMINATIONS, MATERIALS *(continued)*

ophthalmodynamometry — ODN t.
ophthalmoscopy direct t.
ophthalmoscopy indirect t.
ophthalmoscopy red free light t.
optotype
Ortho-Rater
over-refraction
P&C — prism and cover t.
parallax t.
Parks-Bielschowsky three-step head-tilt t.
passive forced duction t.
PAT — prism adaptation t.
Perkins tonometer
phoropter t.
pilocarpine t.
Pinhole and Dominance t.
pinhole vision t.
Polaroid vectograph slide
primary position of gaze
prism adaptation t.
prism and cover t.
projection t.
provocative t.
pseudoisochromatic plates
Randot chart
reading chart
red glare t.
red glass t.
Red-Green t.
refined refraction
refraction
regurgitation t.

TESTS, EXAMINATIONS, MATERIALS *(continued)*

- retinal correspondence
- retinoscopy
- Reuss color chart
- Rochat t.
- Rosenbaum t.
- saccadic velocity t.
- Schiotz tonometry t.
- Schirmer tear quality t.
- Schweigger hand perimeter
- screen and cover t.
- secondary dye t.
- Seidel t.
- separate image t.
- serologic t.
- serology t.
- shadow t.
- Sheridan-Gardiner Letter Matching t.
- simultaneous finger-count t.
- simultaneous prism and cover t.
- skein t.
- skiascopy bar
- slip lamp t.
- Snellen chart
- SPC t.
- specular reflection
- Spherical Twirl
- static perimetry
- stereo campimeter
- stereopsis t.
- stigmometric test card
- Stilling color t.
- subjective refraction t.
- sunburst dial chart
- swinging flashlight t.
- swinging light t.
- synoptophore t.

TESTS, EXAMINATIONS, MATERIALS *(continued)*

- T3, T4, TSH — thyroid function t.
- taco t.
- tangent screen
- tear film stability
- tear quality
- tear quantity
- tear secretion
- telebinocular
- Tensilon t.
- tension t.
- test card
- test letter
- test type
- Three-character test
- three-step t.
- thyroid function t.
- Titmus t.
- TNO t.
- tonography t.
- TPI — treponema pallidum immobilization
- traction
- transillumination t.
- University of Waterloo chart
- ultrasonography
- vectograph chart
- VER — Visual Evoked Response
- visual acuity t.
- visual field t.
- Visuscope motor
- Visuscope sensory
- W4D t.
- water provocative t.
- Welland t.
- Westcott t.
- Wilbrand t.
- Wing t.

TESTS, EXAMINATIONS, MATERIALS *(continued)*
- Wirt four dot t.
- Wirt stereopsis t.
- Wolff-Eisner t.
- Worth t.

Theobald's probe
Thomas Kapsule Instruments
Thomas's
- brush
- calipers
- cannula
- cryoptor
- cryoretractor
- fixation forceps
- forceps
- retractor
- scissors

Thorpe's
- caliper
- forceps
- scissors

Thorpe-Castroviejo
- caliper
- corneal forceps
- fixation forceps
- goniolens
- scissors
- vitreous foreign body forceps

Thorpe-Westcott scissors
Thrasher's lens implant forceps
3-M small aperature Steri-Drape
Ticho's
- pliable iris retractor
- zonule sweeper

tie-over dressing
Tilderquist's needle holder
Tillyer's bifocal lens
tire
- 276 t.
- implant t.

tire *(continued)*
- silicone t.
- Watzke's t.

titanium needle
Titmus t.
TNO stereotest
Todd's
- cautery
- gouge

Tolentino's ring
Tolentino's vitreous cutter
Tomas'
- iris hook
- suture hook

tomogram
tonometer
- air puff contact t.
- Alcon's t.
- Allen-Schiotz t.
- applanation t.
- Aus Jena-Schiotz t.
- Berens' t.
- Carl Zeiss t.
- Challenger t.
- Coburn's t.
- Digilab t.
- Goldmann's applanation t.
- Harrington's t.
- impression t.
- indentation t.
- Intermedics intraocular t.
- Keeler's t.
- Lombert's t.
- MacKay-Marg t.
- McLean's t.
- noncontact t.
- Perkins' applanation t.
- pneumotonometer t.
- Pulsair t.
- Reichert's t.
- Rosner's t.
- Ruedemann's t.

tonometer *(continued)*
- Schiotz t.
- Sklar-Schiotz t.
- Storz t.
- Tono-Pen t.

Tooke's
- knife
- spatula

Tooke-Johnson corneal knife

Topcon
- aspheric lens
- camera
- chart projector
- lensometer
- LM P5 digital lensmeter
- perimeter
- refractor
- refractometer
- slit lamp
- vision tester

toric lens

trabeculotome
- Allen-Burian t.
- Harms' t.
- McPherson's t.

Tracor Northern

Tracoustic RV275

Transpore eye tape

trephine
- Arruga's lacrimal t.
- automatic t.
- Bard-Parker t.
- Barraquer's t.
- Barron's epikeratophakia t.
- Bonaccolto's t.
- Boston's t.
- Brown-Pusey corneal t.
- Castroviejo's corneal transplant t.
- chalazion t.
- corneal t.
- Davis' t.

trephine *(continued)*
- Dimitry's chalazion t.
- Elliot's t.
- Elschnig's t.
- Gradle's corneal t.
- Green's t.
- Grieshaber's corneal t.
- Guyton's corneal transplant t.
- Hessburg-Barron vacuum t.
- Iliff's lacrimal t.
- Katena's t.
- King's corneal t.
- lacrimal t.
- Lichtenberg's corneal t.
- Martinez disposable corneal t.
- Mueller's electric corneal t.
- Paton's corneal t.
- Paufique's t.
- Scheie's t.
- Searcy's chalazion t.

triple facet tip needle

Troncoso's
- gonioscope
- gonioscopic lens implant

tropometer

troposcope

Troutman's
- bladebreaker
- cannula
- conjunctiva scissors
- corneal knife
- implant
- lens loupe
- microsurgical scissors
- needle holder
- punch
- rectus forceps
- suture scissors
- tenotomy trephine

Troutman's *(continued)*
 trephine
 tying forceps
Troutman-Barraquer corneal fixation forceps
Troutman-Castroviejo corneal section scissors
Troutman-Katzin corneal transplant scissors
Troutman-Llobera fixation forceps
T-tube
 Houser cul-de-sac irrigator T.
 lacrimal duct T.
 polyethylene T.
 Pyrex T.
 Silastic T.
 vinyl T.
tube
 Bowman t.
 fil d'Arion t.
 Guibor Silastic t.
 Houser cul-de-sac irrigator t.
 Jones Pyrex t.
 L. T. Jones tear duct t.
 Luer t.
 Moulton lacrimal duct t.
 polyethylene t.
 Quickert-Dryden t.
 silicone t.
 vinyl t.
Tubingen perimeter
tucker
 Burch-Greenwood t.
 Green's muscle t.
 Green's strabismus t.
Tulevech's cannula
tunable dye laser
tunneled implant
Twisk micro scissors
twist fixation hook
twisted virgin silk suture
two-angled polypropylene loop
two-way
 cataract aspirating cannula
 syringe
 towel clip
Tycos' manometer
Tyrell's
 iris hook
 tympanic membrane hook

U

Ulanday's double cannula
Ultex lens implant
Ultra-Image
 A scan
 SCAN
Ultramatic
 Project-O-Chart
 Rx Master Phoroptor
Ultrascan Digital B System
ultrasonic
 cataract removal lancet
 Micrometer
ultrasonogram
 A scan u.
 B scan u.
 gray-scale u.
ultrasonography
 Doppler u.
UltraThin surgical blades
unit
 Bovie u.
 Mira u.
United Sonics J shock phaco fragmentor system

Universal
- conformer
- eye shield

Uribe's orbital implant
UV Nova Curve

V

Vactro perilimbal suction apparatus
Vaiser sponge
Vaiser-Cibis muscle retractor
Valilab cautery
VA magnet orbital implant
Vannas' scissors
Vari bladebreaker
Varilux lens implant
Vasco-Posada orbital retractor
vectis
- Anis' irrigating v.
- irrigating/aspirating v.
- Pierce irrigating v.

VECP — visual evoked cortical potential
vectograph
velonoskiascopy
VEP — visual evoked potential
VER — visual evoked response
Verhoeff's
- expressor
- forceps
- scissors

VG slit lamp
vibrating scissors
Vicker's needle holder
Vickerall round ringed forceps
Vicrosurgery
Vicryl suture
video specular microscope
Viers'
- cannula
- erysiphake
- needle
- trocar

Vieth-Mueller horopter
Villasensor ultrasonic pachymeter
vinyl T-tube
virgin silk suture
VISC — vitreous infusion suction cutter
VISCOFLOW cannula
Visitec
- angled lens hook
- aspiration unit
- capsule polisher curet
- corneal shield
- cortex extractor
- cystotome
- double cutting cystotome
- intraocular lens dialer
- iris retractor
- irrigating/aspirating cannula
- lens pusher
- micro double iris hook
- micro hook
- micro iris hook
- nucleus removal loop
- RK zone marker
- straight lens hook
- vico manipulator

Visual-Tech machine
Visulab System
Visulas
- argon C laser
- argon/YAG laser
- YAG C laser
- YAG E laser
- YAG S laser

visuometer
Visuscope ophthalmoscope

Vitallium implant
vitrector
- Alcon v.
- Charles v. with sleeve
- CILCO v.
- CooperVision v.
- Frigitronic v.
- Kaufman v.
- Microvit v.
- Peyman v.
- SITE Guillotine v.
- Storz Microvit v.

vitreoretinal infusion cutter
vitreous
- v. aspirating cannula
- v. aspirating needle
- v. cutter
- v. forceps
- v. pencil
- v. strand scissors
- v. sweep spatula
- v. transplant needle

vitreous cutter
- Buettner-Parel v.c.
- Douvas' v.c.
- infusion suction cutter
- Kloti's v.c.
- Maguire-Harvey v.c.
- O'Malley-Heintz v.c.
- Parel-Crock v.c.
- Tolentino's v.c.

Vitrophage-Peyman unit
V-lance
- V. blade
- V. knife
- V. Sharpoint

Vogt-Barraquer corneal needle
Volk's coronoid lens
von Graefe's
- cataract knife
- cautery
- cystotome
- fixation forceps

von Graefe's *(continued)*
- iris forceps
- knife
- knife needle
- muscle hook
- strabismus hook
- tissue forceps

von Mondak's forceps
V-slit lamp
Vuero Meter
Vygantas-Wilder retinal drainage probe

W

W4D test
Wadsworth's lid forceps
Wadsworth-Todd cautery
Wainstock's suturing forceps
Waldeau's forceps
Walker's
- coagulator
- electrode
- lid everter
- micro pin
- pin
- scissors
- trephine

Walker-Apple scissors
Walker-Atkinson scissors
Walker-Lee sclerotome
Wallach's cryosurgical pencil
Walser's corneoscleral punch
Walter's spud
Walton's
- punch
- spud

water
- w. drinking test
- w. provocative test

X

Y

Z